Molecular Imaging and Precision Medicine, Part I

Editor

RATHAN M. SUBRAMANIAM

PET CLINICS

www.pet.theclinics.com

Consulting Editor
ABASS ALAVI

January 2017 • Volume 12 • Number 1

ELSEVIER

1600 John F. Kennedy Boulevard • Suite 1800 • Philadelphia, Pennsylvania, 19103-2899

http://www.pet.theclinics.com

PET CLINICS Volume 12, Number 1
January 2017 ISSN 1556-8598, ISBN-13: 978-0-323-48266-0

Editor: John Vassallo (j.vassallo@elsevier.com)
Developmental Editor: Meredith Clinton

PET Clinics (ISSN 1556-8598) is published quarterly by Elsevier Inc., 360 Park Avenue South, New York, NY 10010-1710. Months of issue are January, April, July, and October. Periodicals postage paid at New York, NY, and additional mailing offices. Subscription prices per year are $232.00 (US individuals), $381.00 (US institutions), $100.00 (US students), $263.00 (Canadian individuals), $428.00 (Canadian institutions), $140.00 (Canadian students), $268.00 (foreign individuals), $428.00 (foreign institutions), and $140.00 (foreign students). To receive student and resident rate, orders must be accompanied by name of affiliated institution, date of term, and the signature of program/residency coordinator on institution letterhead. Orders will be billed at individual rate until proof of status is received. Foreign air speed delivery is included in all Clinics subscription prices. All prices are subject to change without notice. POSTMASTER: Send address changes to PET Clinics, Elsevier Health Sciences Division, Subscription Customer Service, 3251 Riverport Lane, Maryland Heights, MO 63043. **Customer Service: 1-800-654-2452 (U.S. and Canada); 314-447-8871 (outside U.S. and Canada). Fax: 314-447-8029. E-mail: journalscustomerservice-usa@elsevier.com (for print support); journalsonlinesupport-usa@elsevier.com (for online support).**

Reprints. For copies of 100 or more of articles in this publication, please contact the Commercial Reprints Department, Elsevier Inc., 360 Park Avenue South, New York, NY 10010-1710. Tel.: 212-633-3874; Fax: 212-633-3820; E-mail: reprints@elsevier.com.

PET Clinics is covered in MEDLINE/PubMed (Index Medicus).

Contributors

CONSULTING EDITOR

ABASS ALAVI, MD, MD (Hon), PhD (Hon), DSc (Hon)
Professor, Division of Nuclear Medicine, Department of Radiology, Hospital of the University of Pennsylvania, University of Pennsylvania Perelman School of Medicine, Philadelphia, Pennsylvania

EDITOR

RATHAN M. SUBRAMANIAM, MD, PhD, MPH
Russell H. Morgan Department of Radiology and Radiological Sciences, Johns Hopkins School of Medicine, Johns Hopkins University, Baltimore, Maryland; Robert W. Parkey MD Distinguished Professor in Radiology; Professor and Chief, Division of Nuclear Medicine; Departments of Radiology, Clinical Sciences, and Biomedical Engineering, University of Texas Southwestern Medical Center, Dallas, Texas; Advanced Imaging Research Center, University of Texas Southwestern Medical Center, Dallas, Texas

AUTHORS

SANDIP BASU, MBBS (Hons), DRM, DNB, MNAMS
Consultant Physician & Head, Nuclear Medicine Academic Programme, Radiation Medicine Centre, Bhabha Atomic Research Centre, Tata Memorial Hospital Annexe, Bombay, India

PAOLO CASTELLUCCI, MD
Service of Nuclear Medicine, S. Orsola-Malpighi University Hospital, University of Bologna, Bologna, Italy

FRANCESCO CECI, MD, PhD
Service of Nuclear Medicine, S. Orsola-Malpighi University Hospital, University of Bologna, Bologna, Italy

AMY V. CHUDGAR, MD
Division of Nuclear Medicine, Department of Radiology, Hospital of the University of Pennsylvania, University of Pennsylvania, Philadelphia, Pennsylvania

ALEXANDER DRZEZGA, MD
Director, Department of Nuclear Medicine, University Hospital of Cologne; German Center for Neurodegenerative Diseases (DZNE), Cologne, Germany

STEFANO FANTI, MD
Service of Nuclear Medicine, S. Orsola-Malpighi University Hospital, University of Bologna, Bologna, Italy

MICHELANGELO FIORENTINO, MD
Department of Pathology, S. Orsola-Malpighi University Hospital, University of Bologna, Bologna, Italy

JAMES R. GALT, PhD
Associate Professor, Division of Research, Department of Radiology and Imaging Sciences, Emory University School of Medicine, Atlanta, Georgia

VICTOR H. GERBAUDO, PhD, MSHCA
Division of Nuclear Medicine and Molecular Imaging, Department of Radiology, Brigham and Women's Hospital, Harvard Medical School, Boston, Massachusetts

RAGHUVEER HALKAR, MD
Professor, Division of Nuclear Medicine and Molecular Imaging, Department of Radiology and Imaging Sciences, Emory University School of Medicine, Atlanta, Georgia

A. TUBA KENDI, MD
Assistant Professor, Division of Nuclear Medicine and Molecular Imaging, Department of Radiology and Imaging Sciences, Emory University School of Medicine, Atlanta, Georgia

MICHAEL V. KNOPP, MD, PhD
Professor; Novartis Chair of Imaging Research, Wright Center of Innovation in Biomedical Imaging, Division of Imaging Science, Department of Radiology, The Ohio State University Wexner Medical Center, Columbus, Ohio

ATUL K. MALLIK, MD, PhD
Neuroradiology Fellow, Department of Radiology and Imaging Sciences, University of Utah, Salt Lake City, Utah

JOSEPH J. MALY, MD
Fellow and Clinical Instructor, Division of Hematology, Department of Internal Medicine, The Ohio State University Wexner Medical Center, Columbus, Ohio

DAVID A. MANKOFF, MD, PhD
Division of Nuclear Medicine, Department of Radiology, Hospital of the University of Pennsylvania, University of Pennsylvania, Philadelphia, Pennsylvania

ESTHER MENA, MD
Russell H. Morgan Department of Radiology and Radiological Sciences, Johns Hopkins School of Medicine, Johns Hopkins University, Baltimore, Maryland

SATOSHI MINOSHIMA, MD, PhD
Chair, Department of Radiology and Imaging Sciences, University of Utah, Salt Lake City, Utah

VALERIA M. MONCAYO, MD
Assistant Professor, Division of Nuclear Medicine and Molecular Imaging, Department of Radiology and Imaging Sciences, Emory University School of Medicine, Atlanta, Georgia

JONATHON A. NYE, PhD
Assistant Professor, Division of Research, Department of Radiology and Imaging Sciences, Emory University School of Medicine, Atlanta, Georgia

RAHUL VITHALRAO PARGHANE, MBBS, MD
Consultant Physician, Radiation Medicine Centre, Bhabha Atomic Research Centre, Tata Memorial Hospital Annexe, Bombay, India

PUSKAR PATTANAYAK, MD
Russell H. Morgan Department of Radiology and Radiological Sciences, Johns Hopkins School of Medicine, Johns Hopkins University, Baltimore, Maryland

SIDDALING REDY, MD
Russell H. Morgan Department of Radiology and Radiological Sciences, Johns Hopkins School of Medicine, Johns Hopkins University, Baltimore, Maryland

DAVID M. SCHUSTER, MD
Professor, Division of Nuclear Medicine and Molecular Imaging, Department of Radiology and Imaging Sciences, Emory University School of Medicine, Atlanta, Georgia

SARA SHEIKHBAHAEI, MD, MPH
Russell H. Morgan Department of Radiology and Radiological Sciences, Johns Hopkins School of Medicine, Johns Hopkins University, Baltimore, Maryland

LILJA B. SOLNES, MD
Russell H. Morgan Department of Radiology and Radiological Sciences, Johns Hopkins School of Medicine, Johns Hopkins University, Baltimore, Maryland

RATHAN M. SUBRAMANIAM, MD, PhD, MPH
Russell H. Morgan Department of Radiology and Radiological Sciences, Johns Hopkins School of Medicine, Johns Hopkins University, Baltimore, Maryland; Robert W. Parkey MD Distinguished Professor in Radiology; Professor and Chief, Division of Nuclear Medicine; Departments of Radiology, Clinical Sciences, and Biomedical Engineering, University of Texas Southwestern Medical Center, Dallas, Texas; Advanced Imaging Research Center, University of Texas Southwestern Medical Center, Dallas, Texas

MEHDI TAGHIPOUR, MD
Russell H. Morgan Department of Radiology and Radiological Sciences, Johns Hopkins School of Medicine, Johns Hopkins University, Baltimore, Maryland

SHWETHA THIPPSANDRA, MD
Russell H. Morgan Department of Radiology and Radiological Sciences, Johns Hopkins School of Medicine, Johns Hopkins University, Baltimore, Maryland

CHADWICK L. WRIGHT, MD, PhD
Assistant Professor, Wright Center of Innovation in Biomedical Imaging, Division of Imaging Science, Department of Radiology, The Ohio State University Wexner Medical Center, Columbus, Ohio

ANUSHA YANAMADALA, MD
Russell H. Morgan Department of Radiology and Radiological Sciences, Johns Hopkins School of Medicine, Johns Hopkins University, Baltimore, Maryland

JUN ZHANG, PhD
Assistant Professor, Wright Center of Innovation in Biomedical Imaging, Division of Imaging Science, Department of Radiology, The Ohio State University Wexner Medical Center, Columbus, Ohio

KATHERINE A. ZUKOTYNSKI, MD, FRCPC
Division of Nuclear Medicine and Molecular Imaging, Departments of Medicine and Radiology, McMaster University, Hamilton, Ontario, Canada

Contributors

SARA SHEIKHBAHAEI, MD, MPH
Russell H. Morgan Department of Radiology and Radiological Sciences, Johns Hopkins School of Medicine, Johns Hopkins University, Baltimore, Maryland

LILJA B. SOLNES, MD
Russell H. Morgan Department of Radiology and Radiological Sciences, Johns Hopkins School of Medicine, Johns Hopkins University, Baltimore, Maryland

RATHAN M. SUBRAMANIAM, MD, PhD, MPH
Russell H. Morgan Department of Radiology and Radiological Sciences, Johns Hopkins School of Medicine, Johns Hopkins University, Baltimore, Maryland; Robert W. Parkey MD Distinguished Professor in Radiology; Professor and Chief, Division of Nuclear Medicine, Departments of Radiology; Clinical Sciences, and Biomedical Engineering, University of Texas Southwestern Medical Center, Dallas, Texas; Advanced Imaging Research Center, University of Texas Southwestern Medical Center, Dallas, Texas

MEHDI TAGHIPOUR, MD
Russell H. Morgan Department of Radiology and Radiological Sciences, Johns Hopkins School of Medicine, Johns Hopkins University, Baltimore, Maryland

SHWETHA THIPSANDRA, MD
Russell H. Morgan Department of Radiology and Radiological Sciences, Johns Hopkins School of Medicine, Johns Hopkins University, Baltimore, Maryland

CHADWICK L. WRIGHT, MD, PhD
Assistant Professor, Wright Center of Innovation in Biomedical Imaging, Division of Imaging Science, Department of Radiology, The Ohio State University Wexner Medical Center, Columbus, Ohio

ANUSHA YANAMADALA, MD
Russell H. Morgan Department of Radiology and Radiological Sciences, Johns Hopkins School of Medicine, Johns Hopkins University, Baltimore, Maryland

JUN ZHANG, PhD
Assistant Professor, Wright Center of Innovation in Biomedical Imaging, Division of Imaging Science, Department of Radiology, The Ohio State University Wexner Medical Center, Columbus, Ohio

KATHERINE A. ZUKOTYNSKI, MD, FRCPC
Division of Nuclear Medicine and Molecular Imaging, Departments of Medicine and Radiology, McMaster University, Hamilton, Ontario, Canada

Contents

Precision Medicine is about selecting the right therapy for the right patient, at the right time, specific to the molecular targets expressed by disease or tumors, in the context of patient's environment and lifestyle. Some of the challenges for delivery of precision medicine in oncology include biomarkers for patient selection for enrichment-precision diagnostics, mapping out tumor heterogeneity that contributes to therapy failures, and early therapy assessment to identify resistance to therapies. PET/computed tomography offers solutions in these important areas of challenges and facilitates implementation of precision medicine.

The concept of using tumor genomic profiling information has revolutionized personalized cancer treatment. Head and neck (HN) cancer management is being influenced by recent discoveries of activating mutations in epidermal growth factor receptor and related targeted therapies with tyrosine kinase inhibitors, targeted therapies for Kristen Rat Sarcoma, and MET proto-oncogenes. Molecular imaging using PET plays an important role in assessing the biologic behavior of HN cancer with the goal of delivering individualized cancer treatment. This review summarizes recent genomic discoveries in HN cancer and their implications for functional PET imaging in assessing response to targeted therapies, and drug resistance mechanisms.

This communication enumerates the current uses and potential areas where PET could be clinically utilized for developing "precision medicine" type model in thyroid carcinoma. (1) In routine clinics, PET imaging (with fluorodeoxyglucose [FDG]) is utilized to investigate patients of differentiated thyroid carcinoma (DTC) with high thyroglobulin and negative iodine scintigraphy (TENIS) and in medullary carcinoma thyroid (MCT) when the tumor markers (eg, calcitonin and carcino embryonic antigen [CEA]) are raised postoperatively (PET with FDG, ^{68}Ga-DOTA-NOC/TATE, FDOPA). Both are examples of management personalization, where PET-computed tomography (CT) has been found substantially useful in detecting sites of metastatic disease and making decision with regard to feasibility and planning of surgery on an individual patient basis. (2) The next important area of management personalization is in patients of TENIS with metastatic disease not amenable to surgery through examining FDG-PET findings in tandem with radio iodine scan and ^{68}Ga-DOTA-TATE/NOC PET/CT. Heterogeneous behavior of the metastatic lesions is frequently observed clinically: analyzing the findings of three studies aids in sub-segmenting patients into subgroups and thereby deciding upon the best approach (observation with LT4 suppression vs PRRT vs tyrosine kinase inhibitors) that could be individualized in a given case. (3) In metastatic/inoperable MCT, ^{68}Ga-DOTA-TATE/NOC PET-CT helps in deciding upon feasibility of targeted PRRT in an individual patient and helps in follow-up and response evaluation. (4) Disease prognostification with FDG-PET is evolving both in DTC and MCT, where FDG avidity would indicate an aggressive biology, though the implication of this from treatment viewpoint is unclear at this point. Conversely, a negative FDG-PET in DTC and TENIS would suggest a favorable prognosis in an individual. (5) Iodine-124 PET/CT has the added potential of obtaining lesional dosimetry compared to the SPECT approach, and could help in selecting appropriate doses on an individual basis.

The aim of the present review is to discuss about the role of new probes for molecular imaging in the evaluation of prostate cancer (PCa). This review focuses particularly on the role of new promising radiotracers for the molecular imaging with PET/computed tomography in the detection of PCa recurrence. The role of these new imaging techniques to guide lesion-target therapies and the potential application of these molecular probes as theranostics agents is discussed. Finally, the molecular mechanisms underlying resistance to castration in PCa and the maintenance of active androgen receptor are discussed.

This article reviews recent advances and applications of radionuclide therapy. Individualized precision medicine, new treatments, and the evolving role of radionuclide therapy are discussed.

A variety of methods have been developed to assess tumor response to therapy. Standardized qualitative criteria based on 18F-fluoro-deoxyglucose PET/computed tomography have been proposed to evaluate the treatment effectiveness in specific cancers and these allow more accurate therapy response assessment and survival prognostication. Multiple studies have addressed the utility of the volumetric PET biomarkers as prognostic indicators but there is no consensus about the preferred segmentation methodology for these metrics. Heterogeneous intratumoral uptake was proposed as a novel PET metric for therapy response assessment. PET imaging techniques will be used to study the biological behavior of cancers during therapy.

Precision medicine (PM) has been defined as "prevention and treatment strategies that take individual variability into account." Molecular imaging (MI) is an ideally suited tool for PM approaches to neurodegenerative dementia and movement disorders (MD). Here we review PM approaches and discuss how they may be applied to other associated neurodegenerative dementia and MD. With ongoing major therapeutic research initiatives that include the use of molecular imaging, we look forward to established interventions targeted to specific molecular pathophysiology and expect the potential benefit of MI PM approaches in neurodegenerative dementia and MD will only increase.

PET CLINICS

PROGRAM OBJECTIVE

The goal of the *PET Clinics* is to keep practicing radiologists and radiology residents up to date with current clinical practice in positron emission tomography by providing timely articles reviewing the state of the art in patient care.

TARGET AUDIENCE

Practicing radiologists, radiology residents, and other health care professionals who provide patient care utilizing radiologic findings.

LEARNING OBJECTIVES

Upon completion of this activity, participants will be able to:
1. Review molecular imaging and precision medicine in movement disorders.
2. Discuss the use of molecular imaging and precision medicine in providing personalized care.
3. Recognize developments in molecular imaging and precision medicine in cancer care.

ACCREDITATION

The Elsevier Office of Continuing Medical Education (EOCME) is accredited by the Accreditation Council for Continuing Medical Education (ACCME) to provide continuing medical education for physicians.

The EOCME designates this enduring material for a maximum of 15 *AMA PRA Category 1 Credit*(s)™. Physicians should claim only the credit commensurate with the extent of their participation in the activity.

All other health care professionals requesting continuing education credit for this enduring material will be issued a certificate of participation.

DISCLOSURE OF CONFLICTS OF INTEREST

The EOCME assesses conflict of interest with its instructors, faculty, planners, and other individuals who are in a position to control the content of CME activities. All relevant conflicts of interest that are identified are thoroughly vetted by EOCME for fair balance, scientific objectivity, and patient care recommendations. EOCME is committed to providing its learners with CME activities that promote improvements or quality in healthcare and not a specific proprietary business or a commercial interest.

The planning committee, staff, authors and editors listed below have identified no financial relationships or relationships to products or devices they or their spouse/life partner have with commercial interest related to the content of this CME activity:

Abass Alavi, MD, MD (Hon), PhD (Hon), DSc (Hon); Sandip Basu, MBBS (Hons), DRM, DNB, MNAMS; Paolo Castellucci, MD; Francesco Ceci, MD, PhD; Amy V. Chudgar, MD; Alexander Drzezga, MD; Stefano Fanti, MD; Michelangelo Fiorentino, MD; James R. Galt, PhD; Victor H. Gerbaudo, PhD, MSHCA; Raghuveer Halkar, MD; A. Tuba Kendi, MD; Micahel V. Knopp, MD, PhD; Atul K. Mallik, MD, PhD; Joseph J. Maly, MD; David A. Mankoff, MD, PhD; Satoshi Minoshima, MD, PhD; Valeria M. Moncayo, MD; Jonathon A. Nye, PhD; Rahul Vithalrao Parghane, MBBS, MD; Puskar Pattanayak, MD; Siddaling Redy, MD; Erin Scheckenbach; David M. Schuster, MD; Sara Sheikhbahaei, MD, MPH; Lilja B. Solnes, MD; Rathan M. Subramaniam, MD, PhD, MPH; Megan Suermann; Mehdi Taghipour, MD; Shwetha Thippsandra, MD; John Vassallo; Rajakumar Venkatesan; Chadwick L. Wright, MD, PhD; Anusha Yanamadala, MD; Jun Zhang, PhD; Katherine A. Zukotynski, MD, FRCPC.

The planning committee, staff, authors and editors listed below have identified financial relationships or relationships to products or devices they or their spouse/life partner have with commercial interest related to the content of this CME activity:
Esther Mena, MD has research support from the National Institute for Basic Biology and the National Institutes of Health.

UNAPPROVED/OFF-LABEL USE DISCLOSURE

The EOCME requires CME faculty to disclose to the participants:
1. When products or procedures being discussed are off-label, unlabelled, experimental, and/or investigational (not US Food and Drug Administration [FDA] approved); and
2. Any limitations on the information presented, such as data that are preliminary or that represent ongoing research, interim analyses, and/or unsupported opinions. Faculty may discuss information about pharmaceutical agents that is outside of FDA-approved labelling. This information is intended solely for CME and is not intended to promote off-label use of these medications. If you have any questions, contact the medical affairs department of the manufacturer for the most recent prescribing information.

TO ENROLL

To enroll in the PET Clinics Continuing Medical Education program, call customer service at 1-800-654-2452 or sign up online at http://www.theclinics.com/home/cme. The CME program is available to subscribers for an additional annual fee of USD $235.

METHOD OF PARTICIPATION

In order to claim credit, participants must complete the following:

1. Complete enrolment as indicated above.
2. Read the activity.
3. Complete the CME Test and Evaluation. Participants must achieve a score of 70% on the test. All CME Tests and Evaluations must be completed online.

CME INQUIRIES/SPECIAL NEEDS

For all CME inquiries or special needs, please contact elsevierCME@elsevier.com.

Preface
Precision Medicine and PET/Computed Tomography: Time Has Arrived

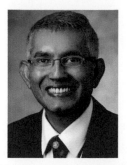

Rathan M. Subramaniam, MD, PhD, MPH
Editor

The time has arrived for the imaging community to take responsibility and deliver how imaging will be a valuable asset and how it will become an integral part in the implementation of precision medicine.

Precision medicine is about *selecting the right type of treatment for the right disease, at the right time, and for right patient*. The focus is on identifying which approach will be effective for which patient based on genetic, environmental, and lifestyle factors. Some of the challenges for implementing precision medicine include biomarkers for patient selection—precision diagnostics, biomarkers for tumor heterogeneity, which contributes to therapy failure, and biomarkers for early management decisions, which lead to an early identification of the therapies that are unlikely to be successful.

In this first issue of a two-part series of *PET Clinics*, which is dedicated to collate the immense value of PET/computed tomography (CT) for implementation of precision medicine, we cover the definition of precision medicine and the national imperatives, the role and value of PET/CT for implementing precision medicine in head and neck cancer, thyroid cancer, breast cancer, lung cancer, lymphoma, prostate cancer, radionuclide therapies, therapy assessment, dementia, and movement disorders.

Unlike other imaging modalities, PET/CT is unique in its quantitative nature and its ability to target small molecules, which play critical roles in biologic mechanisms of disease processes. This reveals the functional status of disease process at an earlier stage, in vivo, allowing the opportunity to enrich the population for a particular therapy or identify therapy resistance earlier in the treatment paradigm. For PET/CT to be valuable, these studies must be performed in a standardized manner so that the PET-based imaging biomarkers are reliable, precise, and deployable from academic centers to community practices. Significant efforts are now devoted to achieving standardization of PET/CTs, both in clinical trials and in clinical practices, advancing the implementation of precision medicine.

Let's keep advancing the field of PET/CT, which is impactful in implementing the precision medicine and influencing patient outcomes.

Rathan M. Subramaniam, MD, PhD, MPH
Robert W. Parkey MD Distinguished Professor in Radiology
Professor and Chief, Division of Nuclear Medicine
Department of Radiology
UT Southwestern Medical Center
5323 Harry Hines Boulevard
Dallas, TX 75390-8896, USA

E-mail address:
rathan.subramaniam@UTsouthwestern.edu

PET Clin 12 (2017) xiii
http://dx.doi.org/10.1016/j.cpet.2016.10.001
1556-8598/17/© 2016 Published by Elsevier Inc.

Precision Medicine and PET/Computed Tomography
Challenges and Implementation

Rathan M. Subramaniam, MD, PhD, MPH[a,b,c,d,e,]*

KEYWORDS

- Precision medicine • PET/computed tomography • Biomarker • Patient selection

KEY POINTS

- Precision Medicine is about selecting the right therapy for the right patient, at the right time, specific to the molecular targets expressed by disease or tumors, in the context of patient's environment and lifestyle.
- Some of the challenges for delivery of precision medicine in oncology include biomarkers for patient selection for enrichment-precision diagnostics, mapping out tumor heterogeneity that contributes to therapy failures, and early therapy assessment to identify resistance to therapies.
- PET/computed tomography (CT) offers solutions in these important areas of challenges and facilitates implementation of precision medicine.
- Early therapy assessment using PET/CT for precision medicine is highly influenced by (1) the biology or molecular subtype of the tumor, (2) therapy selected, (3) timing of early therapy assessment PET/CT, and (4) standardization of PET/CT procedures.

The National Institutes of Health (NIH) defines precision medicine as "an emerging approach for disease treatment and prevention that takes into account individual variability in genes, environment, and lifestyle for each person." This approach will allow doctors and researchers to predict more accurately which treatment and prevention strategies for a particular disease will work and in which groups of people. It is about selecting the right type of treatment for the right disease, at the right time, and for the right patient. The focus is on identifying which approach will be effective for which patient based on genetic, environmental, and lifestyle factors. It is in contrast to the current therapy paradigm of "one-size-fits-all" approach, in which disease treatment and prevention strategies are developed for the "average" patient, with less consideration for the differences between patients.

"Precision Medicine" also can be differentiated from "personalized medicine," which may imply

Disclosure: The author has nothing to disclose.
The author is supported by National Institutes of Health (U10 CA180870, HHSN268201500021C [E], and HHSN268201500021C [B]).

[a] Department of Radiology, University of Texas Southwestern Medical Center, 5323 Harry Hines Boulevard, Dallas, TX 75390-8896, USA; [b] Department of Clinical Sciences, University of Texas Southwestern Medical Center, 5323 Harry Hines Boulevard, Dallas, TX 75390-8896, USA; [c] Department of Biomedical Engineering, University of Texas Southwestern Medical Center, 5323 Harry Hines Boulevard, Dallas, TX 75390-8896, USA; [d] Advanced Imaging Research Center, University of Texas Southwestern Medical Center, 5323 Harry Hines Boulevard, Dallas, TX 75390-8896, USA; [e] Russell H. Morgan Department of Radiology and Radiological Sciences, Johns Hopkins School of Medicine, Johns Hopkins University, 601 North Caroline Street, Baltimore, MD 21287, USA
* Department of Radiology, University of Texas Southwestern Medical Center, 5323 Harry Hines Boulevard, Dallas, TX 75390-8896.
E-mail address: rathan.subramaniam@UTsouthwestern.edu

PET Clin 12 (2017) 1–5
http://dx.doi.org/10.1016/j.cpet.2016.08.010
1556-8598/17/© 2016 Elsevier Inc. All rights reserved.

that treatment and prevention strategies are developed uniquely for each individual. Medicine has been practiced for centuries as personalized medicine, tailoring treatments to each patient. In contrast, precision medicine is about therapies that are more precisely tailored to specific molecular targets.

In 2015, President Obama, as part of his State of the Union address, announced the Precision Medicine initiative—a research effort that focuses on bringing precision medicine to many aspects of health care. The budget for fiscal year 2016 included $216 million in funding for the NIH, the National Cancer Institute (NCI), and the US Food and Drug Administration (FDA). Specifically, the funding provides $130 million to the NIH to assemble a data set (genomic data, lifestyle information, biologic samples linking to health care records) with a cohort of at least 1 million volunteers, $70 million to the NCI for efforts to identify genes that contributes to tumors, $10 million for the FDA, and $5 million to the National Coordinator for Health Information Technology to develop the information technology infrastructure.[1] The President's initiative addresses the need for multifaceted data about patients (lifestyle, environment, and genomic information), the tools needed to work with large patient data sets, building infrastructure and interoperability of these systems, and finally, the stakeholders who will use the information.

In this context, oncology is at the forefront of precision medicine, today. There has been progress toward the discovery and development of targeted therapeutic agents with evidence in clinical trials of the improvement of therapeutic efficacy. More and more patients are receiving targeted and biologically rational therapies based on patients' cancer genome analysis and on the basis of deeper biologic understanding of the disease than unselected therapies based on a simple phenotypic marker. Selection of targeted therapies avoids overtreatment or undertreatment and unnecessary toxicities, morbidities, and therapy failure. For example, (1) the targeting of HER2 overexpression with the monoclonal antibody, trastuzumab, to improve outcome in metastatic breast cancer was the first example of targeted treatment[2]; (2) the tyrosine kinase inhibitor, imatinib, developed to target the BCR-ABL fusion gene, a consequence of the Philadelphia chromosome and pathognomonic of chronic myeloid leukemia, transformed the care of patients, changing this aggressive, life-threatening disease to a manageable chronic disease[3]; and (3) the epidermal growth factor receptor (EGFR) pathway has been targeted for the treatment of patients with somatic EGFR mutant non–small cell lung carcinoma (NSCLC). EGFR tyrosine kinase inhibitors, such as erlotinib and gefitinib, have confirmed significant improvements in the progression-free survival, in advanced EGFR-mutated NSCLC[4,5]; (4) immune checkpoint inhibitors (eg, anti-CTLA4 or PD-1 monoclonal antibody agents, ipilimumab, nivolumab, atezolizuumab) for melanoma, NSCLC, renal cell cancer, Hodgkin lymphoma, and head and neck squamous cell cancer (HNSCC). Most of the therapeutic targets are in critical molecular signaling pathways associated with development of disease. Targeting specific molecular or effectors of different diseases has shown therapeutic advantages and great potential as an important aspect of precision medicine. Next-generation drugs would be designed for disease subtypes with more specificity, efficacy, and lower toxicity.

However, there are many challenges delivering the promises of precision medicine for oncologic patients. Some of these challenges, pertinent to imaging, include biomarkers for patient selection: precision diagnostics, biomarkers for tumor heterogeneity, which contributes to therapy failure, and biomarkers for early management decisions, which leads to identifying early the therapies that are unlikely to be successful. PET/computed tomography (CT) has a vital role in each of these domains or challenges and has potential to add value in the promise of delivery of precision medicine.

BIOMARKER FOR PATIENT SELECTION: PRECISION DIAGNOSTICS

A good biomarker for patient selection is key to achieving an acceptable cost/benefit ratio for any novel therapeutic agent—to avoid unnecessary side effects for patients in whom the therapy may not be successful and to avoid the cost to patients and health care systems. It is necessary to have companion diagnostic predictive markers, when a novel targeted therapy is developed to select the right patients. Ideally, a biomarker should enable the identification of subpopulations in whom to test new agents where they have the best chance of working, thus enriching the study population. For example, Tirapazamine (TPZ) is a bioreductively activated, hypoxia-selective antitumor agent of the benzotriazine series. For phase III trials using TPZ as therapy agent, a PET/CT with hypoxic radiopharmaceutical, such as fluorine-18-labeled fluoromisonidazole (^{18}F-FMISO) or ^{18}F fluoroazomycin arabinoside (FAZA) or ^{18}F HX-4,[6] can be deployed to enrich the study population as a companion diagnostic marker. Other examples include enriching the patient with metastatic breast cancer with ^{18}F-fluoroestradiol (^{18}F-FES)

PET/CT for estrogen receptor (ER) expression before treating with hormonal therapies or enriching the neuroendocrine tumor patients with ^{68}Ga DOTATATE PET/CT, before therapy with ^{177}Lu-DOTATATE[7] or enriching the patients with ^{68}Ga-PSMA PET/CT before therapy with ^{177}Lu-PSMA therapy.[8] It is vital to develop new PET radiopharmaceuticals with specific molecular targets, which are likely to be coupled with therapy agents and facilitate the companion diagnostic-therapy paradigm that is critical for precision medicine.

TUMOR HETEROGENEITY

Tumor heterogeneity is one of the most significant challenges for implementing precision medicine in oncology.[9] Tumor heterogeneity can be (1) intertumoral heterogeneity within a patient: patient may have tumors or lesions that may appear similar from a histologic point of view but varies significantly by molecular subtype and malignant potential; (2) intratumor heterogeneity: cancer cells within a tumor may have varied functional heterogeneity and spatial heterogeneity. Spatial heterogeneity of subclones within a primary lesion or metastasis provides a challenge for precision medicine as sequencing a portion of the tumor may miss important therapeutically relevant information. Lesions may be at locations that render getting a tissue biopsy practically impossible. In addition, after therapy, clones can change with selective pressure from a targeted therapy and as a result of mutagenic activity of radiation and chemotherapy. Usually the patient outcomes are poor when biomarkers found in the primary tumor and metastatic lesions are varied. Thus, precision medicine requires the development of approaches to detect and deal with intratumor and intertumor heterogeneity in a patient.

PET/CT can provide information about intratumor spatial heterogeneity as well as intrapatient intertumoral heterogeneity because it is a whole body examination and can image the primary lesion as well as metastases in a single study. In addition, the availability of multiple molecular-specific PET radiopharmaceuticals provides feasible probing of intratumor and intertumor heterogeneity. For example, studies have shown that PET with ^{18}F-FES can be used to noninvasively assess regional ER expression[10] and has the potential to overcome the sampling errors that arise from disease heterogeneity. PET can simultaneously measure the in vivo delivery and binding of estrogens and thus ER expression at multiple tumor sites. Earlier studies showed that ^{18}F-FES uptake at a tumor site correlates with ER expression assayed in vitro by radioligand

binding[10] and that the level of uptake predicts the likelihood of a response to tamoxifen and aromatase inhibitor treatment.[11–13] FES-PET has shown promise for assessment of heterogeneity of ER expression in individual patients.[14] In a recent study, the ^{18}F-FES PET/CT resulted in a change in the management plan in 48.5% of patients. In detecting ER status in the metastasis group (n = 27), ^{18}F-FES PET/CT showed increased ^{18}F-FES uptake in all metastatic lesions in 11 patients; absence in all lesions in 13 patients, and the remaining 3 patients had both ^{18}F-FES positive and negative lesions. In total, on the basis of the ^{18}F-FES PET/CT results, investigators found changes in the treatment plans in 16 patients (48.5%, 16/33).[15] Another example is modifying radiation therapy delivery based on heterogeneity of tumor hypoxia within tumors based on ^{18}F-FMISO PET/CT.[16] In this study, heterogeneous distribution of ^{18}F-FMISO within the gross tumor volume (GTV) demonstrated variable levels of hypoxia within the tumor. Plans directed at performing ^{18}F-FMISO PET/CT-guided intensity modulated radiotherapy (IMRT) for 10 patients with head and neck cancer achieved 84 Gy to the GTV(h) and 70 Gy to the GTV, without exceeding the normal tissue tolerance. Investigators also attempted to deliver 105 Gy to the GTV(h) for 2 patients and were successful in 1, with normal tissue sparing.[16]

EARLY THERAPY ASSESSMENT

Current therapy assessment methods, based on tumor anatomic changes, are insensitive or late markers for novel and targeted therapies. Because identifying therapy resistance early is a priority for delivering precision medicine, PET/CT plays an invaluable role for delivering precision medicine. Using PET/CT successfully for early therapy assessment highly influenced (1) the biology of the tumors or molecular subtypes, (2) therapy selection, (3) timing of early therapy assessment PET/CT, and (4) performing PET/CT in a standardized manner.

Biology of the Tumors/Molecular Subtypes

The avidity of PET radiopharmaceutical at baseline (before any therapy) is an important determinant of how PET/CT can be deployed in early assessment of therapy. A good example is Hodgkin disease, which is intensely FDG avid; an early therapy assessment with PET/CT is now standard of care, performed after 2 or 3 cycles of therapy, which predicts outcome of patients and impacts therapy decisions. Another example, most of the HNSCC are intensely FDG avid before therapy, and the FDG avidity diminishes rapidly with successful therapy. Hence, an early therapy FDG PET/CT can be performed after 2 cycles of induction chemotherapy or 2 weeks of concurrent chemoradiation therapy, and the change in FDG avidity between the baseline imaging and early therapy assessment imaging can separate the responders and nonresponders,[17] reliably. Not all tumors are intensely FDG avid, such as lobular breast cancer and bronchioalveolar cancer of the lung, and it would be difficult to implement FDG PET/CT–based early therapy assessment for these cancers. However, a novel PET radiopharmaceutical such as fluciclovine,[18] which demonstrates intense uptake in lobular breast cancer, can be successfully deployed. Therefore, selecting a tumor type or molecular subtype, which has moderate to intense avidity for the PET radiopharmaceutical, is fundamentally important.

Therapy Selection

Therapies that induce an inflammatory response early can interfere with the intensity of FDG uptake, which can lead to errors in early therapy assessment. Radiation-induced inflammatory FDG uptake can be noticeable after the second week of therapy until at least 12 weeks after therapy completion or even later.[19] Inflammatory uptake due to immunotherapy can be seen early during the first 2 cycles and then usually subsides over many months. It is also known that chemotherapy in combination with Rituximab induces inflammatory FDG uptake. In addition, rate of decline in FDG avidity depends on the effectiveness of the therapy against the tumor. Novel therapy assessment methods for immunotherapy assessment using FDG PET/CT or other novel PET radiopharmaceuticals must be developed in the future. It is important to use FDG PET/CT in an appropriate therapy context for early therapy assessment.

Timing of PET/Computed Tomography

The early therapy assessment by PET/CT is usually performed after the first or second cycle of therapy, which allows time for adaptation to modify the therapy as well as minimize the nonspecific inflammatory uptake induced by therapy. Early therapy assessment is important to avoid the unnecessary cost of expensive therapies and side effects associated with the therapies soon after 2 cycles.

Standardization of PET/Computed Tomography

Implementing standardized and structured qualitative therapy assessment methods such as Lugano classification for lymphoma[20] and Hopkins criteria for solid tumors[21,22] and quantitative methods such as standardized uptake values (SUVmax or SUVpeak) or tumor volumetric markers such as metabolic tumor volume or total lesion glycolysis or tumor heterogeneity indices requires standardization of PET/CT procedures. The standardization of methods for PET/CT calibration, patient preparation, image acquisition, and image analysis are essential for precision therapy assessment. European Association of Nuclear Medicine (EANM) guidelines[23] or the Quantitative Imaging Biomarker Alliance FDG PET/CT profile (version 1.0)[24] must be followed to standardize the PET/CT procedures. EANM guidelines recommend a blood glucose level of 200 mg/dL for clinical and 150 mg/dL for research studies and an uptake time of 60 minutes for FDG PET/CT. When therapy assessment PET/CT is performed, the uptake time is recommended to be within 10 minutes of the baseline study.[23] In addition, patients need to be scanned in the same PET/CT system, and the same reconstruction methods and analysis are used when a patient has multiple PET/CT studies.

In conclusion, Precision Medicine is about selecting the right therapy for the right patient, at the right time, specific to the molecular targets expressed by disease or tumors, in the context of patient's environment and lifestyle. Some of the challenges for delivery of precision medicine in oncology include biomarkers for patient selection for enrichment: precision diagnostics, mapping out tumor heterogeneity that contributes to therapy failures, and early therapy assessment to identify resistance to therapies. PET/CT offers solutions in these important areas of challenges and facilitates implementation of precision medicine.

REFERENCES

1. Office of the Press Secretary. FACT SHEET: President Obama's precision medicine initiative. The White House; 2015. Available at: https://www.whitehouse.gov/the-press-office/2015/01/30/fact-sheet-president-obama-s-precisionmedicine- initiative. Accessed August 14, 2016.
2. Slamon DJ, Leyland-Jones B, Shak S, et al. Use of chemotherapy plus a monoclonal antibody against HER2 for metastatic breast cancer that overexpresses HER2. N Engl J Med 2001;344(11):783–92.
3. Hughes TP, Kaeda J, Branford S, et al. Frequency of major molecular responses to imatinib or interferon alfa plus cytarabine in newly diagnosed chronic myeloid leukemia. N Engl J Med 2003;349(15):1423–32.

4. Mitsudomi T, Morita S, Yatabe Y, et al. Gefitinib versus cisplatin plus docetaxel in patients with non-small-cell lung cancer harbouring mutations of the epidermal growth factor receptor (WJTOG3405): an open label, randomised phase 3 trial. Lancet Oncol 2010;11(2):121–8.

5. Rosell R, Carcereny E, Gervais R, et al. Erlotinib versus standard chemotherapy as first-line treatment for European patients with advanced EGFR mutation-positive non-small-cell lung cancer (EURTAC): a multicentre, open-label, randomised phase 3 trial. Lancet Oncol 2012;13(3):239–46.

6. Zegers CM, van Elmpt W, Szardenings K, et al. Repeatability of hypoxia PET imaging using [(1)(8)F]HX4 in lung and head and neck cancer patients: a prospective multicenter trial. Eur J Nucl Med Mol Imaging 2015;42(12):1840–9.

7. Strosberg J, Wolin E, Chasen B, et al. 177-Lu-dotatate significantly improves progression-free survival in patients with midgut neuroendocrine tumours: results of the phase III NETTER-1 trial. Available at: https://www.nanets.net/nanets_cd/2015/pdfs/C39.pdf. Accessed August 14, 2016.

8. Baum RP, Kulkarni HR, Schuchardt C, et al. 177Lu-labeled prostate-specific membrane antigen radioligand therapy of metastatic castration-resistant prostate cancer: safety and efficacy. J Nucl Med 2016;57(7):1006–13.

9. Burrell RA, McGranahan N, Bartek J, et al. The causes and consequences of genetic heterogeneity in cancer evolution. Nature 2013;501(7467): 338–45.

10. Mintun MA, Welch MJ, Siegel BA, et al. Breast cancer: PET imaging of estrogen receptors. Radiology 1988;169(1):45–8.

11. Mortimer JE, Dehdashti F, Siegel BA, et al. Metabolic flare: indicator of hormone responsiveness in advanced breast cancer. J Clin Oncol 2001;19(11): 2797–803.

12. Mortimer JE, Dehdashti F, Siegel BA, et al. Positron emission tomography with 2-[18F]fluoro-2-deoxy-D-glucose and 16alpha-[18F]fluoro-17beta-estradiol in breast cancer: correlation with estrogen receptor status and response to systemic therapy. Clin Cancer Res 1996;2(6):933–9.

13. Linden HM, Stekhova SA, Link JM, et al. Quantitative fluoroestradiol positron emission tomography imaging predicts response to endocrine treatment in breast cancer. J Clin Oncol 2006;24(18):2793–9.

14. Kurland BF, Peterson LM, Lee JH, et al. Between-patient and within-patient (site-to-site) variability in estrogen receptor binding, measured in vivo by 18F-fluoroestradiol PET. J Nucl Med 2011;52(10):1541–9.

15. Sun Y, Yang Z, Zhang Y, et al. The preliminary study of 16alpha-[18F]fluoroestradiol PET/CT in assisting the individualized treatment decisions of breast cancer patients. PLoS One 2015;10(1):e0116341.

16. Lee NY, Mechalakos JG, Nehmeh S, et al. Fluorine-18-labeled fluoromisonidazole positron emission and computed tomography-guided intensity-modulated radiotherapy for head and neck cancer: a feasibility study. Int J Radiat Oncol Biol Phys 2008;70(1):2–13.

17. Yu J, Cooley T, Truong MT, et al. Head and neck squamous cell cancer (stages III and IV) induction chemotherapy assessment: value of FDG volumetric imaging parameters. J Med Imaging Radiat Oncol 2014;58(1):18–24.

18. Tade FI, Cohen MA, Styblo TM, et al. Anti-3-18F-FACBC (18F-Fluciclovine) PET/CT of breast cancer: an exploratory study. J Nucl Med 2016;57:1357–63.

19. Subramaniam R, Truong M, Peller P, et al. Fluorodeoxyglucose–positron-emission tomography imaging of head and neck squamous cell cancer. Am J Neuroradiol 2010;31(4):598–604.

20. Cheson BD, Fisher RI, Barrington SF, et al. Recommendations for initial evaluation, staging, and response assessment of Hodgkin and non-Hodgkin lymphoma: the Lugano classification. J Clin Oncol 2014;32(27):3059–68.

21. Marcus C, Ciarallo A, Tahari AK, et al. Head and neck PET/CT: therapy response interpretation criteria (Hopkins Criteria)-interreader reliability, accuracy, and survival outcomes. J Nucl Med 2014; 55(9):1411–6.

22. Sheikhbahaei S, Mena E, Marcus C, et al. 18F-FDG PET/CT: therapy response assessment interpretation (Hopkins criteria) and survival outcomes in lung cancer patients. J Nucl Med 2016;57(6):855–60.

23. Boellaard R, Delgado-Bolton R, Oyen WJ, et al. FDG PET/CT: EANM procedure guidelines for tumour imaging: version 2.0. Eur J Nucl Med Mol Imaging 2015;42(2):328–54.

24. Available at: www.rsna.org/uploadedFiles/RSNA/Content/Science_and_Education/QIBA/QIBA_FDG-PET_Profile_v105_Publicly_Reviewed_Version_FINAL_11Dec2013.pdf. Accessed August 14, 2016.

Molecular Imaging and Precision Medicine in Head and Neck Cancer

 CrossMark

Esther Mena, MD[a], Shwetha Thippsandra, MD[a], Anusha Yanamadala, MD[a], Siddaling Redy, MD[a], Puskar Pattanayak, MD[a], Rathan M. Subramaniam, MD, PhD, MPH[a,b,c,d,e],*

KEYWORDS

- Head and neck cancer • Tumor genetic profiling • Molecular imaging • Targeted therapy

KEY POINTS

- Human papillomavirus (HPV) in head and neck squamous cell carcinoma (HNSCC), Epstein-Barr virus in nasopharyngeal carcinoma (EBV), and PET imaging features provide robust prognostic biomarkers that are being incorporated into clinical trials.
- Patients with HPV-positive HNSCCs have a better prognosis than patients with HPV-negative tumors; the HPV-positive status has facilitated efforts to de-intensify therapy in a subset of patients with a more favorable prognosis; FDG-PET/CT plays a role in safely de-intensifying therapy.
- Understanding the molecular and genetic alterations in the pathogenesis of head and neck cancer will help elucidate the mechanisms involved in tumor growth as well as identify potential targets for improved treatment.
- Novel drug developments focused on molecular targeting therapeutic agents for patients with genomically defined head and neck cancer have brought a new, exciting approach in the response assessment of head and neck cancer; this may open new strategies for using PET imaging to identify treatment response, and manage secondary resistances.
- Development of prognostic biomarkers using PET imaging could potentially predict early identification of responders/nonresponders, leading to improvement in clinical management and individualizing therapy decisions.

INTRODUCTION

Head and neck (HN) cancer is a heterogeneous malignancy that involves multiple sites and cellular origins, commonly arising from the oral cavity, oropharynx, hypopharynx, larynx, sinonasal tract, and nasopharynx.[1] HN cancer accounts for 650,000 cases annually worldwide and is the sixth most common neoplasm.[2,3]

Disclosure: Dr R.M. Subramaniam receives National Cancer Institute/National Institutes of Health (NIH) support under the award 1UO1CA140204-01A2. Dr E. Mena receives National Institute of Biomedical Imaging and Bioengineering (NIBIB)/NIH support under the award T32EB006351. Drs S. Thippsandra, A. Yanamadela, S. Redy, and P. Pattanayak have nothing to disclose.

[a] Russell H. Morgan Department of Radiology and Radiological Sciences, Johns Hopkins School of Medicine, Johns Hopkins University, 601 North Caroline Street, Baltimore, MD 21287, USA; [b] Department of Radiology, University of Texas Southwestern Medical Center, 5323 Harry Hines Boulevard, Dallas, TX 75390-8896, USA; [c] Department of Clinical Sciences, University of Texas Southwestern Medical Center, 5323 Harry Hines Boulevard, Dallas, TX 75390-9096, USA; [d] Department of Biomedical Engineering, University of Texas Southwestern Medical Center, 5323 Harry Hines Boulevard, Dallas, TX, 75390-8896, USA; [e] Advanced Imaging Research Center, University of Texas Southwestern Medical Center, Dallas, TX, 75390-8896, USA
* Corresponding author. Department of Radiology, UT Southwestern Medical Center, 5323 Harry Hines Boulevard, Dallas, TX 75390-8896.
E-mail address: rathan.subramaniam@UTsouthwestern.edu

PET Clin 12 (2017) 7–25
http://dx.doi.org/10.1016/j.cpet.2016.08.009
1556-8598/17/© 2016 Elsevier Inc. All rights reserved.

According to American Cancer Society, 47,000 new cases of HN cancers are diagnosed every year in the United States, constituting 3% of all cancers.[4] Squamous cell carcinoma (SCC) is the commonest type of HN cancer, accounting for 95% of cancers, and the remaining 5% includes non-SCC.[5] The most important risk factors for developing HN cancer include carcinogens (tobacco and alcohol) and human papillomavirus (HPV). Although the prevalence of traditional carcinogen risk factors–related HN cancers have reduced, there is an increased incidence of HPV-related HN cancers.[6] Despite the advances in management of HN cancer, the prognosis of patients with locally advanced HNSCC is poor, with 5-year survival rate of 40% to 50%,[7] without much change in the survival rates over the past decades, mainly due to the inability to control locoregional recurrences and distant metastases. Currently the treatment decisions are based on clinical and imaging diagnostics. Understanding the molecular carcinogenesis, individual genetic differences, and pharmaco-genetics may help in formulating new tailored therapeutic approaches; hence, improving the disease outcome. Identification of biological markers predictive of treatment failure also allows the use of more targeted therapies. This is illustrated in the use of novel targeted therapies focusing on epidermal growth factor receptor (EGFR). EGFR is overexpressed in nearly 80% to 90% of the HNSCC and correlates with poor prognosis and resistance to radiation therapy.[8] Evidence showed that treatment with inhibitors of EFGR offers better survival benefits when compared with standard therapies.[9]

The use of molecular imaging using PET offers unique insights in the field of oncology, helping early disease detection, localization, monitoring treatment responses, and identification of tumor recurrence. This review summarizes the recent genomic discoveries in HN cancer and their implications in imaging, highlighting the evolving role of PET imaging in HN cancer, with the use of ^{18}F-Fluorodeoxy-glucose (FDG) and other novel PET tracers designed to characterize the specific biological behavior of the cancer, and follow-up response assessment to a specific therapy.

MOLECULAR GENETICS IN HEAD AND NECK CANCER: VALUE OF PET IMAGING

The molecular origins of HN cancer lie on the interaction between environmental factors and host genetic susceptibility. Classically, HN cancer was driven by habitual exposure to tobacco and alcohol; however, in the past decades, there has been an alarming rise in the number of HN cancer cases arising from the oropharynx (tonsil and base of the tongue) as a result of oral infection with human papillomavirus (HPV), especially serotype 16. Tumor HPV status has been shown to be the single strongest predictor factor for oropharyngeal squamous cell cancer (OPSCC) (**Fig. 1**). HPV-positive tumors have a favorable prognosis, responding better to chemotherapy, radiation, and chemoradiation. Although currently HPV status does not influence treatment choices, increasingly clinical trials are exploring whether HPV-positive tumors may require less therapy in the goal of reducing long-term side-effects in a younger patient population. Emerging insights into the genetic differences between HPV-positive and HPV-negative HN cancers may eventually guide treatment choices; that is, HPV-negative tumors consistently show lower expression levels of EGFR and other kinase amplifications, whereas HPV-positive tumors have higher rates of PI3K-pathway alterations.[10] Genetic abnormalities have been extensively studied in HN cancer, suggesting the existence of several different molecular types of HNSCC based on the biological characteristics of differentially expressed genes.[11,12] Among others, the most reported genes and their molecular pathways involved in the development and progression of HNSCC are TP53, PI3K, EGFR, p16, and NOTCH1.[13] Recently, Chung and colleagues[14] investigated the genomic profile among HPV-positive and HPV-negative tumors including DNA samples from 252 HNSCCs, concluding that the most common genes with genomic alterations were PIK3CA and phosphatase and tensin homolog (PTEN) for HPV-positive tumors and TP53 and CDKN2A/B for HPV-negative tumors. In the pathway analysis, the PI3K pathway in HPV-positive tumors and DNA repair-p53 and cell cycle pathways in HPV-negative tumors were frequently altered. Moreover, the HPV-positive oropharynx and HPV-positive nasal cavity/paranasal sinus carcinoma shared similar mutational profiles.

Understanding the role of viral mechanisms, epigenetics, and genetics in HN cancer could play a role in developing a robust personalized medicine approach by identifying individuals whose tumors harbor specific characteristics that can guide more appropriate treatment selection; and as a direct result, developing new strategies for tumor imaging, using PET imaging as an early biomarker to identify responders/nonresponders and ultimately to accelerate personalized drug development for patients with HN cancer.

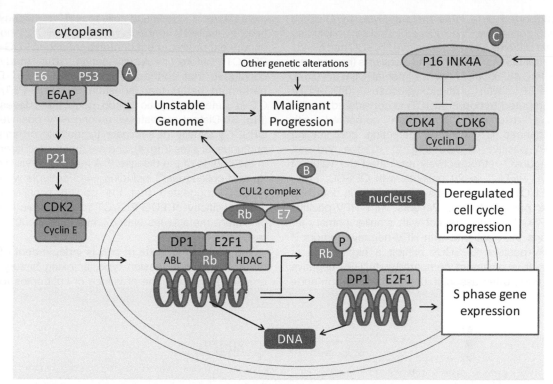

Fig. 1. Role of molecular genetics in HPV OPC. (A) The cancer regulatory gene, p53 undergoes ubiquitination from viral protein E6 and ubiquitin ligase, E6AP which makes the genome unstable resulting in malignant transformation. (B) Another cancer regulatory gene -Rb, undergoes ubiquitination with HPV viral protein, E7 and ubiquitination ligand-CUL-2 complex resulting in unstable Rb gene. (C) Degradation of Rb gene resulting in increased gene expression in S phase resulting in increased expression of p16INK4A. CDK, cyclin-dependant kinase; CUL-2, cullin-2; HDAC, histone deacetylase; OPC, oropharyngeal carcinoma; Rb, retinoblastoma protein. (*Adapted from* Kang H, Kiess, A, Chung C. Emerging biomarkers in head and neck cancer in the era of genomics. Nat Rev Clin Oncol 2015;12(1):13; with permission.)

The Human Papilloma Virus

In the past decades, several epidemiologic studies have shown increased incidence of OPCin North America and Europe, due to the emerging risk factor of HPV infection.[6] HPV, in particular HPV 16, is a causal factor for oropharyngeal (40%–67%) and hypopharynx (13%–25%) carcinoma, and least often for oral cavity (12%–18%) and larynx carcinoma (3%–7%).[15–18] With an increasing incidence of HPV-positive OPSCCs in the past decade, research has shed light on the molecular mechanisms to better understand the pathogenesis of HNSCC.[19] HPV-positive OPSCCs differ from HPV-negative tumors by distinct histologic features and gene expressions.[19] HPV-mediated cancers are more common among young (40–50 years), nonsmoking white men, and is strongly associated with sexual behaviors and HPV-16 type, different from HPV-negative group related to tobacco exposure and alcohol consumption.[20,21] Histologically, HPV-positive OPSCCs are poorly differentiated, nonkeratinizing tumors with high mitotic rates in contrast to HPV-negative tumors, which are moderately differentiated and keratinizing.[22]

HPV-positive OPSCCs have better overall survival (OS) and progression-free survival (PFS) when compared with HPV-negative tumors.[23,24] Studies have shown that HPV-positive patients have considerably reduced risk of death by 40% to 80% or relapse by 60% to 70%, when compared with HPV-negative patients. Fakhry and colleagues[23] retrospectively demonstrated that patients with HPV-positive OPSCC had significantly longer OS rates than patients with HPV-negative tumors, with a median OS of 2.6 years versus 0.8 years. Ang and colleagues[24] retrospectively assessed the association of HPV status and survival in OPSCC reporting that 206 of 323 HPV-positive patients were found to have a better 3-year OS than the HPV-negative group (82.4% vs 57.1%); the HPV-positive group had a 58% reduction in the risk of death. This was further supported by a large meta-analysis by O'Rorke and colleagues[25] including 42 studies, concluding that patients with HPV-positive HNSCC had a 54% better OS than HPV-negative patients (hazard ratio [HR] 0.46, 95% confidence interval [CI] 0.37–0.57).

PET with fludeoxyglucose (FDG-PET)/ computed tomography (CT) is considered a valuable diagnostic tool when compared with enhanced CT alone in detecting and staging HPV-positive OPSCC (**Fig. 2**). Krabbe and colleagues[26] retrospectively evaluated the value of FDG-PET/CT in 20 patients with OPSCC; FDG-PET/CT showed a sensitivity of 96% in detecting the primary tumor. Patients with HPV-positive OPSCC usually present with smaller primary lesions than patients with HPV-negative tumors.[24] HPV-positive OPSCCs exhibit a higher rate of nodal involvement compared with HPV-negative tumors, often associated with cystic lymph node

metastases.[22] Haerle and colleagues[27] retrospectively evaluated 34 patients with tonsilar SCC, who underwent pretreatment contrast-enhanced FDG-PET/CT before neck dissection. The study concluded that contrast-enhanced FDG-PET/CT performed better than nonenhanced FDG-PET/CT in detecting cystic lymph node metastases (**Fig. 3**). Distant metastases among HPV-positive OPSCCs usually disseminate to multiple organs and unusual sites (**Fig. 4**), and are manifested later in the course of the disease.[28] A meta-analysis by Xu and colleagues[29] including 1445 patients with HNSCC suggested that the pooled sensitivity and specificity of FDG-PET/CT for the detection of distant metastases was 87.55% and 95.00%, respectively.

The prognostic value of p16 is independent of tumor stage, progression type, smoking history, or salvage surgery. the presence of antibodies to

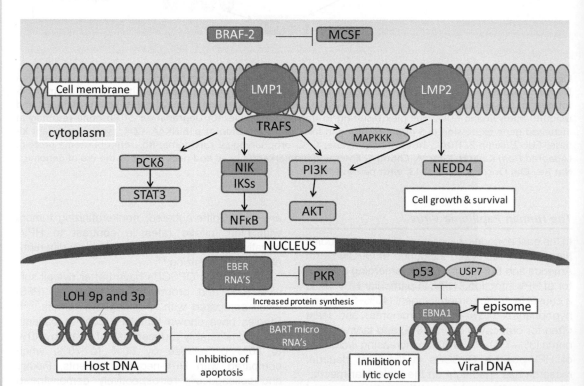

Fig. 2. Role of molecular genetics in EBV-related NPC. LOH (loss of heterozygosity) at 9p and 3p can predispose to EBV-NPC. The various EBV-related genes, highlighted in orange, inhibit regulatory genes of apoptosis and viral regulatory cycle. EBNA1 unstabilizes the oncoregulatory gene p53 by maintaining an episome. LMP1 and LMP2 in the cell membrane signals various cellular pathways, including MAPKKK, STAT3, AKT, and E3 ubiquitin protein ligase–NEDD4 leading to cell growth and survival. BARF-1, Bam H1A reading frame-1; BART, Bam H1A rightward transcript; EBERNAs, EBV-encoded RNAs; EBNA-1, Epstein-Barr nuclear antigen-1; IKKs, inhibitor of nuclear factor κ B kinases; LMP 1/2, latent membrane protein 1,2; MAPKKK, mitogen-activated protein kinase; MCSF, macrophage colony-stimulating factor-1; NFκB, nuclear factor κ B; NIK, NFκB inducing kinase; PI3K, phosphatidylinositol 4,5 bisphosphate kinase; PKCδ, protein kinase C δ; PKR, protein kinase RNA dependent; STAT3, signal transducer and activator-3. (*Adapted from* Kang H, Kiess, A, Chung C. Emerging biomarkers in head and neck cancer in the era of genomics. Nat Rev Clin Oncol 2015;12(1):12; with permission.)

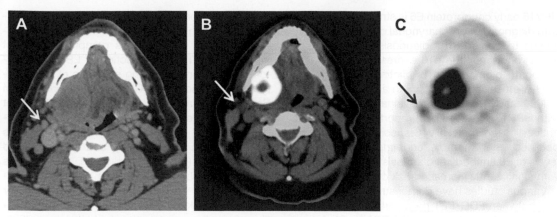

Fig. 3. Contrast-enhanced CT and FDG-PET/CT images performed during the same acquisition: a 58-year-old gentleman with a large right tongue base mass, biopsy-proven SCC, which is better characterized and delineated by the contrast-enhanced CT (*A*), as compared with the axial-fused PET/CT (*B*) and axial PET (*C*) images that demonstrate FDG avidity within the periphery of the tumor, with a cold central necrosis. By contrast, the fused PET/CT (*B*) and PET (*C*) images are able to identify FDG avidity in a small subcentimeter right cervical lymph node (*arrows*), which was subsequently proven to be positive for metastasis.

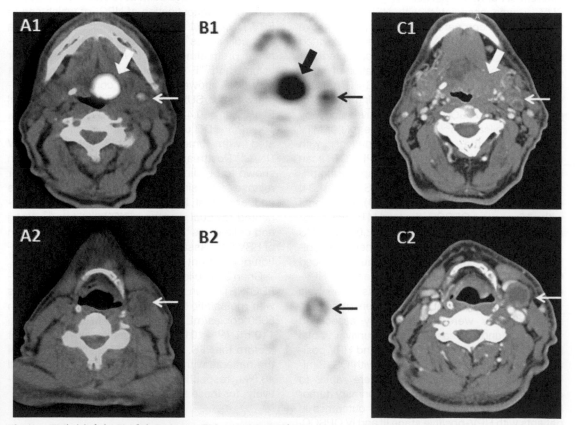

Fig. 4. HPV(+) left base of the tongue SCC, stage T4aN2bM0, with large necrotic cervical lymph node metastasis: 67-year-old gentleman with history of HPV-positive left base of the tongue SCC (T4aN2bM0). Staging FDG-PET/CT scan, including axial fused axial PET/CT (*A1, A2*) and axial PET (*B1, B2*) images, demonstrates intense metabolic activity within the primary malignancy (*A1, B1*) (*arrows*) also seen on the diagnostic contrast-enhanced CT (*C1*). The necrotic left cervical lymph node metastases demonstrate low FDG avidity (*A2, B2*), which are better characterized on the diagnostic contrast-enhanced CT (*C1, C2*) (*thin arrows*).

HPV16 early oncoprotein E6 is strongly associated with diagnosis of oropharyngeal cancer (OPC) and seems to precede the diagnosis by 10 years.[30] More importantly the p16 expression serves as a surrogate biomarker in predicting the prognosis of HPV-positive tumors.[13,22] In a recent study by Fakhry and colleagues[31] evaluating 60 patients with HPV16-positive OPC, reported that levels of antibodies against HPV16-specific oncoproteins declined after therapy, and importantly, higher levels of E6 antibody at diagnosis were associated with significantly increased risk of recurrence.

Various studies have demonstrated the correlation between FDG-PET parameters and HPV and p16 expression status in HNSCC[1,22]; Clark and colleagues[32] prospectively determined the correlation between the FDG uptake using maximum standard uptake value (SUV_{max}) with the p16 positivity in 65 patients with OPSCC, reporting higher levels of SUV_{max} in the primary tumor among the p16-negative cases than those with p16-positive tumors (13.7 vs 10.3) but there was no significant difference. For nodal disease, a significantly higher SUV_{max} was associated with HPV/p16-positive nodes when compared with the p16-negative nodes (SUV_{max} = 10.8 vs 7.9). Thus, an elevated nodal SUV_{max} seemed to be a significant predictor of HPV/p16-positive OPSCC. Calculation of metabolic tumor volume (MTV) using FDG-PET/CT has shown a significant value in predicting the OS of patients with OPSCC. A prospective study by Tang and colleagues[33] assessing the role of MTV in predicting the prognosis of patients with HNSCC, the pretreatment FDG-PET/CT scan before receiving definitive radiotherapy, using primary tumor MTV, predicted PFS (HR 1.94; $P<.0001$) and OS (HR 1.57, $P<.001$). In patients with p16-positive OPSCC, the total MTV was a significant predictor of PFS (HR 4.23, $P<.001$) and OS (HR 3.21, $P<.0029$). In a study by Cheng and colleagues[34] including 70 patients with advanced OPSCC, 13 of them HPV-positive and 57 HPV-negative, a multivariate Cox regression analysis showed that age, total tumor lesion glycolysis, and uniformity were independently associated with PFS and disease-specific survival. Total lesion glycolysis (TLG), uniformity, and HPV positivity were significantly associated with OS. Similarly, Alluri and colleagues[35] were able to demonstrate that total MTV and primary tumor MTV were associated with survival outcomes in patients with HPV-positive stage III and IV OPSCC.

Epstein-Barr Virus

Epstein-Barr virus (EBV) belongs to gamma herpes virus family. Tumorigenesis by EBV occurs only in a small fraction of the infected population, suggesting that the malignant transformation of human cells by EBV involves complex virus-host interactions (**Fig. 5**).[36] Infection of EBV is ubiquitous to the nonkeratinizing subtypes of nasopharyngeal carcinoma (NPC), which are endemic in Southeast Asia.[37] The expression of EBV latent genes is predominantly restricted to EBNA1 nuclear antigen, the latent membrane proteins (LMP1, LMP2, and LMP2B), and virus-encoded small RNAs (EBERs) and BART micro-RNAs (miRNAs).[38] LMP1 enhances the epithelial-mesenchymal transition, expression of cancer stem cell markers, and acquisition of stem-cell–like properties contributing to highly metastatic features of NPC.[6]

Circulating serum EBV DNA has proven to be an independent prognostic factor for patients with NPC. In Hong Kong, pretreatment EBV DNA was found in 96% of patients with NPC, and high EBV DNA levels contributed to advanced-stage disease, relapse, and poor survival.[39] Various blood markers have been developed for the detection and prognostication of NPC, of which serum EBV DNA level is the most validated test.[40] Ma and colleagues[41] evaluated the relationship between pretreatment EBV DNA (pEBV) levels, tumor volume and ^{18}F-FDG uptake in NPC. Pretreatment EBV DNA showed significant correlation with primary tumor SUV_{max} (r = 0.276), regional nodal SUV_{max} (r = 0.434) and total SUV_{max} (r = 0.457). Thus, ^{18}F-FDG uptake was independently associated with tumor volume but not with pEBV DNA.[41] Posttreatment EBV DNA levels have been shown to be clinically useful for monitoring tumor relapse.[42] Persistently elevated EBV DNA levels and abnormal PET scans after treatment suggested residual disease in NPC patients.[43] Wang and colleagues[44] also investigated the implication of EBV DNA assay and ^{18}F-FDG-PET in the detection of recurrent NPC.

Chan and colleagues[40] evaluated the role of ^{18}F-FDG-PET/CT in predicting survival in 56 patients with metastatic NPC. EBV DNA titer greater than 5000 copies/mL ($P = .001$) and MTV greater than 110 mL ($P = .013$) were found to be independent factors for PFS. The 2-year PFS and OS rates of the patients with MTV $\leq$110 mL were 23.2% and 43.0%, respectively and 0% and 9.1%, respectively, for those with MTV greater than 110 mL.

Epidermal Growth Factor Receptor Mutation

EGFR is a transmembrane glycoprotein, member of the HER family of cell-surface receptor tyrosine kinases, involved in signaling cell pathways. EGFR plays an important role in several radiation

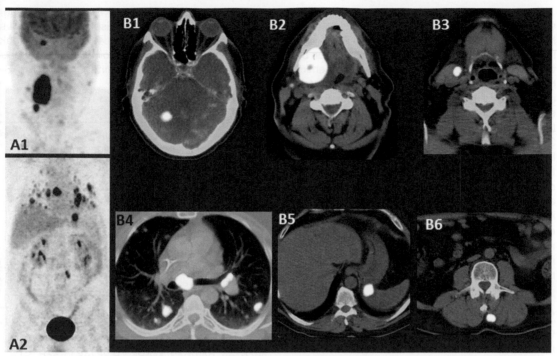

Fig. 5. Multiple locoregional and distant metastasis in a patient newly diagnosed with SCC of the right tongue base: a 58-year-old gentleman newly diagnosed with SCC of the right tongue base. Staging FDG-PET/CT scan including maximum intensity projection of the HN field of view (A1) and of the whole body (A2) demonstrate a large intense FDG-avid mass within the right tongue base (B2), with several FDG-avid ipsilateral cervical lymph nodes (B2, B3). Unexpected multiple additional FDG-avid foci are identified throughout the body, as seen in a right occipital lobe lesion (B1), in multiple mediastinal lymphadenopathy and bilateral pulmonary nodules (B4), in a splenic lesion (B5) and in the posterior left musculature of the thoraco-lumbar region (B6), consistent with metastatic disease, which changed patient management.

resistance mechanisms, as it steers the pathways related to DNA damage repair, cancer cell proliferation, hypoxia, and apoptosis. EGFR is overexpressed in nearly 80% to 90% of cases of HNSCC and correlates with unfavorable outcomes and resistance to radiation.[45,46] Feldman and colleagues[47] retrospectively analyzed the molecular profiling of 735 patients with advanced HNSCC using multiple platforms, such as gene sequencing, gene copy number, and protein expression, concluding that 90% of patients with HNSCC showed overexpression of EGFR and 21% patients showed increased gene copy numbers.

Furthermore, HPV positivity has been associated with a lack of EGFR expression in several studies.[8] In a gene expression analysis including 134 patients with locoregional advanced HNSCC (44% HPV-positive tumors), Keck and colleagues[48] concluded that patients with HPV-positive tumors had low expression and no copy number events for EGFR/HER ligands. In HPV-positive patients, high EGFR expression was associated with decreased response and survival in comparison with those with low EGFR expression.[49,50] These findings suggest that EGFR expression is an independent negative prognostic marker in HNSCC.[49,50]

Presence of genetic alteration of activating EGFR signaling pathway have proven to be relevant in patient stratification for treatment with EGFR inhibitors.[51] EGFR targeted therapies either with tyrosine kinase inhibitors (TKIs) such as gefitinib, erlotinib, or lapatinib, or monoclonal antibodies (mAbs) against the extracellular domain of EGFR, such as cetuximab (IMC-C225, Erbitux) and panitumumab (ABX-EGF, Vectibix).[52,53] Cetuximab is the only targeted therapy for HNSCC approved by the Food and Drug Administration with overall response rates of 10% to 13%.[47] In a phase III trial, cetuximab combined with radiotherapy was proven the mainstay of treatment for locally advanced HNSCC and cetuximab as a single agent is used in recurrent or metastatic disease, prolonging the median progression-free survival from 3.3 to 6.0 months.[6,52]

Radionuclide molecular imaging to noninvasively assessed EGFR target expression levels has been conducted. Rasmussen and colleagues[45] retrospective studied the correlation between the expression of immune-histochemical biomarkers and the maximum FDG-PET uptake in patients with HNSCC; primary tumor SUV_{max} showed positive correlation with EGFR mutation (r = 0.24, P = .021). In a meta-analysis including 37 studies with more than 3000 patients with HNSCC, Keren and colleagues[54] reported that the overexpression of EGFR was associated with reduced OS, whereas, EGFR expression was not associated with disease-free survival, after adjusting for publication bias. Furthermore, EGFR expression has the potential to noninvasively monitor anti-EGFR antibody treatment with cetuximab and its analogs to steer individualized treatment regimens.

KRAS Mutation

Oncogenes of RAS family are strongly implicated in pathogenesis of cancer. RAS gene encodes for a family of related proteins called p21s, which participate in signal transduction involved in cellular growth and differentiation.[4] KRAS mutations are extremely rare in patients with HNSCC, accounting for fewer than 5% of the cases.[55] Overexpression of RAS gene product p21 has been reported in patients with HNSCC.[56] Although it is a well-established biomarker for colorectal cancer, it has limited prognostic value in patients with HNSCC. Studies have shown that the presence of KRAS-variant predicts poor outcome in HN cancer.[55] The mechanism of activation of KRAS was attributed to tobacco carcinogens, as 35% of smokers in India had mutation of codons 12, 13, and 61 in the RAS gene.[51,57] A study by Bissada and colleagues[4] suggested that 3.5% of patients with locally advanced HNSCC showed KRAS mutations at codon 12.

KRAS mutations in patients with HNSCC have shown resistance to chemotherapy and radiotherapy.[51] In a retrospective study conducted by Chung and colleagues[55] including 103 patients with HNSCC, KRAS-variant status was determined in 92% of the patients. The study showed that PFS significantly improved in KRAS-variant patients who received the combination of cisplatin and cetuximab when compared to those who received placebo, with median time of 1.9 months for cisplatin + placebo versus 3.9 months for cisplatin + cetuximab (log rank, P = .03). However, the combination of cetuximab plus cisplatin had no significant effect on OS (Kras-variant group median: 5.4 months in cisplatin + placebo vs 8.0 months in

cisplatin + cetuximab, log-rank P = .37; non-variant group median: 8.1 months in cisplatin + placebo vs 8.2 months in cisplatin + cetuximab, log-rank P = .96).[55] The study also showed that recurrent/metastatic patients with HNSCC with KRAS-variant had worse prognosis.

C-MET Mutation

C-MET is a receptor tyrosine kinase for hepatocyte growth factor (HGF) that enhances migration, invasion, and angiogenesis when overexpressed in cancer.[58] The C-MET gene is overexpressed in 80% of patients with HNSCC when assessed by immunohistochemistry.[59] Di Renzo and colleagues[60] identified 2 somatic active c-met mutations in lymph node metastases of patients with HNSCC, whereas primary tumors were barely detectable, suggesting that c-met mutations are highly increased in metastatic sites. Increased serum level of HGF is associated with higher tumor stage progression and poor outcome.[61] C-MET mutated tumors amplify EGFR because both of them share the common signal intermediates, such as p44/p42 MAPK, PI3K/AKT, and STAT. This signal redundancy has facilitated therapy with EGFR TKIs in patients with HNSCC with MET mutations.[59]

TP53 Mutation

TP53 is a tumor suppressor gene located on the short arm (p) of chromosome 17, which induces growth arrest and cell death when activated in cancers. It is a commonly mutated gene in HNSCC, accounting for 40% to 50% of the cases.[62] Expression of p53 is most commonly seen in heavy drinkers and smokers.[62] Loss of heterozygosity, interaction with HPV viral protein E6, and overexpression of MDM2 are the common molecular alterations in HNSCC.[39] In a prospective study by Poeta and colleagues[63] including 560 patients with surgically treated HNSCC, 53.3% patients had TP53 mutations. The presence of TP53 mutations was associated with decreased OS when compared with wild-type TP53 (HR = 1.4, P = .009) and had a much stronger association with disruptive TP53 mutations (HR = 1.7, P<.001). Five-year OS rate in patients with TP53 mutations was 40.7% and median survival was 3.2 years.

TP53 mutations are rare in HPV-positive HNSCC and correlates with poor prognosis. Inactivation of TP53 by binding of HPV to E6 protein attributes to low frequency of these mutations.[63] Licitra and colleagues[64] retrospective studied 90 patients with oropharyngeal cancer, who were treated surgically, and concluded that patients with

HPV-positive tumors with TP53 mutations had a shorter time to disease progression and OS.

Tumor Heterogeneity

The importance of personalized medicine in cancer therapy has been more widely accepted in recent years, as we increasingly recognize that tumors, even of the same subtype, are different in different patients. Tumors are heterogeneous at microscopic level. Tumor cells show diversity in origin, clonally, and regulation of genomic and proteomic pathways. Heterogeneity not only varies in different pathologic subtypes of cancer but also within the same tumor stage. Multiple environmental factors and molecular characteristics contribute to tumor heterogeneity, such as hypoxia, necrosis, angiogenesis, cellular proliferation and growth rate, gene mutation, and expression of specific receptors. Tumor heterogeneity within the same histopathological subtype of malignancy is referred to as intratumoral heterogeneity.[65] Even a small subpopulation of tumor cells with different phenotypic or genetic characteristics may eventually cause treatment failure and poor survival rates.[66] ^{18}F-FDG-PET/CT has been recently proposed for the assessment of intratumoral metabolic heterogeneity and, thus, potentially aid to predict the patient's prognosis (**Figs. 6** and **7**). Various metabolic parameters, such as the SUV, MTV, and TLG provide accurate assessment of tumor heterogeneity and better prognostic value. SUV_{max} is a semiquantitative measure of tumor ^{18}F-FDG uptake, whereas MTV refers to volumetric measurement of tumor cells with high glycolytic activity, and TLG is the sum of SUVs within the tumor, calculated as MTV × SUV_{mean}.

The intratumoral ^{18}F-FDG uptake is represented as heterogeneity index (HF), defined as a derivative (dV/dT) of volume-threshold function for a primary tumor. Kwon and colleagues[67] evaluated the prognostic significance of intratumoral heterogeneity in oral cavity cancer; the HF was significantly correlated with SUV_{max} (r = −0.353, P = .017), MTV (r = −0.708, P<.0001), and TLG (r = −0.709, P<.0001). A multivariate analysis revealed HF to be an independent predictor of OS. Patients with HF <−0.13 showed a worse prognosis than those with HF ≥ −0.13 (P = .005). A study by Henriksson and colleagues[68] demonstrated that intratumoral heterogeneity corresponded to heterogeneous metabolic activity measured with FDG-PET. It was found that distribution of tracer to the tumor is dependent on blood flow, which varies due to tumor growth, necrosis, and intratumoral pressure. Metabolic activity of tumor was influenced by glycolytic status of tumor cells, which is upregulated in malignant transformation. Tumor stage and grade influence the metabolism of tumor. The larger the tumor, and lower the grade, the higher was the FDG uptake.

FDG-PET textural features have been successfully used for predicting clinical outcome and treatment response in a variety of malignancies. Zone-size nonuniformity (ZSNU) was proven to be a significant prognostic factor in patients with advanced oropharyngeal SCC (OPSCC). In a retrospective study by Cheng and colleagues[69] including 88 patients with T3 or T4 OPSCC with completion of primary treatment, investigators concluded that MTV and TLG were significantly associated with ZSNU, also demonstrating that ZSNU served as an independent predictor of PFS and disease-specific survival (DSS) in advanced T-stage OPSCC.

PET IMAGING IN ASSESSING RESPONSE TO THERAPY

Selection of the most appropriate treatment strategies varies depending on disease stage and primary site of HN cancer. Surgery, radiotherapy, chemotherapy, or combinations of these are accepted treatment options for patients with HN cancer[70,71]; single-treatment modalities can be used for early-stage disease, but advanced-staged disease typically requires combination of therapies.[3] Studies have also reported that HPV-positive HN tumors respond better to chemotherapy or radiation than HPV-negative tumors.[72]

FDG-PET/CT scans have been proven to be a useful modality for assessing treatment response[73] and have become the modality of choice for therapy response assessment. In a large meta-analysis involving 2335 patients, Gupta and colleagues[73] reported sensitivity, specificity, positive predictive value (PPV) and negative predictive value (NPV) of PET/CT for detection of residual primary tumor after treatment of 94%, 82%, 75%, and 95%, respectively. The PPV is low, due to the high number of false-positive results related to posttreatment changes, such as inflammation and fibrosis causing distortion of the anatomy and preventing accurate response assessment.[74] Hence, a positive FDG-PET/CT result in the posttreatment phase needs careful correlation with clinical information and corresponding CT/MR imaging findings and consider biopsy of positive sites. To reduce the number of false-positive findings, it is crucial to accurately select high-risk patients, such as HPV-negative tumors, to know radiation treatment volume and set the optimal timing for performing the PET/CT

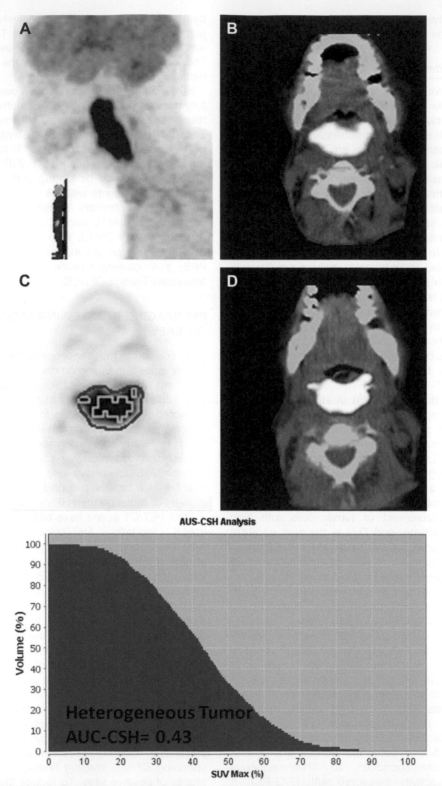

AUS-CSH Analysis

Heterogeneous Tumor
AUC-CSH= 0.43

Fig. 6. HPV(+) OPSCC with a primary metabolic heterogeneous tumor: a 72-year-old woman with an HPV(+) base of the tongue SCC (T4N2cM0). Staging PET/CT scan at the top row includes (*A*) maximum intensity projection, (*B*) fused axial PET/CT images, (*C*) PET images, and (*D*) CT images with superimposed FDG-PET uptake subtracting background, demonstrating intense metabolic activity within the base of the tongue tumor with SUV_{max} of

imaging. There is general consensus of performing FDG-PET/CT scans at 12 weeks after radiation therapy, as results may be inconclusive if performed too early,[75] no sooner than 2 months.[76]

FDG-PET imaging has been proven to be better than either PET or CT with high NPV, and an SUV_{max} of 2 was shown to able to predict the response to radiation therapy (RT) with a high NPV of 100% avoiding unnecessary neck dissections in 77 patients with HPV-positive OPSCC.[71] In a recent retrospective study (n = 78), Kim and colleagues[77] stated that a post-SUV_{max} value of 4.4 was the optimum cutoff value for predicting immediate treatment failure in patients with HNSCC undergoing chemoradiation therapy (CRT) with a sensitivity, specificity, NPV, and PPV of 90%, 84%, 98%, and 45%, respectively. In addition, Isles and colleagues[78] in a meta-analysis, including 27 studies, reported that FDG-PET had sensitivity, specificity, PPV, and NPV of 94%, 82%, 75%, and 95%, respectively, for evaluating treatment response of HNSCC. This was further supported by Sjovall and colleagues[79] who evaluated 82 patients with HNSCC with 85% being OPSCC and reported the sensitivity and specificity of FDG-PET/CT to be 100% and 78%, respectively.

To improve the accuracy and reliability of imaging in therapy assessment, standardizing interpretation criteria is one of the most important factors to decrease the interobserver variability across institutions. Recently, Marcus and colleagues[80] proposed the Hopkins criteria for HN PET/CT imaging, which demonstrated excellent interreader reliability, accuracy, and survival prediction. This method has been adapted and included in multicenter clinical trials sponsored by the National Cancer Institute[81] and has been validated as a secondary analysis of randomized, multicenter HN trial in the United Kingdom.[82]

PET/CT is valuable for assessing treatment response after CRT; however, there are small number of studies evaluating the role and timing of performing an FDG-PET/CT after surgical treatment of patients with HN cancer. Recently, Taghipour and colleagues[83] investigated a large series of 98 patients with HNSCC treated with surgical resection of the primary tumor with or without CRT, concluding that posttreatment FDG-PET/CT had a high NPV, added value to clinical assessment in 35% of the patients, influenced in the subsequent patient's management, and were associated with the patient's survival outcome.

Because of the increase use of effective molecular targeting therapy for specific genomic abnormalities in HN cancer, recent investigations have also attempted to address the utility of FDG-PET/CT imaging addressing metabolic response of tumors to targeted therapy. The chimeric anti-EGFR mAb cetuximab was the first molecularly targeted therapy to receive US Food and Drug Administration approval for the treatment of HNSCC, and has been integrated into the standard of care. Cetuximab is approved for use with RT in locally or regionally advanced disease, and in recurrent or metastatic disease as monotherapy after progression on platinum-based therapy or in combination with platinum plus 5-fluorouracil in patients with incurable HNSCC. Per the National Comprehensive Cancer Network guidelines, cetuximab plus platinum (cisplatin or carboplatin) and 5-fluorouracil is a category 1 treatment option for patients with unresectable or recurrent/metastatic non-nasopharyngeal SCC.

^{18}F-FDG-PET had been clinically evaluated as a potential imaging biomarker to monitor response to EGFR-targeting therapies. Schmitz and colleagues[84] reported a partial response to preoperative administration of cetuximab in 18 of 19 patients, which corresponded to a ΔSUV_{max} below 25%, measured between baseline and before surgery. In a similar small sample with 10 patients, Adkins and colleagues[85] showed that a partial response corresponded to a mean decrease of ΔSUV_{max} below 48% as measured before and after 8 weeks of cetuximab infusion. Beyond FDG-PET imaging, recent experiments labeling cetuximab with other radionuclides, such as [124]I, ^{64}Cu, [89]Zr, ^{177}Lu,[86] could potentially address anti-EGFR PET imaging, which is still under investigation in the preclinical setting.

BEYOND FLUDEOXYGLUCOSE-PET: FUNCTIONAL AND MOLECULAR IMAGING WITH NOVEL PET TRACERS

Although ^{18}F-FDG is the most commonly used PET tracer in the routine oncology imaging, there is an increasing interest for testing novel PET tracers to address biological tumor behavior beyond glucose metabolism, including targeting molecules, cell proliferation, hypoxia, and angiogenesis. In this section, we review some of the

---

22.4; MTV of 63.5 mL; TLG of 619.7 by gradient-based segmentation. The calculated intratumoral heterogeneity index (AUC-CSH) was 0.43; that is, indicating a heterogeneous tumor. Patient underwent CRT and developed tumor recurrence 15 months later.

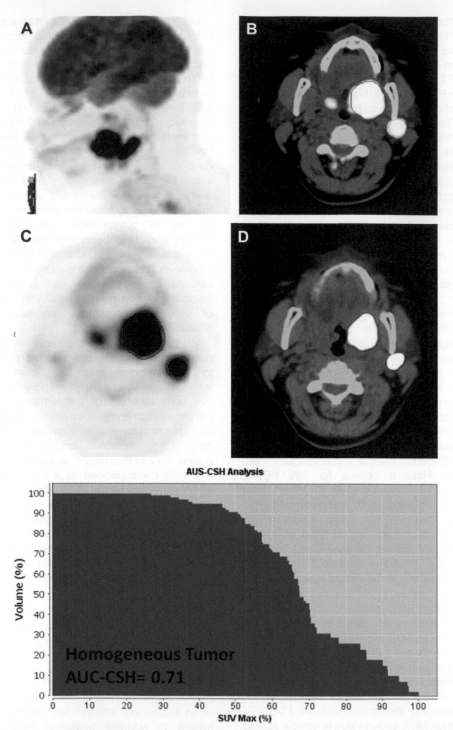

Fig. 7. HPV(+) OPSCC with a primary metabolic homogeneous tumor: 57-year-old woman with an HPV(+) left tonsil SCC (T2N2bM0). Staging PET/CT scan includes (*A*) maximum intensity projection, (*B*) fused axial PET/CT images, (*C*) PET images with volumes of interest, and (*D*) CT images with superimposed FDG-PET uptake subtracting background, demonstrating intense metabolic activity within the primary tumor in the left tonsil, and nodal lesions, with SUV$_{max}$ of 19.0, MTV of 35.8 mL, and TLG of 221.1 g, by gradient-based segmentation. The calculated primary AUC-CSH was 0.71; that is, indicating a homogeneous tumor. Patient underwent CRT, being free of disease 5 years after diagnosis.

novel PET tracers currently under research for HN cancer.

Molecular Targeting Imaging

Molecularly targeted agents could provide clinical benefits in patients with HNSCC with specific molecular features or particular mutations using PET imaging based on radiolabeling mAbs, small antibody fragments (immunoPET), or small-molecule inhibitors that target EGFR and could aid in visualizing tumor EGFR expression. Various PET tracers, such as ^{64}Cu (half-life [T1/2] = 12.7 hours), ^{86}Y (T1/2 = 14.7 h), and ^{89}Zr (T1/2 = 78.4 h) have been used to determine EGFR levels.[87] Most of the studies so far have been carried out in animal models. Perk and colleagues[86] labeled cetuximab with ^{124}I, ^{64}Cu, ^{89}Zr, and ^{177}Lu and found that the biodistribution of radiolabels in mice with A431 xenografts was similar. A study was conducted to evaluate PET imaging with ^{64}Cu-DOTA-cetuximab in detecting overexpression of EGFR in tumor-bearing mice; the EGFR-positive tumor cell line showed high accumulation of ^{64}Cu-DOTA-cetuximab in PET imaging, whereas relatively lower uptake was seen in EGFR-negative tumors.[88] Li and colleagues[52] conducted a preclinical study to evaluate a novel PET tracer, ^{18}F-FBEM, for molecular imaging of EGFR in a human HN squamous carcinoma UM-SCC1 cell line. Positive EGFR tumors were clearly visualized with significantly higher uptake using ^{18}F-FBEM-cEGF. Aerts and colleagues[89] demonstrated that cetuximab uptake in mice tumors also could be assessed using ^{89}Zr-labeled cetuximab, although the results indicated a disparity between the antibody uptake and the EGFR expression levels of the target tumor, as the intermediate EGFR-expressing tumors had a higher uptake of ^{89}Zr-cetuximab than those with high EGFR expression. Ultimately, the application of these novel PET tracers targeting EFGR would be treatment monitoring and response prediction.

Imaging Hypoxia

The presence of tumor hypoxia is a common contributing factor of HNSCC, known to be associated with tumor progression and resistance to RT.[90] Hypoxic imaging with PET has been achieved using ^{18}F-misonidazole (FMISO), a 2-nitroimidazole molecule that accumulates selectively in hypoxic conditions. In the setting of patients with HN cancer, various studies with small cohorts have suggested the value of ^{18}F-FMISO as a potential maker for predicting outcome following therapy. Thus, Eschmann and colleagues[91] evaluated 26 patients with HN cancers before curative RT

treatment, concluding that patients' outcome could be predicted on the basis of kinetic behavior of FMISO in tumor tissue, thus an accumulation-type curve, high SUV_{max}, and high tumor-background ratios at 4 hours postinjection. were highly suggestive of an incomplete response to treatment and might be used to select patients for intensified therapy protocols. Similarly, Dirix and colleagues[92] showed in 15 patients with HNSCC that tumor-to-blood ratios measured before and during CRT correlated negatively with disease-free survival. Rischin and colleagues[93] also demonstrated that in patients receiving nontirapazamine-containing CRT for advanced, stage III or IV HN tumors, hypoxia levels on FMISO-PET imaging was associated with a higher rate of locoregional failure. Furthermore, the strongest prognostic value was found after 1 and 2 weeks of RT in patients with stage III/IV HN cancer at 4 time points before and during concomitant CRT, stressing the potential benefit of early imaging during treatment to select patients who might benefit from RT dose escalation or hypoxia modifiers.[94] Indeed, Sato and colleagues[95] also emphasized the advantage of FMISO-PET over FDG-PET for predicting histologic response before preoperative chemotherapy in a prospective study with 22 patients with oral SCC. A "good" histologic response was significantly more prevalent in patients with negative FMISO results compared with those with positive FMISO uptake, whereas the FDG uptake was not significantly correlated with the chemotherapy response.

Despite the widely applicability of ^{18}F-FMISO for research purposes, it has not gained general acceptance for routine clinical use due to its slow pharmacokinetic profile, with limited clearance from normal tissue and blood, resulting in modest hypoxic-to-normoxic tissue ratios. Another hypoxia PET agent, ^{18}F-fluoroazomycin-arabinofuranoside (^{18}F-FAZA), more hydrophilic than ^{18}F-FMISO, has shown more favorable kinetics, resulting in better tumor-to-background ratios, thus allowing a 1-hour uptake interval. Mortensen and colleagues[96] investigated the prognostic value of ^{18}F-FAZA PET in 40 patients with HN cancer before RT. In 63% of the patients, a hypoxic volume could be delineated using a tumor-to-muscle ratio in the range of 1.1 to 2.9, median 1.5 before RT. After a median follow-up of 19 months, the disease-free survival rate was significantly lower among patients with a hypoxic volume than among patients without (60% vs 93%, P = .04). In a recent study, hypoxic ^{18}F-FAZA PET imaging was also used to perform the semiquantitative assessment of hypoxic volume before and during intensity-modulated RT (IMRT) for 12 patients with locally advanced HN cancer.[97]

Another group of hypoxia-avid PET tracers, with a more stable but also more complex labeling chemistry, is represented by ^{18}F-2-nitroimidazol-pentafluoropropyl acetamide (^{18}F-EF5) and ^{18}F-2 nitroimidazol-trifluoropropyl acetamide (^{18}F-EF3), which are slightly more lipophilic than the formerly described compounds and have been investigated in animal models as well as in clinical studies on HN cancer.[98,99] In a small cohort of 22 patients with HNSCC, Komar and colleagues[99] reported that a high uptake of the hypoxia tracer ^{18}F-EF5 showed a stronger correlation with a poor clinical outcome than F-FDG uptake.

Another alternative class of agents for the study of hypoxia with PET is based on a complex of Cu with diacetyl-bis (N4-methylthiosemicarbazone) (ATSM) ligands, among which ATSM is the prototype. Due to its lipophilicity and low molecular weight, Cu-ATSM is characterized by high membrane permeability and therefore rapid diffusion into cells. Tumor-specific Cu-ATSM retention has been demonstrated for HN cancer.[100,101] In a pilot study, Minagawa and colleagues[100] reported that ^{62}Cu-ATSM PET uptake before initiation of chemoradiation was predictive of response to therapy in patients with locally advanced HN cancers. In 15 of the 17 cases, the investigators assessed the relationship between clinical outcome and ^{62}Cu-ATSM uptake. The SUV_{max} differed significantly in patients free of disease at 2 years' follow-up postradiation versus those with residual/recurrent disease. More specifically, all cured patients had an SUV_{max} less than 5.0 and all patients with persistent disease had an SUV_{max} greater than 5.0. In a slightly larger study comparing 62Cu-ATSM and FDG-PET imaging, Sato and colleagues[102] reported that pretreatment ^{62}Cu-ATSM PET imaging was able to predict outcome in 25 patients with stage II to IV HN cancer, whereas F-FDG-related indices did not show any significant difference in either PFS or cause-specific survival.

All these results show a promising potential application of hypoxia PET imaging for guidance of hypoxia-modifying therapies in the future; however, larger clinical trials are still necessary to validate their utility in HN cancer.

Imaging Assessing Cell Proliferation (Fluorothymidine)

Over recent years, the most extensively studied PET tracer to image tumor proliferation is ^{18}F-fluorothymidine (^{18}F-FLT), a thymidine analog that gets trapped inside proliferating cells through specific phosphorylation by thymidine kinase-1 (TK-1), the key enzyme of the salvage pathway of DNA synthesis.[103,104] In the setting of HNSCC, ^{18}F-FLT has been shown to be able to detect early changes in tumor metabolism after therapy with significant correlation between these changes and clinical outcome. This was addressed by Hoeben and colleagues[105] in 48 patients with HNSCC scanned before and during the second and fourth week of therapy; the magnitude of decrease in SUV_{max} between baseline and the second-week scan was found to be of predictive value for 3-year disease-free survival. In another study, 28 patients with HNSCC were scanned with ^{18}F-FDG and ^{18}F-FLT-PET at baseline, after the fourth week of RT and 5 weeks after completion of treatment. Image analysis was, however, based on visual assessment rather than SUV analysis. No correlation was found between the presence of residual ^{18}F-FLT or ^{18}F-FDG uptake after 4 weeks of radiation and local control of disease at a median follow-up of 39 months.[106] Based on these results, there is not yet enough evidence to identify a clear quantifier to be used in future clinical studies for treatment modification or risk group stratification.

Imaging of Angiogenesis

Visualization of tumor angiogenesis by using novel targeting angiogenesis PET agents would be of great importance for patient selection and monitoring of response to antiangiogenic drug therapies. Several molecular targets for in vivo imaging of angiogenesis have been developed, such as metalloproteinases, $\alpha v \beta 3$ integrins, and vascular endothelial growth factor (VEGF) and its receptor (VEGFR).[107] ^{18}F-Galacto-RGD-PET is a promising PET angiogenesis radiotracer consisting of peptides containing arginine-glycine-aspartic acid (RGD) sequences, which bind to $\alpha v \beta 3$ integrins, for imaging of tumor angiogenesis and metastasis, with potential utility for planning and response to avB3-targeted therapy. HN cancer was successfully identified using ^{18}F-Galato-RGD PET imaging.[108] In a recent pilot study, Chen and colleagues,[109] was able to image 9 patients with advanced HN cancer using another novel PET tracer targeting $\alpha v \beta 3$ integrins, named RGD-K5 PET, which was able to identify patients with incomplete responses to CRT.

SUMMARY

HN cancer comprises a group of highly heterogeneous tumors. Their management is likely to change in the near future, moving from treatment as a single disease to tailoring the therapy based on both patient and tumor characteristics. Identification of specific genetic, epigenetic, and metabolic aberrations, together with the more traditional techniques in diagnosis, staging, and prognostication, would aid in addressing the individual treatment strategy. Understanding of molecular biology through the developments in high-throughput technology heralds a future of personalized medicine. Furthermore, numerous novel molecules are showing promise for personalized care, newer drugs, and disease response assessment, which would potentially tailor treatment strategies for individual patients depending on tumor behavior.

REFERENCES

1. Paidpally V, Chirindel A, Lam S, et al. FDG-PET/CT imaging biomarkers in head and neck squamous cell carcinoma. Imaging Med 2013;4(6):633–47.
2. Sheikhbahaei S, Marcus C, Hafezi-Nejad N, et al. Value of FDG PET/CT in patient management and outcome of skeletal and soft tissue sarcomas. PET Clin 2015;10(3):375–93.
3. Tantiwongkosi B, Yu F, Kanard A, et al. Role of (18) F-FDG PET/CT in pre and post treatment evaluation in head and neck carcinoma. World J Radiol 2014; 6(5):177–91.
4. Bissada E, Abboud O, Abou Chacra Z, et al. Prevalence of K-RAS codons 12 and 13 mutations in locally advanced head and neck squamous cell carcinoma and impact on clinical outcomes. Int J Otolaryngol 2013;2013:848021.
5. Abgral R, Querellou S, Potard G, et al. Does 18F-FDG PET/CT improve the detection of posttreatment recurrence of head and neck squamous cell carcinoma in patients negative for disease on clinical follow-up? J Nucl Med 2009;50(1):24–9.
6. Pezzuto F, Buonaguro L, Caponigro F, et al. Update on head and neck cancer: current knowledge on epidemiology, risk factors, molecular features and novel therapies. Oncology 2015;89(3):125–36.
7. Leemans CR, Braakhuis BJ, Brakenhoff RH. The molecular biology of head and neck cancer. Nat Rev Cancer 2010;11(1):9–22.
8. Alorabi M, Shonka NA, Ganti AK. EGFR monoclonal antibodies in locally advanced head and neck squamous cell carcinoma: what is their current role? Crit Rev Oncol Hematol 2015;99:170–9.
9. van Dijk LK, Boerman OC, Kaanders JH, et al. PET imaging in head and neck cancer patients to monitor treatment response: a future role for EGFR-targeted imaging. Clin Cancer Res 2015; 21(16):3602–9.
10. Seiwert T. Accurate HPV testing: a requirement for precision medicine for head and neck cancer. Ann Oncol 2013;24(11):2711–3.
11. Walter V, Yin X, Wilkerson MD, et al. Molecular subtypes in head and neck cancer exhibit distinct patterns of chromosomal gain and loss of canonical cancer genes. PLoS One 2013;8(2):e56823.
12. Pickering CR, Zhang J, Yoo SY, et al. Integrative genomic characterization of oral squamous cell carcinoma identifies frequent somatic drivers. Cancer Discov 2013;3(7):770–81.
13. Friedland P, Thomas A, Naran A, et al. Human papillomavirus and gene mutations in head and neck squamous carcinomas. ANZ J Surg 2011; 82(5):362–6.
14. Chung CH, Guthrie VB, Masica DL, et al. Genomic alterations in head and neck squamous cell carcinoma determined by cancer gene-targeted sequencing. Ann Oncol 2015;26(6):1216–23.
15. Adelstein DJ, Ridge JA, Gillison ML, et al. Head and neck squamous cell cancer and the human papillomavirus: summary of a National Cancer Institute State of the Science Meeting, November 9-10, 2008, Washington, DC. Head Neck 2009; 31(11):1393–422.
16. Gillison ML, D'Souza G, Westra W, et al. Distinct risk factor profiles for human papillomavirus type 16-positive and human papillomavirus type 16-negative head and neck cancers. J Natl Cancer Inst 2008;100(6):407–20.
17. Shaikh MH, McMillan NA, Johnson NW. HPV-associated head and neck cancers in the Asia Pacific: a critical literature review & meta-analysis. Cancer Epidemiol 2015;39(6):923–38.
18. Gillison ML, Chaturvedi AK, Anderson WF, et al. Epidemiology of human papillomavirus-positive head and neck squamous cell carcinoma. J Clin Oncol 2015;33(29):3235–42.
19. Cheng NM, Chang JT, Huang CG, et al. Prognostic value of pretreatment (1)(8)F-FDG PET/CT and human papillomavirus type 16 testing in locally advanced oropharyngeal squamous cell carcinoma. Eur J Nucl Med Mol Imaging 2012;39(11): 1673–84.
20. Pytynia KB, Dahlstrom KR, Sturgis EM. Epidemiology of HPV-associated oropharyngeal cancer. Oral Oncol 2014;50(5):380–6.
21. Kalyankrishna S, Grandis JR. Epidermal growth factor receptor biology in head and neck cancer. J Clin Oncol 2006;24(17):2666–72.
22. Subramaniam RM, Alluri KC, Tahari AK, et al. PET/CT imaging and human papilloma virus-positive oropharyngeal squamous cell cancer: evolving clinical imaging paradigm. J Nucl Med 2014; 55(3):431–8.
23. Fakhry C, Zhang Q, Nguyen-Tan PF, et al. Human papillomavirus and overall survival after progression of oropharyngeal squamous cell carcinoma. J Clin Oncol 2014;32(30):3365–73.
24. Ang KK, Harris J, Wheeler R, et al. Human papillomavirus and survival of patients with oropharyngeal cancer. N Engl J Med 2014;363(1):24–35.

25. O'Rorke MA, Ellison MV, Murray LJ, et al. Human papillomavirus related head and neck cancer survival: a systematic review and meta-analysis. Oral Oncol 2012;48(12):1191–201.

26. Krabbe CA, Balink H, Roodenburg JL, et al. Performance of 18F-FDG PET/contrast-enhanced CT in the staging of squamous cell carcinoma of the oral cavity and oropharynx. Int J Oral Maxillofac Surg 2011;40(11):1263–70.

27. Haerle SK, Strobel K, Ahmad N, et al. Contrast-enhanced (1)(8)F-FDG-PET/CT for the assessment of necrotic lymph node metastases. Head Neck 2011;33(3):324–9.

28. Huang SH, Perez-Ordonez B, Weinreb I, et al. Natural course of distant metastases following radiotherapy or chemoradiotherapy in HPV-related oropharyngeal cancer. Oral Oncol 2013;49(1): 79–85.

29. Xu GZ, Zhu XD, Li MY. Accuracy of whole-body PET and PET-CT in initial M staging of head and neck cancer: a meta-analysis. Head Neck 2011; 33(1):87–94.

30. Kreimer AR, Johansson M, Waterboer T, et al. Evaluation of human papillomavirus antibodies and risk of subsequent head and neck cancer. J Clin Oncol 2013;31(21):2708–15.

31. Fakhry C, Qualliotine JR, Zhang Z, et al. Serum antibodies to HPV16 early proteins warrant investigation as potential biomarkers for risk stratification and recurrence of HPV-associated oropharyngeal cancer. Cancer Prev Res (Phila) 2016;9(2):135–41.

32. Clark J, Jeffery CC, Zhang H, et al. Correlation of PET-CT nodal SUVmax with p16 positivity in oropharyngeal squamous cell carcinoma. J Otolaryngol Head Neck Surg 2015;44:37.

33. Tang C, Murphy JD, Khong B, et al. Validation that metabolic tumor volume predicts outcome in head-and-neck cancer. Int J Radiat Oncol Biol Phys 2012;83(5):1514–20.

34. Cheng NM, Fang YH, Chang JT, et al. Textural features of pretreatment 18F-FDG PET/CT images: prognostic significance in patients with advanced T-stage oropharyngeal squamous cell carcinoma. J Nucl Med 2013;54(10):1703–9.

35. Alluri KC, Tahari AK, Wahl RL, et al. Prognostic value of FDG PET metabolic tumor volume in human papillomavirus-positive stage III and IV oropharyngeal squamous cell carcinoma. AJR Am J Roentgenol 2014;203(4):897–903.

36. Tsang CM, Tsao SW. The role of Epstein-Barr virus infection in the pathogenesis of nasopharyngeal carcinoma. Virol Sin 2015;30(2):107–21.

37. Raab-Traub N. Epstein-Barr virus in the pathogenesis of NPC. Semin Cancer Biol 2002;12(6): 431–41.

38. Yoshizaki T, Kondo S, Wakisaka N, et al. Pathogenic role of Epstein-Barr virus latent membrane protein-1 in the development of nasopharyngeal carcinoma. Cancer Lett 2013;337(1):1–7.

39. Kang H, Kiess A, Chung CH. Emerging biomarkers in head and neck cancer in the era of genomics. Nat Rev Clin Oncol 2015;12(1):11–26.

40. Chan SC, Hsu CL, Yen TC, et al. The role of 18F-FDG PET/CT metabolic tumour volume in predicting survival in patients with metastatic nasopharyngeal carcinoma. Oral Oncol 2012;49(1):71–8.

41. Ma BB, King A, Lo YM, et al. Relationship between pretreatment level of plasma Epstein-Barr virus DNA, tumor burden, and metabolic activity in advanced nasopharyngeal carcinoma. Int J Radiat Oncol Biol Phys 2006;66(3):714–20.

42. Chang KP, Tsang NM, Liao CT, et al. Prognostic significance of 18F-FDG PET parameters and plasma Epstein-Barr virus DNA load in patients with nasopharyngeal carcinoma. J Nucl Med 2012;53(1):21–8.

43. Makitie AA, Reis PP, Irish J, et al. Correlation of Epstein-Barr virus DNA in cell-free plasma, functional imaging and clinical course in locally advanced nasopharyngeal cancer: a pilot study. Head Neck 2004;26(9):815–22.

44. Wang WY, Twu CW, Lin WY, et al. Plasma Epstein-Barr virus DNA screening followed by 18F-fluoro-2-deoxy-D-glucose positron emission tomography in detecting posttreatment failures of nasopharyngeal carcinoma. Cancer 2011;117(19):4452–9.

45. Rasmussen GB, Vogelius IR, Rasmussen JH, et al. Immunohistochemical biomarkers and FDG uptake on PET/CT in head and neck squamous cell carcinoma. Acta Oncol 2015;54(9):1408–15.

46. Temam S, Kawaguchi H, El-Naggar AK, et al. Epidermal growth factor receptor copy number alterations correlate with poor clinical outcome in patients with head and neck squamous cancer. J Clin Oncol 2007;25(16):2164–70.

47. Feldman R, Gatalica Z, Knezetic J, et al. Molecular profiling of head and neck squamous cell carcinoma. Head Neck 2016;38(Suppl 1):E1625–38.

48. Keck MK, Zuo Z, Khattri A, et al. Integrative analysis of head and neck cancer identifies two biologically distinct HPV and three non-HPV subtypes. Clin Cancer Res 2015;21(4):870–81.

49. Kumar B, Cordell KG, Lee JS, et al. EGFR, p16, HPV Titer, Bcl-xL and p53, sex, and smoking as indicators of response to therapy and survival in oropharyngeal cancer. J Clin Oncol 2008;26(19): 3128–37.

50. Kong CS, Narasimhan B, Cao H, et al. The relationship between human papillomavirus status and other molecular prognostic markers in head and neck squamous cell carcinomas. Int J Radiat Oncol Biol Phys 2009;74(2):553–61.

51. Smilek P, Neuwirthova J, Jarkovsky J, et al. Epidermal growth factor receptor (EGFR)

expression and mutations in the EGFR signaling pathway in correlation with anti-EGFR therapy in head and neck squamous cell carcinomas. Neoplasma 2012;59(5):508–15.

52. Li W, Niu G, Lang L, et al. PET imaging of EGF receptors using [18F]FBEM-EGF in a head and neck squamous cell carcinoma model. Eur J Nucl Med Mol Imaging 2012;39(2):300–8.

53. Psyrri A, Seiwert TY, Jimeno A. Molecular pathways in head and neck cancer: EGFR, PI3K, and more. Am Soc Clin Oncol Educ Book 2013;246–55.

54. Keren S, Shoude Z, Lu Z, et al. Role of EGFR as a prognostic factor for survival in head and neck cancer: a meta-analysis. Tumour Biol 2014;35(3): 2285–95.

55. Chung CH, Lee JW, Slebos RJ, et al. A 3'-UTR KRAS-variant is associated with cisplatin resistance in patients with recurrent and/or metastatic head and neck squamous cell carcinoma. Ann Oncol 2014;25(11):2230–6.

56. Hoa M, Davis SL, Ames SJ, et al. Amplification of wild-type K-ras promotes growth of head and neck squamous cell carcinoma. Cancer Res 2002;62(24):7154–6.

57. Wang WY, Chien YC, Wong YK, et al. Effects of KRAS mutation and polymorphism on the risk and prognosis of oral squamous cell carcinoma. Head Neck 2011;34(5):663–6.

58. Peruzzi B, Bottaro DP. Targeting the c-Met signaling pathway in cancer. Clin Cancer Res 2006;12(12):3657–60.

59. Knowles LM, Stabile LP, Egloff AM, et al. HGF and c-Met participate in paracrine tumorigenic pathways in head and neck squamous cell cancer. Clin Cancer Res 2009;15(11):3740–50.

60. Di Renzo MF, Olivero M, Martone T, et al. Somatic mutations of the MET oncogene are selected during metastatic spread of human HNSC carcinomas. Oncogene 2000;19(12):1547–55.

61. Zhao D, Wang SH, Feng Y, et al. Intratumoral c-Met expression is associated with vascular endothelial growth factor C expression, lymphangiogenesis, and lymph node metastasis in oral squamous cell carcinoma: implications for use as a prognostic marker. Hum Pathol 2011;42(10):1514–23.

62. Nylander K, Dabelsteen E, Hall PA. The p53 molecule and its prognostic role in squamous cell carcinomas of the head and neck. J Oral Pathol Med 2000;29(9):413–25.

63. Poeta ML, Manola J, Goldwasser MA, et al. TP53 mutations and survival in squamous-cell carcinoma of the head and neck. N Engl J Med 2007;357(25): 2552–61.

64. Licitra L, Perrone F, Bossi P, et al. High-risk human papillomavirus affects prognosis in patients with surgically treated oropharyngeal squamous cell carcinoma. J Clin Oncol 2006;24(36):5630–6.

65. Basu S, Kwee TC, Gatenby R, et al. Evolving role of molecular imaging with PET in detecting and characterizing heterogeneity of cancer tissue at the primary and metastatic sites, a plausible explanation for failed attempts to cure malignant disorders. Eur J Nucl Med Mol Imaging 2011;38(6):987–91.

66. Saunders NA, Simpson F, Thompson EW, et al. Role of intratumoural heterogeneity in cancer drug resistance: molecular and clinical perspectives. EMBO Mol Med 2012;4(8):675–84.

67. Kwon SH, Yoon JK, An YS, et al. Prognostic significance of the intratumoral heterogeneity of (18) F-FDG uptake in oral cavity cancer. J Surg Oncol 2014;110(6):702–6.

68. Henriksson E, Kjellen E, Wahlberg P, et al. 2-Deoxy-2-[18F] fluoro-D-glucose uptake and correlation to intratumoral heterogeneity. Anticancer Res 2007; 27(4B):2155–9.

69. Cheng NM, Fang YH, Lee LY, et al. Zone-size nonuniformity of 18F-FDG PET regional textural features predicts survival in patients with oropharyngeal cancer. Eur J Nucl Med Mol Imaging 2015; 42(3):419–28.

70. Iyer NG, Tan DS, Tan VK, et al. Randomized trial comparing surgery and adjuvant radiotherapy versus concurrent chemoradiotherapy in patients with advanced, nonmetastatic squamous cell carcinoma of the head and neck: 10-year update and subset analysis. Cancer 2015;121(10):1599–607.

71. Chan JY, Sanguineti G, Richmon JD, et al. Retrospective review of positron emission tomography with contrast-enhanced computed tomography in the posttreatment setting in human papillomavirus-associated oropharyngeal carcinoma. Arch Otolaryngol Head Neck Surg 2012; 138(11):1040–6.

72. Wang MB, Liu IY, Gornbein JA, et al. HPV-positive oropharyngeal carcinoma: a systematic review of treatment and prognosis. Otolaryngol Head Neck Surg 2015;153(5):758–69.

73. Gupta T, Master Z, Kannan S, et al. Diagnostic performance of post-treatment FDG PET or FDG PET/CT imaging in head and neck cancer: a systematic review and meta-analysis. Eur J Nucl Med Mol Imaging 2011;38(11):2083–95.

74. Bussink J, van Herpen CM, Kaanders JH, et al. PET-CT for response assessment and treatment adaptation in head and neck cancer. Lancet Oncol 2010;11(7):661–9.

75. Nakamura S, Toriihara A, Okochi K, et al. Optimal timing of post-treatment [18F]fluorodeoxyglucose-PET/CT for patients with head and neck malignancy. Nucl Med Commun 2013;34(2):162–7.

76. Leung AS, Rath TJ, Hughes MA, et al. Optimal timing of first posttreatment FDG PET/CT in head and neck squamous cell carcinoma. Head Neck 2016;38(Suppl 1):E853–8.

77. Kim R, Ock CY, Keam B, et al. Predictive and prognostic value of PET/CT imaging post-chemoradiotherapy and clinical decision-making consequences in locally advanced head & neck squamous cell carcinoma: a retrospective study. BMC Cancer 2016;16(1):116.

78. Isles MG, McConkey C, Mehanna HM. A systematic review and meta-analysis of the role of positron emission tomography in the follow up of head and neck squamous cell carcinoma following radiotherapy or chemoradiotherapy. Clin Otolaryngol 2008;33(3):210–22.

79. Sjovall J, Brun E, Almquist H, et al. Radiotherapy response in head and neck cancer - evaluation of the primary tumour site. Acta Otolaryngol 2014; 134(6):646–51.

80. Marcus C, Ciarallo A, Tahari AK, et al. Head and neck PET/CT: therapy response interpretation criteria (Hopkins Criteria)-interreader reliability, accuracy, and survival outcomes. J Nucl Med 2014; 55(9):1411–6.

81. ClinicalTrials.gov. Reduced-dose intensity-modulated radiation therapy with or without cisplatin in treating patients with advanced oropharyngeal cancer. 2016. Available at: https://clinicaltrials.gov/ct2/show/NCT02254278?term=NRG+HN002&rank=1. Accessed June 28, 2016.

82. Mehanna H, Wong WL, McConkey CC, et al. PET-CT surveillance versus neck dissection in advanced head and neck cancer. N Engl J Med 2016;374(15):1444–54.

83. Taghipour M, Sheikhbahaei S, Wray R, et al. FDG PET/CT in patients with head and neck squamous cell carcinoma after primary surgical resection with or without chemoradiation therapy. AJR Am J Roentgenol 2016;206(5):1093–100.

84. Schmitz S, Hamoir M, Reychler H, et al. Tumour response and safety of cetuximab in a window pre-operative study in patients with squamous cell carcinoma of the head and neck. Ann Oncol 2013;24(9):2261–6.

85. Adkins D, Ley J, Dehdashti F, et al. A prospective trial comparing FDGPET/CT and CT to assess tumor response to cetuximab in patients within curable squamous cell carcinoma of the head and neck. Cancer Med 2014;3(6):1493–501.

86. Perk LR, Visser GW, Vosjan MJ, et al. (89)Zr as a PET surrogate radioisotope for scouting biodistribution of the therapeutic radiometals (90)Y and (177)Lu in tumor-bearing nude mice after coupling to the internalizing antibody cetuximab. J Nucl Med 2005;46(11):1898–906.

87. Garousi J, Andersson KG, Mitran B, et al. PET imaging of epidermal growth factor receptor expression in tumours using 89Zr-labelled ZEGFR:2377 affibody molecules. Int J Oncol 2016;48(4): 1325–32.

88. Koppikar P, Choi SH, Egloff AM, et al. Combined inhibition of c-Src and epidermal growth factor receptor abrogates growth and invasion of head and neck squamous cell carcinoma. Clin Cancer Res 2008;14(13):4284–91.

89. Aerts HJ, Dubois L, Perk L, et al. Disparity between in vivo EGFR expression and 89Zr-labeled cetuximab uptake assessed with PET. J Nucl Med 2009;50(1):123–31.

90. Brizel DM, Sibley GS, Prosnitz LR, et al. Tumor hypoxia adversely affects the prognosis of carcinoma of the head and neck. Int J Radiat Oncol Biol Phys 1997;38(2):285–9.

91. Eschmann SM, Paulsen F, Reimold M, et al. Prognostic impact of hypoxia imaging with 18F-misonidazole PET in non-small cell lung cancer and head and neck cancer before radiotherapy. J Nucl Med 2005;46(2):253–60.

92. Dirix P, Vandecaveye V, De Keyzer F, et al. Dose painting in radiotherapy for head and neck squamous cell carcinoma: value of repeated functional imaging with (18)F-FDG PET, (18)F-fluoromisonidazole PET, diffusion-weighted MRI, and dynamic contrast-enhanced MRI. J Nucl Med 2009;50(7): 1020–7.

93. Rischin D, Hicks RJ, Fisher R, et al. Prognostic significance of [18F]-misonidazole positron emission tomography-detected tumor hypoxia in patients with advanced head and neck cancer randomly assigned to chemoradiation with or without tirapazamine: a substudy of Trans-Tasman Radiation Oncology Group Study 98.02. J Clin Oncol 2006; 24(13):2098–104.

94. Zips D, Zöphel K, Abolmaali N, et al. Exploratory prospective trial of hypoxia-specific PET imaging during radiochemotherapy in patients with locally advanced head-and-neck cancer. Radiother Oncol 2012;105(1):21–8.

95. Sato J, Kitagawa Y, Yamazaki Y, et al. Advantage of FMISO-PET over FDG-PET for predicting histological response to preoperative chemotherapy in patients with oral squamous cell carcinoma. Eur J Nucl Med Mol Imaging 2014;41(11):2031–41.

96. Mortensen LS, Johansen J, Kallehauge J, et al. FAZA PET/CT hypoxia imaging in patients with squamous cell carcinoma of the head and neck treated with radiotherapy: results from the DAHANCA 24 trial. Radiother Oncol 2012;105(1): 14–20.

97. Servagi-Vernat S, Differding S, Hanin FX, et al. A prospective clinical study of (1)(8)F-FAZA PET-CT hypoxia imaging in head and neck squamous cell carcinoma before and during radiation therapy. Eur J Nucl Med Mol Imaging 2014;41(8):1544–52.

98. Komar G, Seppänen M, Eskola O, et al. 18F-EF5: a new PET tracer for imaging hypoxia in head and neck cancer. J Nucl Med 2008;49(12):1944–51.

99. Komar G, Lehtiö K, Seppänen M, et al. Prognostic value of tumour blood flow, [(1)(8)F]EF5 and [(1)(8)F]FDG PET/CT imaging in patients with head and neck cancer treated with radiochemotherapy. Eur J Nucl Med Mol Imaging 2014;41(11):2042–50.

100. Minagawa Y, Shizukuishi K, Koike I, et al. Assessment of tumor hypoxia by 62Cu-ATSM PET/CT as a predictor of response in head and neck cancer: a pilot study. Ann Nucl Med 2011;25(5):339–45.

101. Nyflot MJ, Harari PM, Yip S, et al. Correlation of PET images of metabolism, proliferation and hypoxia to characterize tumor phenotype in patients with cancer of the oropharynx. Radiother Oncol 2012;105(1):36–40.

102. Sato Y, Tsujikawa T, Oh M, et al. Assessing tumor hypoxia in head and neck cancer by PET with (6)(2)Cu-diacetyl-bis(N(4)-methylthiosemicarbazone). Clin Nucl Med 2014;39(12):1027–32.

103. Shields AF, Grierson JR, Dohmen BM, et al. Imaging proliferation in vivo with [F-18]FLT and positron emission tomography. Nat Med 1998;4(11):1334–6.

104. Chalkidou A, Landau DB, Odell EW, et al. Correlation between Ki-67 immunohistochemistry and 18F-fluorothymidine uptake in patients with cancer: a systematic review and meta-analysis. Eur J Cancer 2012;48(18):3499–513.

105. Hoeben BA, Troost EG, Span PN, et al. 18F-FLT PET during radiotherapy or chemoradiotherapy in head and neck squamous cell carcinoma is an early predictor of outcome. J Nucl Med 2013;54(4):532–40.

106. Kishino T, Hoshikawa H, Nishiyama Y, et al. Usefulness of 3'-deoxy-3'-18F-fluorothymidine PET for predicting early response to chemoradiotherapy in head and neck cancer. J Nucl Med 2012;53(10):1521–7.

107. Gaertner FC, Kessler H, Wester HJ, et al. Radiolabelled RGD peptides for imaging and therapy. Eur J Nucl Med Mol Imaging 2012;39(Suppl 1):S126–38.

108. Beer AJ, Grosu AL, Carlsen J, et al. [18F]galacto-RGD positron emission tomography for imaging of alphavbeta3 expression on the neovasculature in patients with squamous cell carcinoma of the head and neck. Clin Cancer Res 2007;13(22 Pt 1):6610–6.

109. Chen SH, Wang HM, Lin CY, et al. RGD-K5 PET/CT in patients with advanced head and neck cancer treated with concurrent chemoradiotherapy: results from a pilot study. Eur J Nucl Med Mol Imaging 2016;43(9):1621–9.

Designing and Developing PET-Based Precision Model in Thyroid Carcinoma
The Potential Avenues for a Personalized Clinical Care

Sandip Basu, MBBS (Hons), DRM, DNB, MNAMS*, Rahul Vithalrao Parghane, MBBS, MD

KEYWORDS

- Differentiated thyroid carcinoma • Thyroglobulin • Radioiodine scan
- Fluorodeoxyglucose-PET/computed tomography
- High thyroglobulin and negative iodine scintigraphy • Radioiodine therapy • PET

KEY POINTS

- PET imaging (with fluorodeoxyglucose [FDG]) is utilized to investigate patients of differentiated thyroid carcinoma (DTC) with high thyroglobulin and negative iodine scintigraphy (TENIS) and in medullary carcinoma thyroid (MCT) when the tumor markers (eg, calcitonin and carcino embryonic antigen [CEA]) are raised postoperatively (PET with FDG, 68Ga-DOTA-NOC/TATE, FDOPA). PET–computed tomography (CT) has been found substantially useful in detecting sites of metastatic disease and making decisions with regard to feasibility and planning of surgery on an individual patient basis.
- Patients with elevated TENIS and metastatic disease are not amenable to surgery through examining FDG-PET findings in tandem with radioiodine scan and 68Ga-DOTA-TATE/NOC PET-CT.
- Managing nonsurgical recurrence/metastasis in TENIS is a challenge to the attending physician.

INTRODUCTION

This article enumerates the current uses and potential areas where PET could be utilized for developing a precision medicine-type model in the management of thyroid carcinoma. For the purpose of a systematic discussion, differentiated thyroid carcinoma (DTC) and medullary thyroid carcinoma (MCT) are discussed separately. In both conditions, the important clinical decision-making steps where PET plays a pivotal role have been dealt with first, with discussion on potentials of management personalization at these steps. Subsequently, the future avenues where PET imaging could be utilized for enhancing a personalized clinical practice have been touched upon. Each aspect is debated and substantiated based upon existing literature evidence under respective subheadings.

DIFFERENTIATED THYROID CARCINOMA
Fluorodeoxyglucose-PET/Computed Tomography in Investigating Thyroglobulin and Negative Iodine Scintigraphy: Detecting Sites of Disease, Assessing Feasibility, and Planning of Surgery on an Individual Basis

In a patient with elevated serum thyroglobulin and negative I-131 whole body scan (popularly known as thyroglobulin and negative iodine scintigraphy

The authors have nothing to disclose.
Radiation Medicine Centre, Bhabha Atomic Research Centre, Tata Memorial Hospital Annexe, Jerbai Wadia Road, Parel, Bombay 400 012, India
* Corresponding author.
E-mail address: drsanb@yahoo.com

PET Clin 12 (2017) 27–37
http://dx.doi.org/10.1016/j.cpet.2016.08.007

[TENIS]), the standard procedure for investigation is an ultrasonography neck and fluorodeoxyglucose-PET/computed tomography (FDG-PET/CT) (Cases 1 and 2, **Figs. 1** and **2**). In a study by Na and colleagues,[1] in a series of 60 patients of TENIS, the sensitivity of PET/CT according to Tg levels was 28.6% when stimulated Tg was between 2 and 5, 57.1% between 5 and 10, 60.0% between 10 and 20, and 85.7% when Tg was equal to or greater than 20 ng/mL subgroups, respectively. There were 3 patients with high anti-Tg Ab level (>70 IU/mL) and low (<2 ng/mL) in this series, in which all cases were positive on FDG-PET/CT. In the study by Vural and colleagues,[2] undertaken in a population of 105 patients with TENIS, the highest accuracy of FDG-PET/CT was reached at Tg greater than 1.9 ng/mL under thyroid stimulating hormone (TSH) suppression and 38.2 ng/mL with TSH stimulation. The other findings in this study included

- Extra-thyroidal spread was an independent risk factor related to FDG-avid recurrence
- Tumor size was significantly higher in PET-positive patients
- Significant correlation was observed between PET positivity and high Tg levels
- Among PET-negative patients, no future recurrence was detected in patients with undetectable/suppressible Tg in on-therapy state

In another study by Ozkan and colleagues,[3] in a total of 59 patients with TENIS or with high level anti-Tg Ab level, FDG PET/CT was found to be a useful imaging modality in defining the recurrence of disease. On receiver operating characteristic analysis, a 4.5 cut-off SUVmax was calculated with 75% sensitivity and 70% specificity for predicting disease recurrence. Trybek and colleagues,[4] in a study population of 19 patients with TENIS, observed on receiver operating

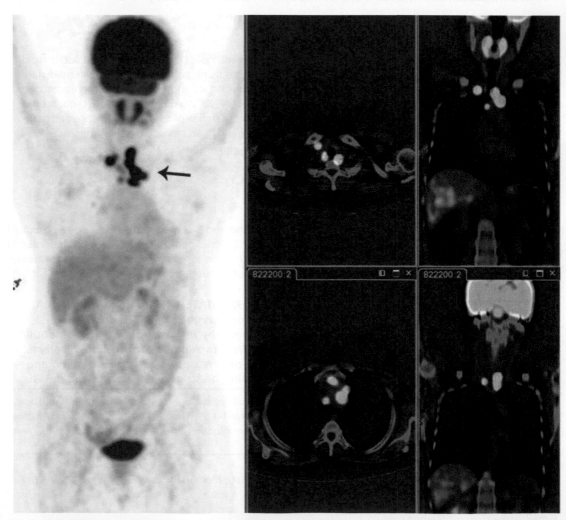

Fig. 1. FDG-PET/CT maximum image projection (MIP) (*left panel*), fused transaxial and coronal images (*right panel*) demonstrating FDG-avid enlarged right supraclavicular and mediastinal lymph nodes.

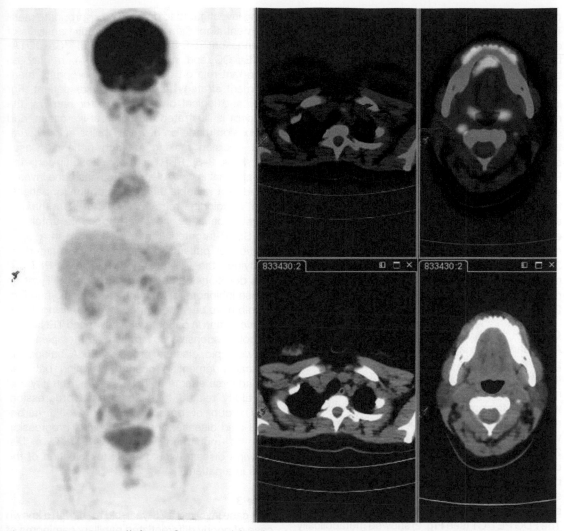

Fig. 2. FDG-PET/CT MIP (*left panel*), transaxial fused and CT images (*right panel*) showing FDG avid right level II cervical and pretracheal lymph nodes.

characteristic curve (ROC) analysis, demonstrated a stimulated Tg cut-off of 28.5 ng/mL with 100% sensitivity and specificity for FDG PET/CT to detect metastases. Asa and colleagues[5] studied 40 DTC patients who were Tg negative and had increased antithyroglobulin antibodies (>40 IU/mL); they found that FDG uptake suspicious for recurrence/metastasis was observed in 20 (50%) of the patients. While this study was primarily focused to demonstrating the value of serum antithyroglobulin antibodies as a tumor marker for DTCs, it also showed the value of FDG-PET in detecting recurrence in this group of patients. Salvatori and colleagues,[6] in their review of the various possible indications of FDG-PET/CT in DTC, studied the recommendations of various thyroid carcinoma-related guidelines pertaining to different societies (such as British Thyroid Association (BTA), American Thyroid Association (ATA), National Comprehensive Cancer Network (NCCN),

Latin American Thyroid Society (LATS), European Society for Medical Oncology (ESMO), European Thyroid Association (ETA)): the most recommendations suggest use of FDG-PET/CT in nonstimulated Tg (ie, on LT4) levels above 10 ng/mL. Additionally, the BTA and ESMO guidelines suggested rising Tg as an important indication, and the NCCN and ETA guidelines suggested a TSH stimulated Tg more than 2 to 5 ng/mL a potential indication.

Although there have been some variations with regard to different studies and the guidelines with regard to the indication of FDG-PET/CT in TENIS, there is uniform agreement about its value in subsequent clinical management, which is detecting sites of recurrent/metastatic disease, differentiating surgical from non-surgical metastatic disease and also planning surgery. In all the aforementioned cases, FDG-PET/CT aids in assessing and deciding on this aspect of the patient on an individual basis.

Case 1

This 43-year-old woman had a known case of differentiated papillary carcinoma thyroid. The patient underwent near total thyroidectomy followed by radioactive iodine (RAI) of 67 mCi in 2002. Twelve years later she presented with recurrence in thyroid bed, for which the patient underwent neck dissection. The histopathology report showed residual differentiated papillary carcinoma thyroid of right thyroid bed with metastases to bilateral neck nodes and tracheal wall infiltration. Postoperative radioiodine whole-body scan showed multifocal neck and mediastinal uptake, for which the patient received 193 mCi I-131 therapy orally. Thereafter, patient was started on tab eltroxin; the repeat radioiodine after 1 year was normal. The stimulated Tg was greater than 300 ng/mL. The FDG PET/CT showed multiple metabolically active right supraclavicular lymph nodes and mediastinal (SUVmax 31.5, largest 2.4 × 1.7 cm in prevascular region).

Case 2

A 34 year old woman had a known case of classical papillary carcinoma of thyroid, and had undergone total thyroidectomy and bilateral central compartmental clearance followed by RAI of 155 mCi with post-therapy scan positive in the neck. The recent follow-up whole-body radioiodine scan was normal, and serum Tg (stimulated) was 23.2 ng/mL. The ultrasonography (USG) neck demonstrated no abnormal focus lesion in thyroid bed; subcentimetric reactive lymph nodes are seen in the bilateral IB, II, and III cervical regions, suggestive of reactive cervical lymphadenopathy. The FDG PET/CT (see **Fig. 2**) showed metabolically active right level II cervical and pretracheal lymph nodes (SUVmax 3.7, measuring 1.2 × 0.6 cm).

Learning point This is an example where FDG-PET/CT demonstrated the disease extent useful for assessing operability and planning surgery in a patient of TENIS on an individual basis. The second case shows it can be useful and serve important goal in detection and characterization of neck nodes when the USG (neck) is otherwise normal.

Assessing and Characterizing Nonsurgical Disease in Thyroglobulin and Negative Iodine Scintigraphy Through Multitracer Molecular Functional Imaging: Individualized Decision on Observation Versus Peptide Receptor Radionuclide Therapy Versus Tyrosine Kinase Inhibitors

Managing non-surgical recurrence/metastasis in TENIS is a challenge to the attending physician, with several routine and experimental approaches being investigated to develop an appropriate management algorithm.[7] The comparative analysis of findings on PET-CT with FDG and ^{68}Ga-DOTA-TATE/NOC and radioiodine scan can play an important role on deciding the appropriate management strategy in each particular patient. For easy and logical understanding for readers, the concept is illustrated through real-life cases, and discussion made on how PET helps in individualized decision making in such patients (Cases 3–5, **Figs. 3–5**). PRRT is a somatostatin-targeted therapy that is well tolerated and has been investigated as a valuable therapeutic option for patients with radioiodine-refractory DTC.[8–10] In the authors' experience, however, adequate uptake of the SSTR-targeted tracer is observed in a small fraction of patients,[11] and it can be guided by studying the ^{68}Ga-GOTATATE/NOC PET-CT; thus decisions can be made individually. Tyrosine kinase inhibitors (TKIs) such as sorafenib and lenvatinib have been described as a promising therapeutic option in patients with advanced TENIS that is not responsive to traditional therapies and shows rapid disease progression. A balance in clinical judgment is needed weighing between the adverse effects of TKIs and the mortality and morbidity related to rapid disease progression. This group of patients typically would harbor FDG-avid disease, and their disease progression can be monitored with FDG-PET/CT; a fast growing disease would argue for initiation of the TKIs in a patient.

Case 3

This case involved a 78-year-old man, with a known case of poorly differentiated papillary carcinoma of thyroid with bilateral pulmonary metastases. The patient had undergone total thyroidectomy followed by radioiodine therapy 190 mCi. Post-therapy-neck and chest scan was positive. The following year, the whole-body radioiodine scan was negative. FDG-PET showed progressively increasing FDG positive lung metastases (initially FDG-PET/CT positive for left lung nodule, see **Fig. 3**A left panel). The recent FDG-PET/CT at 18 months following the previous study (see **Fig. 3**B right panel) show tracer-avid right supraclavicular, mediastinal lymph nodes, and lung nodules. The patient had ^{68}Ga-DOTATATE-negative disease and is a case for consideration for TKI therapy.

Case 4

This was a 56-year-old man with a known case of trabecular variant of papillary carcinoma of thyroid, who had undergone thyroidectomy and subsequently RAI therapy 2 times, showing iodine avid neck and pelvic foci (sacrum). Stimulated serum

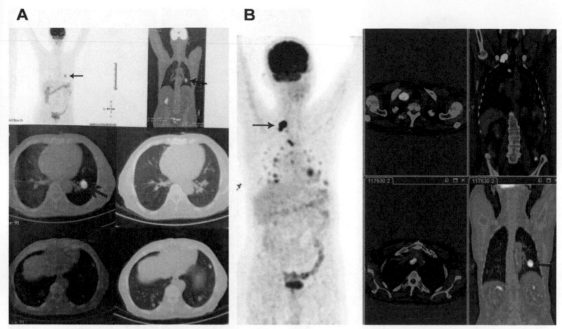

Fig. 3. (*A*) FDG-PET/CT MIP, fused coronal, transaxial fused and CT images showing a few FDG-avid left lung nodules. (*B*) MIP, fused transaxial, and coronal images demonstrating FDG-avid enlarged right supraclavicular lymph node, mediastinal lymph nodes, and lung nodules.

Tg was greater than 300 ng/mL in 2015. Interestingly, FDG-PET/CT at this time demonstrated FDG-avid expansile lytic lesions in right clavicle, right sixth rib, left fifth rib, left ileum, and sacrum. Follow-up whole-body radioiodine scan in 2016 showed faint tracer uptake only in the neck region. ^{68}Ga-DOTATATE (**Fig. 4A, B**) and FDG- (**Fig. 4C, D**)

PET/CT showed tracer-avid lytic–sclerotic lesions with soft tissue component in multiple skeletal sites (right clavicle, bilateral ribs, lumbar vertebrae, pelvic bones, and sacrum). The patient received 146 mCi of ^{177}Lu-DOTATATE therapy; the post-therapy scan (**Fig. 4E**) showed tracer uptake in multiple skeletal sites.

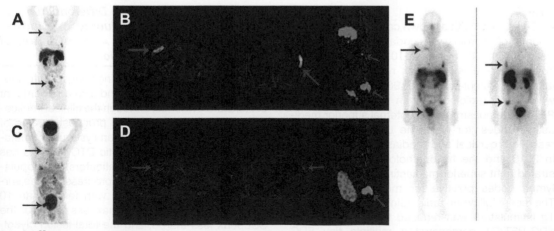

Fig. 4. ^{68}Ga-DOTATATE-PET/CT MIP (*A*), fused transaxial, and sagittal (*B*) images demonstrating somatostatin receptor-avid lytic–sclerotic skeletal lesions involving right clavicle, left side ribs, lumbar vertebrae, and sacrum. FDG-PET/CT MIP (*C*), fused transaxial, and sagittal (*D*) images similarly showing FDG-avid skeletal lesions in previously mentioned skeletal sites. ^{177}Lu-DOTATATE post-therapy whole-body anterior and posterior (*E*) images showing tracer uptake in multiple skeletal lesion sites.

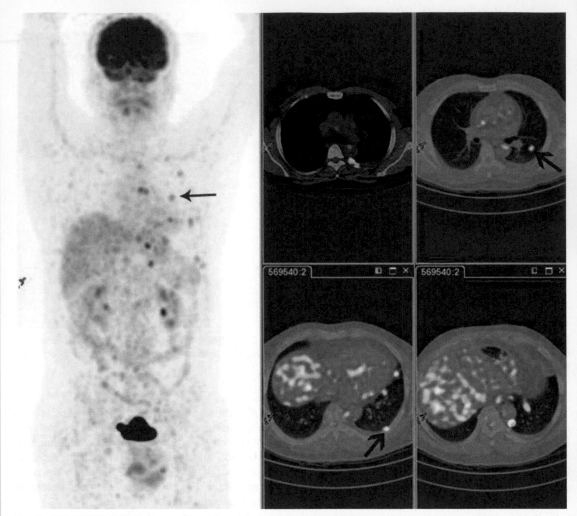

Fig. 5. FDG-PET/CT MIP (*left panel*) and fused transaxial images (*right panel*) demonstrating FDG avid left-sided both pleural and parenchymal-based lung nodules.

Case 5

A 52-year-man with a known case of papillary carcinoma of thyroid with nodal metastases was treated with 98 mCi in 2010; the post-therapy scan was positive for neck residue. Two years later, Tg (stimulated) was 98 ng/mL, and the whole-body radioiodine scan was normal. FDG-PET/CT demonstrated retrosternal superior mediastinal nodes, for which he underwent surgical resection; cervical and mediastinal lymph nodes in 2015 and the histopathology report demonstrated right superior mediastinal and retrosternal lymph nodes positive for metastatic deposits. The recent follow-up radioiodine scan was normal; Tg (stimulated) was reduced to 7.9 ng/mL, and FDG-PET/CT demonstrated multiple tiny FDG avid both pleural and parenchymal lung nodules on the left side (SUVmax 8.0, largest measuring 7.4 mm). It was decided that the patient should be kept under follow-up with TSH suppression.

Disease Prognostication in Differentiated Thyroid Carcinoma with Fluorodeoxyglucose PET Metabolic Parameters: A Potential Area of Management Personalization

This continues to be an evolving concept with substantial clinical experience and also a fair amount of literature evidence, although the clinical implications are not yet clear. The prognostic value of FDG-PET with quantitative analysis using metabolic parameters in metastatic DTC patients has been studied by various investigators. In a population of 37 patients with DTC, progression-free survival was better in patients with fewer than 10 FDG-avid lesions, the SUVmax less than 10, the SULpeak less than 5, and the total lesion glycolysis (TLG) less than 154.[12] The final Cox analyses in this study showed that the result of the PET scan was predictive of survival, with the prognostic factors for progression-free survival and overall survival being SUVmax, the SULpeak, and the TLG. Yoon and colleagues[13] studied the relationship between the BRAFV600E mutation and F-18 FDG uptake in papillary thyroid carcinoma (PTC). They concluded that the presence of the BRAFV600E mutation is independently associated with high F-18 FDG uptake on preoperative PET/CT in patients with overt PTC of greater than 1 cm.

Conversely, the authors observed that elevated Tg but normal ^{18}F-FDG PET exists as a definitive entity, and a negative ^{18}F-FDG PET in the setting of TENIS could be regarded as a favorable prognostic indicator (Case 6, **Fig. 6**) to predict prolonged symptom-free status during the follow-up period.[14]

Case 6

This case involves a 16-year-old boy with a known case of differentiated papillary carcinoma of thyroid with lymph node metastases who underwent total thyroidectomy, central compartmental clearance, and lateral neck dissection in 2012. Chest radiograph showed tiny radio-opacities in bilateral lung fields in 2013, and stimulated serum Tg was greater than 300 ng/mL. He received 2 times

RAI for pulmonary metastases (6475 MBq and 7437 MBq, respectively); the last post-therapy scan showed faint tracer uptake in the chest region. Stimulated Tg was always greater than 300 ng/mL. The latest iodine scan was negative. FDG-PET/CT demonstrated nontracer-avid tiny bilateral lung nodules (see **Fig. 6**). The case suggests a good prognosis commensurate with his excellent general condition, and disease nonprogression over the last 4 years despite radioiodine, was only faintly positive.

Postoperative Fluorodeoxyglucose–PET/ Computed Tomography in Patients with Aggressive Histology of Differentiated Thyroid Cancer

The direct corollary of the aforementioned prognostic implication of FDG-avid thyroid cancer is its potential role in DTCs with aggressive histopathologies. This is an evolving area where FDG-PET/CT could be of potential value in management personalization. Nascimento and colleagues[15] observed that FDG-PET/CT was more sensitive than RAI whole body scan (RAI WBS) for the

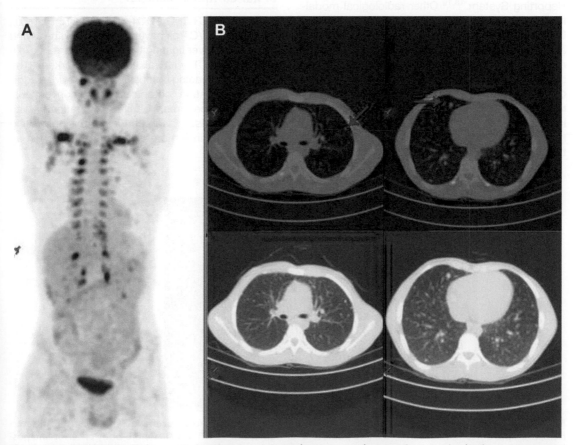

Fig. 6. FDG-PET/CT MIP (*left panel*) showing no abnormal tracer uptake anywhere in the body and transaxial fused and CT images (*right panel*) demonstrating non-FDG avid subcentimetric bilateral lung nodules.

detection of individual lesions (69% vs 59%). Both imaging techniques were complementary, with 41% of the lesions detected only by FDG-PET/ CT and 31% only by RAI WBS. The authors concluded that postoperative FDG-PET/CT should be performed routinely in patients with aggressive histology DTC. These results, however, have not been employed in routine clinics yet, but are very important from an individualized monitoring and disease management standpoint.

Other Potential Areas of Management Personalization

Pretherapeutic [124]I PET/CT-based lesional dosimetry, both for remnant and metastases, is based upon the feasibility of estimation of volume and average lesion absorbed dose (AD), which could enhance the practice of individualized radioiodine therapy more succinctly and be undertaken on an individual patient basis.[16,17] There has been also a resurgence of interest in employing FDG-PET as an adjunct for enhancing diagnostic confidence in intermediate-risk category thyroid nodules on the Bethesda Thyroid Cytopathology Reporting System.[18,19] Other radiological modalities such as ultrasonography elastography and DWI-MRI have also been investigated[19] in this area, and it remains to be seen whether a single modality or a combined approach should be used in this case scenario. The authors have not dealt ^{18}F-fluoride bone PET-CT (as the review is restricted to personalized or precision medicine in thyroid carcinoma), but as per the popular experience and literature bone PET/CT is more sensitive and accurate than conventional bone

scintigraphy for the detection of thyroid cancer bone metastasis[20] (Case 7, **Figs. 7** and **8**).

Case 7

In this case, a 55-year-old man initially presented with metastatic deposit of follicular carcinoma in D8 vertebra. He was then diagnosed with widely invasive follicular carcinoma of thyroid. The patient underwent total thyroidectomy in 2011. He received radioiodine in multiple sessions; the last dose of 231 mCi was in 2016. ^{18}F-fluoride PET/CT scan (see **Fig. 7**A) demonstrated tracer avid lytic lesions in vertebrae and tracer uptake in pelvic bones and left femur; the fusion images (see **Fig. 7**B) are clearly superior in demonstrating the lytic lesions compared with the planar bone scintigraphy with ^{99m}Tc-MDP (see **Fig. 7**C).

Learning point The superior resolution of ^{18}F-fluoride PET/CT makes this preferable to conventional skeletal scintigraphy.

MEDULLARY THYROID CARCINOMA
Detecting Recurrent/Metastatic in the Setting of Raised Tumor Markers

FDOPA PET-CT, ^{68}Ga-DOTA-NOC/TATE PET-CT, and FDG-PET/CT all have been used with varying success for investigating the site of recurrence in a patient of MCT with raised tumor markers. The PET-based imaging is sensitive and provides additional information compared with conventional imaging procedures. Similar to patients with TENIS, their use aids in surgical decision making and planning in a more appropriate fashion in an individual.[21]

Fig. 7. [18]F- fluoride PET/CT MIP (*A*), transaxial fused, and CT (*B*) images show tracer avid lytic lesions in the sternum, multiple dorso-lumbar vertebrae, and pubic and left femur bones. [99m]Tc MDP whole-body anterior and posterior images (*C*) show mildly increased tracer uptake in the left femur with no abnormally increased tracer activity elsewhere in skeleton.

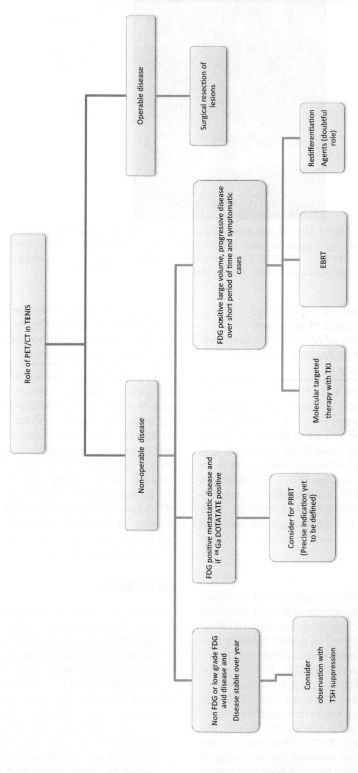

Fig. 8. Flow chart in decision analysis format depicting the potential role of PET/CT in TENIS.

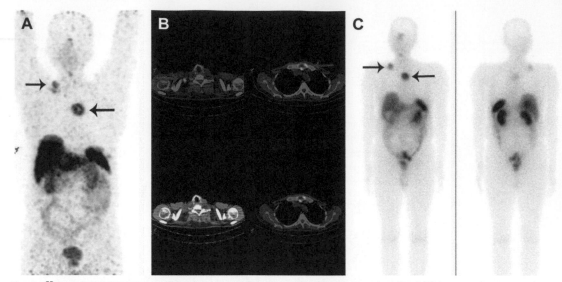

Fig. 9. ^{68}Ga-DOTATATE-PET/CT MIP (*A*), transaxial fused and CT images and sagittal (*B*) images demonstrating somatostatin receptor-avid right supraclavicular lymph nodes and lytic–sclerotic lesion with soft tissue component in the manubrium sternum. ^{177}Lu-DOTATATE post-therapy whole-body anterior and posterior (*C*) images showing tracer uptake in right supraclavicular lymph nodes and manubrium sternal lesion.

^{68}Ga-DOTA-TATE/NOC PET–Computed Tomography in Decision Making and Response Monitoring of Metastatic Medullary Carcinoma Thyroid to Peptide Receptor Radionuclide Therapy

Positive ^{68}Ga-DOTANOC/TATE PET-CT is a prerequisite for considering a patient for somatostatin receptor (SSTR)-targeted PRRT. The SSTR-based PET imaging helps in assessing the tracer avidity on a semiquantitative scale (Krenning score) and thereby helps in individualized clinical decision making in favor of or against PRRT. For treatment response, both FDG (if found positive in baseline scan) and ^{68}Ga-DOTANOC/TATE PET-CT help on an individualized basis and are more sensitive modalities compared with anatomic imaging (Case 8, **Fig. 9**).

Case 8
This was a case of a 65-year-old man with a known case of medullary carcinoma of thyroid, who had undergone total thyroidectomy and right modified neck dissection in 1996. The patient recently presented with sterna swelling and serum calcitonin-1575 pg/mL. ^{68}Ga-DOTATATE PET/CT (see **Fig. 9**A, B) showed tracer-avid right supraclavicular lymph nodes (clinically fixed and hard) and lytic–sclerotic with soft tissue component in manubrium sternum. The patient received ^{177}Lu DOTA-TATE therapy 189 mCi (6993 MBq) recently, and the post-therapy scan showed tracer uptake in the right supraclavicular lymph nodes and manubrium sternum (see **Fig. 9**C).

Immuno-PET Using Anti-Carcino Embryonic Antigen Bispecific Antibody and ^{68}Ga-labeled Peptide for Investigating the Potential of Newer Targeted Therapies

Immuno-PET using anti-carcino embryonic antigen (anti-CEA) bispecific antibody and ^{68}Ga-labeled peptide in metastatic medullary thyroid carcinoma has been recently reported for better identification of patients who could be suitable targets for targeted radionuclide therapies with anti-CEA bispecific antibody. PET-based imaging performs superiorly and provides better contrast compared with ^{111}In or ^{131}I based imaging. This is again an example of PET-based individualized clinical decision making in view of the fact that widely heterogeneous behavior could be encountered in patients with metastatic disease even with same histopathology.

REFERENCES

1. Na SJ, Yoo IeR, O JH, et al. Diagnostic accuracy of (18)F-fluorodeoxyglucose positron emission tomography/computed tomography in differentiated thyroid cancer patients with elevated thyroglobulin and negative (131)I whole body scan: evaluation by thyroglobulin level. Ann Nucl Med 2012;26(1):26–34.
2. Vural GU, Akkas BE, Ercakmak N, et al. Prognostic significance of FDG PET/CT on the follow-up of patients of differentiated thyroid carcinoma with negative 131I whole-body scan and elevated thyroglobulin levels: correlation with clinical and histopathologic characteristics and long-term follow-up data. Clin Nucl Med 2012;37(10):953–9.

3. Ozkan E, Aras G, Kucuk NO. Correlation of 18F-FDG PET/CT findings with histopathological results in differentiated thyroid cancer patients who have increased thyroglobulin or antithyroglobulin antibody levels and negative 131I whole-body scan results. Clin Nucl Med 2013;38(5):326–31.

4. Trybek T, Kowalska A, Lesiak J, et al. The role of 18F-Fluorodeoxyglucose Positron Emission Tomography in patients with suspected recurrence or metastatic differentiated thyroid carcinoma with elevated serum thyroglobulin and negative I-131 whole body scan. Nucl Med Rev Cent East Eur 2014;17(2):87–93.

5. Asa S, Aksoy SY, Vatankulu B, et al. The role of FDG-PET/CT in differentiated thyroid cancer patients with negative iodine-131 whole-body scan and elevated anti-Tg level. Ann Nucl Med 2014;28(10):970–9.

6. Salvatori M, Biondi B, Rufini V. Imaging in endocrinology: 2-[18F]-fluoro-2-deoxy-D-glucose positron emission tomography/computed tomography in differentiated thyroid carcinoma: clinical indications and controversies in diagnosis and follow-up. Eur J Endocrinol 2015;173(3):R115–30.

7. Basu S, Dandekar M, Joshi A, et al. Defining a rational step-care algorithm for managing thyroid carcinoma patients with elevated thyroglobulin and negative on radioiodine scintigraphy (TENIS): considerations and challenges towards developing an appropriate roadmap. Eur J Nucl Med Mol Imaging 2015;42(8):1167–71.

8. Basu S, Parghane RV. Grouping of metastatic thyroid carcinoma by molecular imaging features to allow for individualized treatment, with emphasis on the TENIS syndrome. J Nucl Med Technol 2016;44:184–9.

9. Budiawan H, Salavati A, Kulkarni HR, et al. Peptide receptor radionuclide therapy of treatment-refractory metastatic thyroid cancer using (90)Yttrium and (177)Lutetium labeled somatostatin analogs: toxicity, response and survival analysis. Am J Nucl Med Mol Imaging 2013;4(1):39–52.

10. Czepczyński R, Matysiak-Grześ M, Gryczyńska M, et al. Peptide receptor radionuclide therapy of differentiated thyroid cancer: efficacy and toxicity. Arch Immunol Ther Exp (Warsz) 2015;63(2):147–54.

11. Jois B, Asopa R, Basu S. Somatostatin receptor imaging in non-(131)I-avid metastatic differentiated thyroid carcinoma for determining the feasibility of peptide receptor radionuclide therapy with (177)Lu-DOTATATE: low fraction of patients suitable for peptide receptor radionuclide therapy and evidence of chromogranin A level-positive neuroendocrine differentiation. Clin Nucl Med 2014;39(6):505–10.

12. Masson-Deshayes S, Schvartz C, Dalban C, et al. Prognostic value of (18)F-FDGPET/CT metabolic parameters in metastatic differentiatedthyroidcancers. Clin Nucl Med 2015;40(6):469–75.

13. Yoon S, An YS, Lee SJ, et al. Relation between F-18 FDG uptake ofPET/CT and BRAFV600E mutation in PapillaryThyroid Cancer. Medicine (Baltimore) 2015;94(48):e2063.

14. Ranade R, Kand P, Basu S. Value of 18F-FDG PET negativity and Tg suppressibility as markers of prognosis in patients with elevated Tg and 131I-negative differentiated thyroid carcinoma (TENIS syndrome). Nucl Med Commun 2015;36(10):1014–20.

15. Nascimento C, Borget I, Al Ghuzlan A, et al. Postoperative fluorine-18-fluorodeoxyglucose positron emission tomography/computed tomography: an important imaging modality in patients with aggressive histology of differentiatedthyroid cancer. Thyroid 2015;25(4):437–44.

16. Wierts R, Brans B, Havekes B, et al. Dose-response relationship in differentiated thyroid cancer patients undergoing radioiodine treatment assessed by means of 124I PET/CT. J Nucl Med 2016;57(7):1027–32.

17. Jentzen W, Verschure F, van Zon A, et al. Response assessment of bone metastases from differentiated thyroid Cancer patients in the initial radioiodine treatment using Iodine-124 PET imaging. J Nucl Med 2016 [pii: jnumed.115.170571]. [Epub ahead of print].

18. Buyukdereli G, Aktar Y, Kara E, et al. Role of 18F-fluorodeoxyglucose positron emission tomography/computed tomography in the evaluation of cytologically indeterminate thyroid nodules. Iran J Radiol 2016;13(1):e21186.

19. Basu S, Mahajan A, Arya S. Multimodality molecular imaging (FDG-PET/CT, US Elastography, and DWI-MRI) as complimentary adjunct for enhancing diagnostic confidence in reported intermediate risk category thyroid nodules on Bethesda thyroid Cytopathology reporting System. World J Nucl Med 2016;15(2):130–3.

20. Lee H, Lee WW, Park SY, et al. F-18 Sodium fluoride positron emission tomography/computed tomography for detection of thyroid cancer bone metastasis compared with bone scintigraphy. Korean J Radiol 2016;17(2):281–8.

21. Treglia G, Aktolun C, Chiti A, et al. EANM and the EANM Thyroid Committee. The 2015 Revised American Thyroid Association guidelines for the management of medullarythyroid carcinoma: the "evidence-based" refusal to endorse them by EANM due to the "not evidence-based" marginalization of the role of Nuclear Medicine. Eur J Nucl Med Mol Imaging 2016;43(8):1486–90.

Molecular Imaging and Precision Medicine in Breast Cancer

Amy V. Chudgar, MD[a], David A. Mankoff, MD, PhD[b],*

KEYWORDS

- Breast cancer • Precision medicine • Biomarkers • Fluorodeoxyglucose (FDG)
- 16α-[^{18}F]fluoro-17β-estradiol (FES)

KEY POINTS

- Molecular imaging can serve as a biomarker in breast cancer and provide a complementary, noninvasive global evaluation of the disease process and information to guide treatment.
- Imaging of estrogen, progesterone, and human epidermal growth factor (HER2) receptors may help predict which patients are the most likely to benefit from endocrine or HER2-targeted therapy.
- PET imaging can be used in breast cancer drug development, drug dose optimization, and assessment of early response to therapy.
- Molecular imaging may also provide a key indicator of outcome at later time points in breast cancer treatment.

INTRODUCTION

Breast cancer is the most common malignancy in women, with an estimated 234,000 new cases diagnosed in 2015 and approximately 5% to 9% of patients with metastatic disease at presentation.[1] Biomarkers have become increasingly important in breast cancer treatment for prognosis and for guiding treatment decisions.[2] Precision medicine involves the use of biomarkers to create individualized and targeted treatments.[2] In addition to traditional tissue-based biomarkers, molecular imaging can also serve as a biomarker and provides a complementary, noninvasive global evaluation of the disease process and can provide information to guide treatment, such as prognosis,

drug pharmacodynamics, and response to treatment.

Precision medicine in breast cancer has traditionally been based on results of tissue sampling and assay of the primary breast tumor and metastatic sites, for example, assaying the estrogen receptor (ER) to select patients who may benefit from endocrine therapy.[3] However, there are limitations of biopsy, such as sampling error and invasiveness. Biopsy of the primary neoplasm is not always representative of the entire tumor because of intratumor heterogeneity.[4] Tissue sampling of metastatic lesions is performed when possible, but certain metastatic sites, such as bone and brain, are not always amenable to biopsy, and receptor status is often inferred from the primary

The authors have nothing to disclose.
This work was supported in part by Susan G. Komen SAC130060 and Department of Energy DE-SE0012476 grants.
[a] Division of Nuclear Medicine, Department of Radiology, Hospital of the University of Pennsylvania, University of Pennsylvania, 3400 Spruce Street, Philadelphia, PA 19104, USA; [b] Division of Nuclear Medicine, Department of Radiology, Hospital of the University of Pennsylvania, University of Pennsylvania, Donner 116, 3400 Spruce Street, Philadelphia, PA 19104, USA
* Corresponding author.
E-mail address: david.mankoff@uphs.upenn.edu

tumor. However, receptor status can vary from the primary tumor and metastatic lesions in 25% to 40% of patients.[5] Even when biopsy of metastatic sites is possible, tissue sampling of metastatic lesions is not always representative of the entirety of the disease because of tumor heterogeneity.[4] Monitoring response to targeted treatment to evaluate for changes in the tumor biology would require resampling of primary and metastatic lesions and is invasive and often painful. Furthermore, there are risks associated with biopsy, such as bleeding and infection.

Imaging of biomarkers through PET/computed tomography (CT) offers a complementary, noninvasive method to obtain biological information regarding breast cancer, including tumor burden, tumor metabolic activity, receptor status, and proliferation index. This review focuses on the use of molecular imaging as a biomarker in breast cancer precision medicine, with a focus on (1) imaging as a prognostic biomarker, (2) imaging as a predictive biomarker, (3) imaging to evaluate drug pharmacodynamics, (4) imaging to determine early response to therapy, and (5) imaging to predict biological response (Table 1). Through example of the use of molecular imaging to accomplish each of these tasks, the authors highlight several different PET radiopharmaceuticals used clinically or in clinical trials and describe recent clinical studies that demonstrate the impact and promising future role of imaging in precision medicine.

PROGNOSTIC FACTORS AND BREAST CANCER

Prognostic factors help to distinguish which tumors are most likely to progress to tumor spread and death. Some examples of prognostic factors in breast cancer are ER, progesterone receptor (PR), and human epidermal growth factor type 2 (HER2) receptor status, proliferation index, and Oncotype DX 21-gene panel.[6–8] Most of these prognostic indicators have traditionally been evaluated through tissue assay, typically via immunohistochemistry. An important prognostic factor for breast cancer is the size of the tumor and its extent of spread, that is, staging. As such, imaging serves to help assess breast cancer prognosis by determining the stage of breast cancer. The

Table 1
Sample applications of molecular imaging in breast cancer

	Definition	Sample Applications
Prognostic factors	Indicate which tumors are most likely to progress to tumor spread and death	• FDG-PET/CT for prognostic stratification through staging[10,11] • FDG-PET/CT SUV measurement in primary tumor for histologic grade, triple negative status, proliferation index[11–16]
Predictive factors	Whether treatment is likely to benefit the patient	• FES-PET/CT for evaluation of ER expression to predict response to endocrine therapy[20,22–26] • FFNP-PET/CT for evaluation of PR expression to predict response to endocrine therapy[28–30] • [89]Zr-trastuzumab-PET/CT for HER2 imaging to predict response to trastuzumab-based therapy[41]
Drug binding to target	Evaluates binding of drug to target in the development of new drugs	• FES-PET/CT for evaluation of aromatase inhibitors, tamoxifen, and fulvestrant[45] • FES-PET/CT for optimizing dose of fulvestrant[48] • FES-PET/CT in the evaluation of ARN-810[50] • [89]Zr-trastuzumab-PET/CT in the evaluation of HSP90 inhibitors[52]
Assessment of early response	Indicates some action of the drug on its target and provides an indication of cancer therapy	• FDG-PET/CT showing a "metabolic flare reaction" after treatment with tamoxifen or with estradiol challenge[23,25,53] • FLT-PET/CT for response to chemotherapy and endocrine therapy[58,59]
Biological response	Indicates outcome at later time points in treatment	• FDG-PET/CT to predict outcome is in bone dominant breast cancer[75–78] • FDG-PET/CT in the neoadjuvant setting and post-therapy to predict subsequent relapse and survival[79–82]

National Comprehensive Cancer Network guidelines currently lists fluorodeoxyglucose (FDG)-PET/CT as a consideration in staging clinical stage III or higher breast cancer.[9] FDG-PET/CT has been shown as a tool for prognostic stratification through staging.[10,11] Cochet and colleagues[11] prospectively evaluated 142 patients with at least grade T2 tumor, comparing conventional imaging against FDG-PET/CT and found FDG-PET/CT provided stronger prognostic stratification of progression-free survival compared with conventional imaging ($P<.0001$), and FDG-PET/CT was an independent predictor of recurrence or progression ($P<.001$). Groheux and colleagues[10] showed in a prospective study of 189 patients with clinical stage IIB disease that 47 patients with M1 disease discovered on FDG-PET/CT had statistically significant shorter 3-year disease-specific survival, 57% versus 88% ($P<.001$). In this same group of patients, M1-disease and triple-negative phenotypes were found to be 2 statistically significant independent prognostic variables.[10]

In addition, several studies have also demonstrated that the level of FDG uptake in the primary breast tumor, typically measured as the standardized uptake value (SUV), and in metastases serves as a prognostic factor itself and is indicative of histologic grade, triple negative status, and high proliferation index (Ki-67 expression).[11-16] Although FDG-PET/CT is used for diagnosis and staging, the intensity of FDG uptake on PET/CT in the primary tumor and in metastatic lesions also serves as an important prognostic factor.[11-14] As an analogue of glucose, FDG uptake is a measure of glycolytic rate. Studies using FDG-PET/CT have shown that elevated glycolysis is associated with several aggressive cancer features, such as proliferation and enhanced survival.[17] High FDG uptake in the primary breast tumor has been associated with poor prognostic factors, including high histologic grade, triple negative status, and p53 mutation.[17,18] In the above-mentioned study, Cochet and colleagues[11] found that higher FDG uptake was associated with aggressive features, with a 3:1 ratio of baseline FDG uptake between triple negative and luminal A tumors. Koolen and colleagues[12] found in 203 patients with primary stage II or III breast cancer evaluated with FDG-PET/CT that a higher SUV value was associated with aggressive features, such as distant metastases at time of staging, triple negative tumors, and grade 3 tumors.

Tumor as estimated by tissue sampling and the by Ki-67 immunochemistry index also provides prognostic information. Several studies have demonstrated a correlation between high proliferation index (Ki-67 expression) and higher FDG uptake.[12,15] Furthermore, invasive breast tumors with higher grades demonstrated higher FDG uptake compared with lower-grade tumors.[14,15] Patients with triple negative breast cancer typically have higher FDG avidity.[14,16]

PRECISION MEDICINE AND PREDICTIVE FACTORS

Predictive factors indicate whether a specific treatment is likely to be beneficial to the patient, for example, whether a patient may benefit from endocrine therapy. Predictive biomarkers such as ER, PR, and HER2 based on tissue assays are widely used to direct breast cancer systemic therapy.[4] However, the results may not be reflective of the entire burden of disease due to intratumoral and metastatic heterogeneity. Imaging biomarkers offer an approach that is complementary to tissue sampling to help guide treatment decisions.

Approximately 70% of breast cancers express ERs, and treatment with endocrine therapy has been one of the key factors in improving breast cancer mortality. Endocrine therapy is considered the preferred first-line treatment and is the most effective treatment for metastatic ER+ breast cancer, but only 50% to 75% of ER+ patients with breast cancer will respond to first-line endocrine therapy.[19] Beyond first-line therapy, response to endocrine therapy decreases to 25% due to resistance through various mechanisms.[19]

The PET radiopharmaceutical, 16α-[^{18}F]fluoro-17β-estradiol (FES), an estradiol analogue, is the most researched radioligand for imaging the ER. Measurement of SUV on FES-PET/CT has been shown to correlate with ER expression when compared with immunohistochemistry.[20,21] Several studies have addressed FES as a predictive biomarker. Prior FES studies have shown that FES-PET/CT, using both qualitative and quantitative measures, can identify which patients are most likely to benefit from endocrine therapy.[20,22–24] For example, Dehdashti and colleagues[22] found in 11 patients, a baseline FES SUV in responders was greater than or equal to 2.2 in patients who responded to Tamoxifen therapy at 2 months and less than or equal to 1.7 in the nonresponders. Mortimer and colleagues[25] found in 40 ER+ patients with breast cancer images with FES-PET/CT and FDG-PET/CT before and 7 to 10 days after Tamoxifen therapy; baseline SUV of FES uptake in responders was 4.3 ± 2.4 compared with nonresponders with SUV of 1.8 ± 1.3; $P = .0007$. Linden and colleagues[24] found in 47 pretreated patients with ER+ tumors that 0 of 15 patients with baseline SUV less than

1.5 responded to endocrine therapy versus 11 of 32 patients with SUV greater than 1.5 (*P*<.01) (**Fig. 1**). In assessing studies published across heterogeneous populations, the FES SUV threshold of 1.5 retained predictive value, but with imperfect sensitivity or specificity for predicting response endocrine to therapy.[26] Further studies are necessary to determine the sensitivity and specificity of baseline FES-PET/CT SUV value to predict response to endocrine therapy and identify optimal thresholds. This question is actively being addressed in a phase II trial enrolling patients with ER+ metastatic breast cancer receiving first-line endocrine therapy (NCT02398773).[27]

PR, an estrogen-regulated gene, also serves as a predictive biomarker and is routinely evaluated in immunohistochemical assays. The presence of expression of PR with expression of ER increases the likelihood to respond to endocrine therapy.[7] 21-(^{18}F)F-fluoro-16α,17α-[(R)-(1'-α-furylmethyli-dene)dioxy]-19-norpregn-4-ene-3,20-dione (FFNP) is the radioligand with high affinity and selectivity for the PR and shows the most promise for PR imaging.[28,29] Preclinical breast models have demonstrated decreased uptake of FFNP predicts tumors that will respond to fulvestrant and estrogen-deprivation therapy.[30] Although less research has been performed on FFNP-PET/CT as a predictive biomarker, a current clinical trial (NCT02455453) is addressing this topic.[31] In this trial, FFNP-PET/CT scans are being performed in ER+ postmenopausal patients with breast cancer

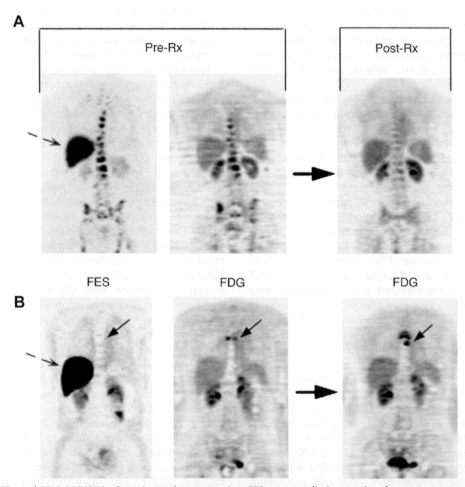

Fig. 1. FES- and FDG-PET/CT in 2 patients demonstrating FES as a predictive marker for response to endocrine therapy (*dashed arrows* show physiologic FES hepatic uptake and *solid arrows* demonstrate osseous metastases). (*A*) Patient with multiple FES- and FDG-avid osseous metastases and posttreatment FDG scan demonstrates a favorable response at 6 months. (*B*) Patient with non-FES avid osseous metastases, which are FDG avid, but does not demonstrate a favorable response to endocrine therapy with progression of hypermetabolic osseous metastases noted on FDG posttreatment scan at 6 months. (*From* Linden HM, Stekhova SA, Link JM, et al. Quantitative fluoroestradiol positron emission tomography imaging predicts response to endocrine treatment in breast cancer. J Clin Oncol 2006;24:2796; with permission.)

before and after the administration of estradiol for 1 day (estrogen challenge) to determine changes in FFNP maximum SUV measurement.

HER2 is overexpressed in approximately 15% to 25% of invasive breast cancer and is associated with aggressive disease.[32–35] HER2 is routinely assayed through immunohistochemistry or fluorescence in situ hybridization to determine which patients may benefit from HER2-directed therapy. However, an estimated 50% of patients with overexpression of HER2 breast cancer do not respond to HER2-directed therapy.[36] The Neoadjuvant Lapatinib and/or Trastuzumab Treatment Optimisation study enrolled 455 women with HER-2-positive breast cancer, of which 77 patients underwent serial FDG-PET/CTs and found that early FDG-PET/CT was able to identify patients more likely to have complete response to neoadjuvant trastuzumab and/or lapatinib with paclitaxel.[37]

Directly imaging HER2 disease has been studied to visualize the tumor burden of HER2+ disease.[38] Several imaging agents have been created to bind to the HER2 receptor, and examples of the positron emitting radionuclides are ^{64}Cu-trastuzumab, ^{64}Cu-DOTA-Z$_{HER2:477}$, ^{68}Ga-trastuzumab F(ab′) b$_2$ fragments, ^{68}Ga-ABY-002, and ^{89}Zr-trastuzumab.[39,40] The ZEPHIR study was the first large prospective trial evaluating ^{89}Zr-trastuzumab-PET/CT (HER2-PET/CT) as a predictive biomarker for advanced HER2+ patients with breast cancer for response to Trastuzumab emtansine, an antibody-drug conjugate to target HER2 receptor in patients who progress after prior line of trastuzumab-based therapy (Fig. 2).[41] They found in 56 patients with advanced HER2-positive breast cancer that pretreatment imaging with HER2-PET/CT and imaging with FDG-PET/CT after 1 month demonstrated a high

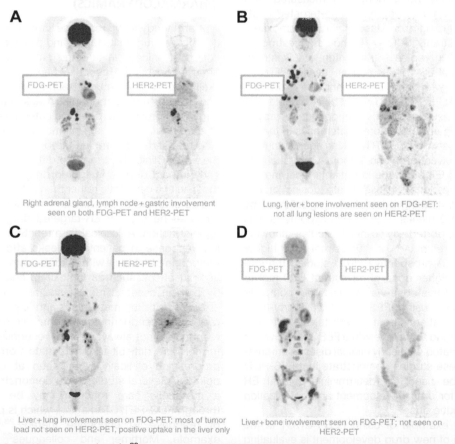

Fig. 2. FDG-PET/CT compared with ^{89}Zr-trastuzumab-PET/CT (HER2-PET/CT) maximum intensity projection (MIP) images in HER2+ patients with breast cancer. (A) Example of similar distribution of metastases on FDG PET and HER2 PET. (B) The dominant portions of the tumor demonstrate uptake on HER2 PET, noting that many of the lung lesions are not seen. (C) Most of the tumor burden does not demonstrate uptake on HER2-PET/CT. (D) None of the tumor demonstrated uptake on the HER2-PET/CT. (From Gebhart G, Lamberts LE, Wimana Z, et al. Molecular imaging as a tool to investigate heterogeneity of advanced HER2-positive breast cancer and to predict patient outcome under trastuzumab emtansine (T-DM1): the ZEPHIR trial. Ann Oncol 2016;27:621; with permission.)

negative predictive value when compared with RECIST1.1 (88%).[41] There are several prospective clinical trials underway to evaluate the clinical utility of HER2 molecular imaging, including 1 study at Institut Jules Bordet (NCT01420146) using [89]Zr-Trastuzumab in HER2+ metastatic breast cancer that correlated to FDG-PET/CT and 2 studies at the University Medical Center Groningen (NCT01832051 and NCT01957332).[42–44]

USING MOLECULAR IMAGING TO EVALUATE DRUG BINDING TO TARGET

Molecular imaging can be used as a tool to evaluate binding of drug to target in the development of new drugs. For example, FES-PET/CT has been shown as an effective tool to assess endocrine therapy on ER binding.[45] A retrospective study of 30 patients with metastatic breast cancer (predominately bone dominant) measured FES uptake before and after endocrine-targeted treatments, including aromatase inhibitors, tamoxifen, and fulvestrant.[45] They found that estrogen-blocking therapies (tamoxifen, fulvestrant) decreased FES binding over serial PET/CTs compared with aromatase inhibitors, demonstrating that FES-PET/CT might be a valuable clinical tool to visualize activity of endocrine therapy.[45] The investigators also noted differences in the ER blockade between the ER blocking agents, tamoxifen and fulvestrant, and hypothesized that the incomplete ER blockade in patients receiving fulvestrant was due to inadequate dosing of this medication (loading dose of 500 mg followed by 250 mg at 2 weeks × 2).[45] This hypothesis was further supported by clinical studies showing increased efficacy of fulvestrant at higher doses.[46,47] A prospective study studied the efficacy of a higher dose of fulvestrant (500 mg) to determine if this dose was sufficient for complete ER blockade using FES-PET/CT.[48] Thirty-eight percent of patients treated with fulvestrant (6 of 16) were found to have residual FES uptake, which was associated with early clinical disease progression.[48] These studies demonstrate that FES-PET/CT can be used for determining optimal ER blockade for drug development and optimization of therapeutic dose.[49]

Another example of using FES-PET/CT in the evaluation of new drug development is evaluating ARN-810, a newer endocrine-directed therapy to treat advanced ER+ breast cancer by blocking and degrading ER.[50,51] A recent multicenter, phase I clinical trial evaluated targeting of ER by ARN-810 in 30 patients with advanced or metastatic ER+ breast cancer. Baseline and subsequent FES PET scans after initiation of ARN-810 demonstrated near complete (>90%) suppression of FES uptake to background levels, indicating successful drug target binding.[50]

HER2 imaging agents have been used in the evaluation of drug binding of HER2-directed therapies.[8] For example, [89]Za-trastuzumab and [89]Zr-bevacizumab PET scans were used for quantitative assessment in the evaluation of NVP-AUY922, a HER2-targeted therapy that inhibits HSP90, a molecular chaperone with client proteins that play a role in metastatic breast cancer through HER2, hypoxia-inducible factor-1α, and ER.[52] [89]Za-trastuzumab PET was found to positively correlate to tumor size after 3 weeks of HSP90 inhibitor treatment, indicating that PET probes such as [89]Za-trastuzumab may be used for evaluation of HER2-targeted therapies.[52]

ASSESSMENT OF EARLY RESPONSE (PHARMACODYNAMICS)

A pharmacodynamic response indicates some action of the drug on its target and provides an indication of efficacy in targeted cancer therapy. A pharmacodynamic response can indicate some likelihood of subsequent response to therapy, and perhaps more importantly, a lack of a pharmacodynamic response often indicates little chance of therapeutic success. Pharmacodynamics may also be used to determine the optimal dosing for therapy.[6] Clinically, it may be difficult to infer the early impact of many targeted drugs, particularly those with a cytostatic rather than cytotoxic effect.

One example of an early pharmacodynamic effect can be seen in ER-targeted drugs with an agonist action. A "clinical flare reaction" is a clinical response in patients 2 weeks after initiating endocrine therapy with drugs with transient agonist effect, such as tamoxifen, characterized by pain in osseous metastases and increase in size of soft tissue metastases and is predictive of response to endocrine treatment.[25] However, this response is not always seen or recognized and is furthermore difficult to differentiate from disease progression clinically when seen at later time points.[23] Several studies have demonstrated that a metabolic flare reaction may be detected through FDG-PET/CT imaging, which is predictive of response to endocrine therapy.[23,25,53] For example, Mortimer and colleagues[25] studied FDG-PET/CT before and after treatment with tamoxifen in postmenopausal ER+ patients with breast cancer and found an increase in tumor FDG uptake after tamoxifen in 20 of 21 responders versus no significant change in tumor FDG uptake in the 19 nonresponders ($P = .0002$). A clinical flare reaction was seen in only 5 of the 21 responders.[25]

Similarly, Dehdashti and colleagues[23] found that a metabolic flare reaction induced by an estradiol challenge could be detected as a significantly higher mean percent change in SUV for responders compared with nonresponders on FDG-PET/CT, and patients with a metabolic flare who were subsequently treated with endocrine therapy had significantly longer overall survival compared with those without a metabolic flare. To further expand on these results, Kurland and colleagues[53] studied the metabolic flare reaction in patients treated with aromatase inhibitors, which decrease circulating estradiol levels, with correlation to proliferation index (Ki-67) assays. They found a decrease in FDG SUV values over a 2-week course of aromatase inhibitor therapy, which corresponded to the lower posttreatment Ki-67.[53] These studies demonstrate that the presence of a metabolic flare response indicates which patients are more likely to respond to endocrine treatment.

Tumor proliferation is most commonly performed by measuring Ki-67 labeling index through immunohistochemistry.[54] 3'Deoxy-3'-^{18}F-fluorothymidine (FLT), a thymidine analogue, is the most widely used proliferation probe that is dependent on the activity of thymidine kinase-1 and correlates with Ki-67 expression.[55–57] An early decline in cellular proliferation assayed by Ki-67 and serial tissue biopsy has been to shown to provide an early indication of successful therapy for both chemotherapy and endocrine therapy, as soon as 1 to 2 weeks after starting treatment.[58,59] Similar findings have been seen using serial FLT-PET/CTs to measure early response to therapy in breast and other cancers.[60,61] A recent multicenter trial performed in the United States has confirmed their early single-center findings (**Fig. 3**).[62]

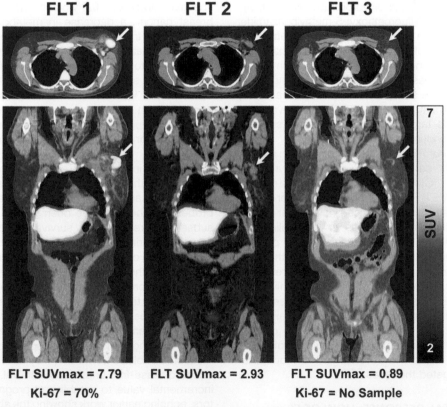

Fig. 3. FLT-PET/CT in a patient undergoing neoadjuvant treatment. The pretherapy scan in column FLT1 (*left*) demonstrates FLT uptake in primary mass in the left breast and left axillary lymph node. Column FLT2 (*middle*) demonstrates decreased tracer uptake after one cycle of neoadjuvant chemotherapy, and column FLT3 (*right*) demonstrates complete metabolic response after completion of neoadjuvant chemotherapy. Pathologic complete response was confirmed surgically (*arrows* indicate site of primary tumor). (*From* Kostakoglu L, Duan F, Idowu MO, et al. A phase II study of 3'-deoxy-3'-18F-fluorothymidine PET in the assessment of early response of breast cancer to neoadjuvant chemotherapy: results from ACRIN 6688. J Nucl Med 2015;56(11):1681–9; with permission.)

FLT PET/CT can also be used to evaluate the pharmacodynamics of drugs impacting components of the thymidine metabolic pathway. For example, *thymidylate synthase (TS)* inhibitor drugs, such as capecitabine, inhibit the de novo thymidine synthesis pathway and have their greatest impact on tumors that rely on this pathway, versus the external (salavage) pathway traced by FLT.[63] Interruption of the de novo pathway by *TS*-targeted drugs can cause a transient increase in thymidine flux through the external pathway, which can be detected by PET proliferation imaging. In a novel study, tumor FLT uptake was found to be increased in patients after treatment with capecitabine, indicating a transient increase in external pathway thymidine flux with *TS* inhibition measured by imaging, and a potential method to measure the pharmacodynamics of *TS* inhibitors.[63]

Another target for imaging proliferation is the sigma-2 receptor, a biomarker of tumor cells that is overexpressed in proliferating tumors.[64–66] The most promising sigma-2 receptor radioligand is N-(4-(6,7-dimethoxy-3,4-dihydroisoquinolin-2(1H)-yl) butyl)-2-(2-(18)F-fluoroethoxy)-5-methylbenzamide, which has been found to correlate with laboratory measures of proliferation status in mouse mammary tumor model and with Ki-67 expression in 13 patients with breast cancer.[67,68] This imaging probe shows promise as a predictive biomarker and may be complementary to FLT-PET/CT in the evaluation of cell cycle–targeted therapies, such as selective cyclin-dependent kinase inhibitors.[69]

Many other PET radiotracers have been studied in breast cancer drug pharmacodynamics, including [11][C]choline and L-methyl-^{11}C-methionine (^{11}C-MET).[54] [11][C]Choline has greater uptake in tumor cells due to increased intracellular choline kinase activity in tumor cells.[54] [11][C]Choline PET uptake decreased over serial scans in patients treated with trastuzumab, indicating that this radiotracer can be used for monitoring response to therapy.[70] L-Methyl-^{11}C-MET is an amino acid used in PET, and a small number of cases were found to have decreased ^{11}C-MET uptake after treatment with endocrine therapy or chemotherapy.[71–73] Numerous others have a potentially important role in the development and optimization of targeted therapies.[7,54]

BIOLOGICAL RESPONSE: HOW DOES IMAGING-BASED RESPONSE PREDICT OUTCOME?

In addition to measuring early response to treatment, molecular imaging may also provide a key indicator of outcome at later time points in breast cancer treatment. Molecular imaging may prove information complementary to size-based measures of response, particularly for disease sites that are difficult to evaluate by anatomic imaging. One primary example of using PET imaging to predict outcome is in bone-dominant breast cancer, a site of disease that has been difficult to evaluate by standard imaging (**Fig. 4**).[74] In bone-dominant metastatic breast cancer, FDG-PET/CT has been established to demonstrate overall time to progression and overall survival.[75–78] In a retrospective study of 253 patients with metastatic breast cancer, there was a strong correlation of maximum SUV of bone metastases on baseline FDG-PET/CT and overall survival.[75] Although not statistically significant, the presence of liver, nodal, and pulmonary metastases were found to have a greater risk of death.[75] A retrospective study of 28 patients undergoing treatment demonstrated that changes in serial FDG-PET/CT scans may predict time to progression and time to first skeletal-related event in bone-dominant metastatic breast cancer.[76] In a retrospective study of 102 women with metastatic breast cancer, a decrease in metabolic activity and increase in CT attenuation of osseous metastases after treatment were found as an independent predictor of response duration.[77] In a retrospective study of 35 patients with 146 identified osseous lesions, FDG uptake was found to correlate with tumor activity independent of the morphologic characteristics.[78] Prospective studies are ongoing to confirm these retrospective studies.

Molecular imaging can also provide a robust indication of the impact of therapy in the neoadjuvant setting, and measures of molecular imaging probes posttherapy have been shown to predict subsequent relapse and survival in several settings. Emmering and colleagues[79] showed that the presence or absence of uptake after neoadjuvant chemotherapy predicted the likelihood of relapse, whereas Dunnwald and colleagues[80] showed that the change in quantitative FDG uptake measures midway through therapy predicted relapse-free and overall survival. Another study by Dunnwald and colleagues[81] also indicated that measures of blood flow from [^{15}O]-water PET predicted disease-free and overall survival, providing incremental value to established prognostic factors, echoing earlier work showing the ability of serial imaging with [^{99m}Tc]-sestamibi to predict similar measures.[82] These examples indicate the ability of molecular imaging to provide biologically based measures of response that are highly predictive of key downstream outcomes such as relapse and survival.

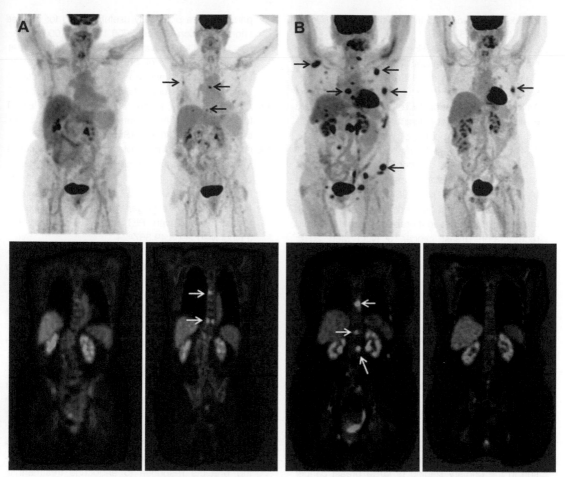

Fig. 4. FDG-PET/CT used for assessing response in 2 patients with osseous-dominant metastatic breast cancer. MIP whole body FDG-PET (*top row*) and fused FDG-PET/CT (*bottom row*). (*A*) Patient on tamoxifen without definite osseous metastases. Follow-up FDG-PET/CT performed 8 months later after switching to aromatase inhibitor (Letrozole) demonstrates new foci of FDG osseous uptake, reflecting progressive metabolic disease (*arrows*). (*B*) Patient with ER + PR+/HER2-metastatic breast cancer with innumerable osseous metastases throughout axial and appendicular skeleton (*arrows*). Follow-up FDG-PET/CT performed after switching treatment to capecitabine demonstrates significant partial metabolic response with near complete resolution of most osseous lesions with a few scattered foci of FDG uptake reflecting residual disease (*arrows*).

SUMMARY

The role of PET in breast cancer continues to evolve with broader applications in diagnostics and therapeutics in patients with metastatic breast cancer. As precision medicine leads to the development of further targeted therapies, PET imaging with new radiotracers provides a complementary and noninvasive method for prognostic and predictive information about tumor burden, tumor metabolic activity, receptor status, and proliferation index. Furthermore, with the development and evolution of targeted treatments, PET imaging offers a method to assess drug binding to the target and optimization of drug dosage and has the potential role for an increasingly important tool in clinical trials. As reviewed, molecular

imaging has shown an important role in the assessment of breast cancer tumor biology, disease burden, and drug development and offers great promise in the future of breast cancer management.

REFERENCES

1. Siegel RL, Miller KD, Jemal A. Cancer statistics, 2015. CA Cancer J Clin 2015;65:5–29.
2. Henry NL, Hayes DF. Cancer biomarkers. Mol Oncol 2012;6:140–6.
3. Hammond MEH, Hayes DF, Wolff AC, et al. American Society of Clinical Oncology/College of American Pathologists guideline recommendations for immunohistochemical testing of estrogen and

progesterone receptors in breast cancer. J Oncol Pract 2010;6:195–7.

4. Gerlinger M, Rowan AJ, Horswell S, et al. Intratumor heterogeneity and branched evolution revealed by multiregion sequencing. N Engl J Med 2012;366:883–92.

5. Amir E, Miller N, Geddie W, et al. Prospective study evaluating the impact of tissue confirmation of metastatic disease in patients with breast cancer. J Clin Oncol 2012;30:587–92.

6. Ulaner GA, Riedl CC, Dickler MN, et al. Molecular imaging of biomarkers in breast cancer. J Nucl Med 2016;57(Suppl 1):53S–9S.

7. Fowler AM, Clark AS, Katzenellenbogen JA, et al. Imaging diagnostic and therapeutic targets: steroid receptors in breast cancer. J Nucl Med 2016;57(Suppl 1):75S–80S.

8. Gebhart G, Flamen P, De Vries EGE, et al. Imaging diagnostic and therapeutic targets: human epidermal growth factor receptor 2. J Nucl Med 2016;57(Suppl 1):81S–8S.

9. Gradishar WJ, Anderson BO, Balassanian R, et al. Invasive Breast Cancer Version 1.2016, NCCN Clinical Practice Guidelines in Oncology. J Natl Compr Canc Netw 2016;14:324–54.

10. Groheux D, Hindié E, Delord M, et al. Prognostic impact of (18)FDG-PET-CT findings in clinical stage III and IIB breast cancer. J Natl Cancer Inst 2012;104(24):1879–87.

11. Cochet A, Dygai-Cochet I, Riedinger JM, et al. ^{18}F-FDG PET/CT provides powerful prognostic stratification in the primary staging of large breast cancer when compared with conventional explorations. Eur J Nucl Med Mol Imaging 2014;41(3):428–37.

12. Koolen BB, Vrancken Peeters MJTFD, Wesseling J, et al. Association of primary tumour FDG uptake with clinical, histopathological and molecular characteristics in breast cancer patients scheduled for neoadjuvant chemotherapy. Eur J Nucl Med Mol Imaging 2012;39:1830–8.

13. Oshida M, Uno K, Suzuki M, et al. Predicting the prognoses of breast carcinoma patients with positron emission tomography using 2-deoxy-2-fluoro [18F]-D-glucose. Cancer 1998;82:2227–34.

14. Groheux D, Giacchetti S, Moretti J-L, et al. Correlation of high 18F-FDG uptake to clinical, pathological and biological prognostic factors in breast cancer. Eur J Nucl Med Mol Imaging 2011;38:426–35.

15. Gil-Rendo A, Martínez-Regueira F, Zornoza G, et al. Association between [18F]fluorodeoxyglucose uptake and prognostic parameters in breast cancer. Br J Surg 2009;96:166–70.

16. Basu S, Chen W, Tchou J, et al. Comparison of triple-negative and estrogen receptor-positive/progesterone receptor-positive/HER2-negative breast carcinoma using quantitative fluorine-18 fluorodeoxyglucose/positron emission tomography imaging parameters: a potentially useful method for disease characterization. Cancer 2008;112:995–1000.

17. Bos R, van Der Hoeven JJM, van Der Wall E, et al. Biologic correlates of (18)fluorodeoxyglucose uptake in human breast cancer measured by positron emission tomography. J Clin Oncol 2002;20:379–87.

18. Avril S, Muzic RF, Plecha D, et al. ^{18}F-FDG PET/CT for monitoring of treatment response in breast cancer. J Nucl Med 2016;57(Suppl 1):34S–9S.

19. Osborne CK, Schiff R. Mechanisms of endocrine resistance in breast cancer. Annu Rev Med 2011;62:233–47.

20. Peterson LM, Mankoff DA, Lawton T, et al. Quantitative imaging of estrogen receptor expression in breast cancer with PET and ^{18}F-fluoroestradiol. J Nucl Med 2008;49:367–74.

21. Mintun MA, Welch MJ, Siegel BA, et al. Breast cancer: PET imaging of estrogen receptors. Radiology 1988;169:45–8.

22. Dehdashti F, Flanagan FL, Mortimer JE, et al. Positron emission tomographic assessment of "metabolic flare" to predict response of metastatic breast cancer to antiestrogen therapy. Eur J Nucl Med 1999;26:51–6.

23. Dehdashti F, Mortimer JE, Trinkaus K, et al. PET-based estradiol challenge as a predictive biomarker of response to endocrine therapy in women with estrogen-receptor-positive breast cancer. Breast Cancer Res Treat 2009;113:509–17.

24. Linden HM, Stekhova SA, Link JM, et al. Quantitative fluoroestradiol positron emission tomography imaging predicts response to endocrine treatment in breast cancer. J Clin Oncol 2006;24:2793–9.

25. Mortimer JE, Dehdashti F, Siegel BA, et al. Metabolic flare: indicator of hormone responsiveness in advanced breast cancer. J Clin Oncol 2001;19:2797–803.

26. van Kruchten M, de Vries EGE, Brown M, et al. PET imaging of oestrogen receptors in patients with breast cancer. Lancet Oncol 2013;14:e465–75.

27. Dehdashti F. [18F]Fluoroestradiol (FES) PET as a predictive measure for endocrine therapy in patients with newly diagnosed metastatic breast cancer. ClinicalTrials.gov [Internet]. Bethesda (MD): National Library of Medicine (US); 2016. Available at: https://clinicaltrials.gov/ct2/show/NCT02398773.

28. Lee JH, Zhou H, Dence CS, et al. Development of [F-18]fluorine-substituted Tanaproget as a progesterone receptor imaging agent for positron emission tomography. Bioconjug Chem 2010;21:1096–104.

29. Dehdashti F, Laforest R, Gao F, et al. Assessment of progesterone receptors in breast carcinoma by PET with 21-^{18}F-fluoro-16α,17α-[(R)-(1'-α-furylmethylidene)dioxy]-19-norpregn-4-ene-3,20-dione. J Nucl Med 2012;53:363–70.

30. Fowler AM, Chan SR, Sharp TL, et al. Small-animal PET of steroid hormone receptors predicts tumor

response to endocrine therapy using a preclinical model of breast cancer. J Nucl Med 2012;53: 1119–26.

31. Dehdashti F. Assessment of functional status of estrogen receptors in breast cancer by positron emission tomography. ClinicalTrials.gov [Internet]. Bethesda (MD): National Library of Medicine (US); 2016. Available at: https://clinicaltrials.gov/ct2/show/NCT02455453.

32. Ross JS, Fletcher JA. The HER-2/neu oncogene in breast cancer: prognostic factor, predictive factor, and target for therapy. Stem Cells 1998;16:413–28.

33. Sjögren S, Inganäs M, Lindgren A, et al. Prognostic and predictive value of c-erbB-2 overexpression in primary breast cancer, alone and in combination with other prognostic markers. J Clin Oncol 1998; 16:462–9.

34. Slamon DJ, Clark GM, Wong SG, et al. Human breast cancer: correlation of relapse and survival with amplification of the HER-2/neu oncogene. Science 1987;235:177–82.

35. Slamon DJ, Godolphin W, Jones LA, et al. Studies of the HER-2/neu proto-oncogene in human breast and ovarian cancer. Science 1989;244:707–12.

36. Slamon DJ, Leyland-Jones B, Shak S, et al. Use of chemotherapy plus a monoclonal antibody against HER2 for metastatic breast Cancer that overexpresses HER2. N Engl J Med 2001;344:783–92.

37. Gebhart G, Gámez C, Holmes E, et al. ^{18}F-FDG PET/CT for early prediction of response to neoadjuvant lapatinib, trastuzumab, and their combination in HER2-positive breast cancer: results from Neo-ALTTO. J Nucl Med 2013;54:1862–8.

38. Potts SJ, Krueger JS, Landis ND, et al. Evaluating tumor heterogeneity in immunohistochemistry-stained breast cancer tissue. Lab Invest 2012;92:1342–57.

39. Mankoff DA, Link JM, Linden HM, et al. Tumor receptor imaging. J Nucl Med 2008;49(Suppl 2): 149S–63S.

40. Linden HM, Dehdashti F. Novel methods and tracers for breast cancer imaging. Semin Nucl Med 2013; 43:324–9.

41. Gebhart G, Lamberts LE, Wimana Z, et al. Molecular imaging as a tool to investigate heterogeneity of advanced HER2-positive breast cancer and to predict patient outcome under trastuzumab emtansine (T-DM1): the ZEPHIR trial. Ann Oncol 2016;27:619–24.

42. Flamen P. Pilot imaging study with [89]Zr-Trastuzumab in HER2-positive metastatic breast cancer patients: correlation with FDG-PET/CT and anatomopathological results. ClinicalTrials.gov [Internet]. Bethesda (MD): National Library of Medicine (US); 2016. Available at: https://clinicaltrials.gov/ct2/show/NCT01420146.

43. Schroder CP. HER2-PET as a diagnostic tool in breast cancer patients with a clinical dilemma.

ClinicalTrials.gov [Internet]. Bethesda (MD): National Library of Medicine (US); 2016. Available at: https://clinicaltrials.gov/ct2/show/NCT01832051.

44. Schroder CP. Towards patient tailored cancer treatment supported by molecular imaging IMPACT: IMaging PAtients for Cancer drug selecTion–metastatic breast cancer. ClinicalTrials.gov [Internet]. Bethesda (MD): National Library of Medicine (US); 2016. Available at: https://clinicaltrials.gov/ct2/show/NCT01957332.

45. Linden HM, Kurland BF, Peterson LM, et al. Fluoroestradiol positron emission tomography reveals differences in pharmacodynamics of aromatase inhibitors, tamoxifen, and fulvestrant in patients with metastatic breast cancer. Clin Cancer Res 2011; 17:4799–805.

46. Robertson JFR, Llombart-Cussac A, Rolski J, et al. Activity of fulvestrant 500 mg versus anastrozole 1 mg as first-line treatment for advanced breast cancer: results from the FIRST study. J Clin Oncol 2009;27:4530–5.

47. Di Leo A, Jerusalem G, Petruzelka L, et al. Results of the CONFIRM phase III trial comparing fulvestrant 250 mg with fulvestrant 500 mg in postmenopausal women with estrogen receptor-positive advanced breast cancer. J Clin Oncol 2010;28: 4594–600.

48. van Kruchten M, de Vries EG, Glaudemans AW, et al. Measuring residual estrogen receptor availability during fulvestrant therapy in patients with metastatic breast cancer. Cancer Discov 2015;5: 72–81.

49. Heidari P, Deng F, Esfahani SA, et al. Pharmacodynamic imaging guides dosing of a selective estrogen receptor degrader. Clin Cancer Res 2015;21: 1340–7.

50. Wang Y, Ulaner G, Manning C, et al. Validation of target engagement using 18F-fluoroestradiol PET in patients undergoing therapy with selective estrogen receptor degrader, ARN-810 (GDC-0810). J Nucl Med 2015;56:565.

51. Lai A, Kahraman M, Govek S, et al. Identification of GDC-0810 (ARN-810), an Orally Bioavailable Selective Estrogen Receptor Degrader (SERD) that demonstrates robust activity in tamoxifen-resistant breast cancer xenografts. J Med Chem 2015;58: 4888–904.

52. Gaykema SBM, Schröder CP, Vitfell-Rasmussen J, et al. 89Zr-trastuzumab and 89Zr-bevacizumab PET to evaluate the effect of the HSP90 inhibitor NVP-AUY922 in metastatic breast cancer patients. Clin Cancer Res 2014;20:3945–54.

53. Kurland BF, Gadi VK, Specht JM, et al. Feasibility study of FDG PET as an indicator of early response to aromatase inhibitors and trastuzumab in a heterogeneous group of breast cancer patients. EJNMMI Res 2012;2:34.

54. Kenny L. The use of novel PET tracers to image breast cancer biologic processes such as proliferation, DNA damage and repair, and angiogenesis. J Nucl Med 2016;57(Suppl 1):89S–95S.

55. Bading JR, Shields AF. Imaging of cell proliferation: status and prospects. J Nucl Med 2008;49(Suppl 2): 64S–80S.

56. Kenny LM, Vigushin DM, Al-Nahhas A, et al. Quantification of cellular proliferation in tumor and normal tissues of patients with breast cancer by [^{18}F] fluorothymidine-positron emission tomography imaging: evaluation of analytical methods. Cancer Res 2005;65:10104–12.

57. Woolf DK, Beresford M, Li SP, et al. Evaluation of FLT-PET-CT as an imaging biomarker of proliferation in primary breast cancer. Br J Cancer 2014;110: 2847–54.

58. Dowsett M, Archer C, Assersohn L, et al. Clinical studies of apoptosis and proliferation in breast cancer. Endocr Relat Cancer 1999;6:25–8.

59. Jones RL, Salter J, A'Hern R, et al. The prognostic significance of Ki67 before and after neoadjuvant chemotherapy in breast cancer. Breast Cancer Res Treat 2009;116:53–68.

60. Kenny L, Coombes RC, Vigushin DM, et al. Imaging early changes in proliferation at 1 week post chemotherapy: a pilot study in breast cancer patients with 3'-deoxy-3'-[^{18}F]fluorothymidine positron emission tomography. Eur J Nucl Med Mol Imaging 2007;34: 1339–47.

61. Contractor KB, Kenny LM, Stebbing J, et al. [18F]-3'Deoxy-3'-fluorothymidine positron emission tomography and breast cancer response to docetaxel. Clin Cancer Res 2011;17:7664–72.

62. Kostakoglu L, Duan F, Idowu MO, et al. A phase II study of 3'-deoxy-3'-18F-fluorothymidine PET in the assessment of early response of breast cancer to neoadjuvant chemotherapy: results from ACRIN 6688. J Nucl Med 2015;56:1681–9.

63. Kenny LM, Contractor KB, Stebbing J, et al. Altered tissue 3'-deoxy-3'-[18F]fluorothymidine pharmacokinetics in human breast cancer following capecitabine treatment detected by positron emission tomography. Clin Cancer Res 2009;15:6649–57.

64. Wheeler KT, Wang LM, Wallen CA, et al. Sigma-2 receptors as a biomarker of proliferation in solid tumours. Br J Cancer 2000;82:1223–32.

65. Mach RH, Smith CR, Al-Nabulsi I, et al. Sigma 2 receptors as potential biomarkers of proliferation in breast cancer. Cancer Res 1997;57:156–61.

66. Vilner BJ, John CS, Bowen WD. Sigma-1 and sigma-2 receptors are expressed in a wide variety of human and rodent tumor cell lines. Cancer Res 1995; 55:408–13.

67. Dehdashti F, Laforest R, Gao F, et al. Assessment of cellular proliferation in tumors by PET using ^{18}F-ISO-1. J Nucl Med 2013;54:350–7.

68. Shoghi KI, Xu J, Su Y, et al. Quantitative receptor-based imaging of tumor proliferation with the sigma-2 ligand [(18)F]ISO-1. PLoS One 2013;8: e74188.

69. McDonald ES, Mankoff DA, Mach RH. Novel strategies for breast cancer imaging: new imaging agents to guide treatment. J Nucl Med 2016;57(Suppl 1): 69S–74S.

70. Kenny LM, Contractor KB, Hinz R, et al. Reproducibility of [11C]choline-positron emission tomography and effect of trastuzumab. Clin Cancer Res 2010;16: 4236–45.

71. Huovinen R, Leskinen-Kallio S, Någren K, et al. Carbon-11-methionine and PET in evaluation of treatment response of breast cancer. Br J Cancer 1993;67:787–91.

72. Jansson T, Westlin JE, Ahlström H, et al. Positron emission tomography studies in patients with locally advanced and/or metastatic breast cancer: a method for early therapy evaluation? J Clin Oncol 1995;13:1470–7.

73. Lindholm P, Lapela M, Någren K, et al. Preliminary study of carbon-11 methionine PET in the evaluation of early response to therapy in advanced breast cancer. Nucl Med Commun 2009;30:30–6.

74. Hamaoka T, Madewell JE, Podoloff DA, et al. Bone imaging in metastatic breast cancer. J Clin Oncol 2004;22:2942–53.

75. Morris PG, Ulaner GA, Eaton A, et al. Standardized uptake value by positron emission tomography/ computed tomography as a prognostic variable in metastatic breast cancer. Cancer 2012;118: 5454–62.

76. Specht JM, Tam SL, Kurland BF, et al. Serial 2-[^{18}F] fluoro-2-deoxy-D-glucose positron emission tomography (FDG-PET) to monitor treatment of bone-dominant metastatic breast cancer predicts time to progression (TTP). Breast Cancer Res Treat 2007; 105:87–94.

77. Tateishi U, Gamez C, Dawood S, et al. Bone metastases in patients with metastatic breast cancer: morphologic and metabolic monitoring of response to systemic therapy with integrated PET/CT. Radiology 2008;247:189–96.

78. Du Y, Cullum I, Illidge TM, et al. Fusion of metabolic function and morphology: sequential [^{18}F]fluoro-deoxyglucose positron-emission tomography/ computed tomography studies yield new insights into the natural history of bone metastases in breast cancer. J Clin Oncol 2007;25:3440–7.

79. Emmering J, Krak NC, Van der Hoeven JJM, et al. Preoperative [^{18}F] FDG-PET after chemotherapy in locally advanced breast cancer: prognostic value as compared with histopathology. Ann Oncol 2008; 19:1573–7.

80. Dunnwald LK, Doot RK, Specht JM, et al. PET tumor metabolism in locally advanced breast cancer

patients undergoing neoadjuvant chemotherapy: value of static versus kinetic measures of fluoro-deoxyglucose uptake. Clin Cancer Res 2011;17: 2400–9.

81. Dunnwald LK, Gralow JR, Ellis GK, et al. Tumor metabolism and blood flow changes by positron emission tomography: relation to survival in patients treated with neoadjuvant chemotherapy for locally advanced breast cancer. J Clin Oncol 2008;26: 4449–57.

82. Dunnwald LK, Gralow JR, Ellis GK, et al. Residual tumor uptake of [^{99m}Tc]-sestamibi after neoadjuvant chemotherapy for locally advanced breast carcinoma predicts survival. Cancer 2005;103:680–8.

Molecular Imaging and Precision Medicine in Lung Cancer

Katherine A. Zukotynski, MD, FRCPC[a,b],
Victor H. Gerbaudo, PhD, MSHCA[c,*]

KEYWORDS

- Lung cancer • Positron emission tomography • Solitary pulmonary nodule • Cancer staging
- Precision medicine • Targeted cancer therapy

KEY POINTS

- PET is essential to accurately stage patients with potentially curable lung cancer.
- PET plays a central role in precision medicine by helping to noninvasively assess molecular pathobiology and genetic make-up of disease so that appropriate therapy is selected and started.
- PET is key for subsequent treatment strategy of patients with lung cancer, including monitoring of therapy response, detection of recurrence, and prediction of patient outcomes.

PRECISION MEDICINE AND LUNG CANCER

Lung cancer is the second most commonly diagnosed malignancy in men and women, estimated to account for approximately 224,390 new cases and 158,080 deaths in 2016 according to the American Cancer Society.[1] Although localized disease may be curable, metastatic lung cancer is the leading cause of cancer-related death. Indeed, it is estimated that one out of four cancer-related deaths are related to manifestations of metastatic lung cancer.[1]

Lung cancer is heterogeneous morphologically and functionally. Furthermore, the genetic profile of the disease evolves with time leading to the development of resistance. Over the past few years, an emerging suite of therapy has become available to treat patients with lung cancer including targeted surgery, radiotherapy, chemotherapy, and immunotherapy. Although historically

the decision-making tools needed to determine appropriate treatment have been elusive, anatomic and metabolic imaging have come to play an important role in evaluating disease extent and biologic behavior, and in monitoring therapy response. Indeed, advances in the understanding of genetic underpinnings and imaging appearance of lung cancer has led to the potential for personalized medicine,[2] identifying a priori the most effective therapy for a specific patient to maximize benefit while limiting futile, toxic treatment.

Positron emission tomography/computed tomography (PET/CT) contributes to precision medicine by interrogating tumor heterogeneity throughout the body. As such, it is extremely helpful, not only to distinguish resectable from nonresectable disease, but also to suggest the most appropriate therapy at a metabolic-molecular level. Furthermore, PET/CT can provide predictive

The authors have nothing to disclose.
a Division of Nuclear Medicine and Molecular Imaging, Department of Medicine, McMaster University, 1200 Main Street West, Hamilton, Ontario L9G 4X5, Canada; b Division of Nuclear Medicine and Molecular Imaging, Department of Radiology, McMaster University, 1200 Main Street West, Hamilton, Ontario L9G 4X5, Canada; c Division of Nuclear Medicine and Molecular Imaging, Department of Radiology, Brigham and Women's Hospital, Harvard Medical School, 75 Francis Street, Boston, MA 02115, USA
* Corresponding author.
E-mail address: gerbaudo@bwh.harvard.edu

PET Clin 12 (2017) 53–62
http://dx.doi.org/10.1016/j.cpet.2016.08.008
1556-8598/17/Crown Copyright © 2016 Published by Elsevier Inc. All rights reserved.

and prognostic insight into therapy response and can identify sites of disease that are developing resistance such that treatment can be modified at an early time point. Thus, the strength of PET/CT lies in its ability to noninvasively evaluate in vivo tumor heterogeneity over time and space.

PET/CT plays an important role in the precision treatment algorithm of patients with lung cancer at the time of initial staging and for subsequent treatment strategy. There are several PET radiotracers, the most common of which is ^{18}F-labeled 2-fluoro-2-deoxy-D-glucose (FDG), a glucose analogue. Because neoplastic cells demonstrate increased glucose metabolism compared with normal tissue,[3,4] FDG-PET/CT is commonly used to detect tumor glucose metabolism throughout the body. Furthermore, because changes in glucose metabolism may precede changes in anatomy, FDG-PET/CT is extremely helpful to monitor early therapy response. It is important to recall that the intensity of FDG uptake depends on several factors including cellular histology, density, aggressiveness, and technical parameters among others. As such, PET/CT should be performed using standardized technical parameters, and images should be evaluated in the correct clinical context. Additional PET/CT radiotracers that may benefit patients with lung cancer and soon should prove to play a significant role in the precision medicine of patients with lung neoplasia include 3'-deoxy-3'-[18F] fluorothymidine (FLT), [18F] fluoromisonidazole 1-(2-nitroimidazolyl)-2-hydroxy-3-fluoropropane (FMISO), [18F] fluoroazomycin arabinofuranoside (FAZA), O-[18F] fluoromethyl-L-tyrosine (FMT), and O-(2-[18F] fluoroethyl)-L-tyrosine (FET) among others. Through the use of these different PET probes, the regional heterogeneous signature of the disease, including differences in cellular proliferation, hypoxia, amino acid transport, and receptor expression, can be studied.[5]

PET/CT IMAGING IN INITIAL STAGING OF THE PATIENT WITH LUNG CANCER

FDG-PET/CT is helpful to (1) characterize a morphologically indeterminate solitary pulmonary nodule (SPN); (2) guide biopsy to the site of most aggressive, intensely FDG-avid, disease; and (3) evaluate disease extent including primary disease, lymph nodes, and distant metastases.

An SPN is a common incidental finding on anatomic imaging done as a part of clinical practice.[6] The differential diagnoses are numerous and include benign and malignant causes, such as infection, inflammation, and lung cancer. FDG-PET/CT has a high sensitivity and specificity to characterize an SPN as malignant, and a high negative predictive value to exclude malignancy, particularly in nodules greater than 8 mm in size.[7-10] However, FDG uptake by an SPN does not always imply malignancy and the standardized uptake value (SUV) should not be relied on to characterize a nodule as benign or malignant. Indeed, certain primary lung malignancies, such as adenocarcinoma in situ, carcinoid, and rarely well-differentiated adenocarcinoma, may have little to no apparent metabolic activity on FDG-PET/CT. Also benign processes, such as pneumonia, tuberculosis, fungal infections, and sarcoidosis, may be highly FDG-avid. Therefore, in patients with an indeterminate SPN on CT, a low probability of lung cancer, and a non-FDG-avid SPN on PET, observation may be entertained. However, in patients with an indeterminate SPN on CT and an FDG-avid SPN on PET, histopathologic evaluation is suggested with surgical resection if this is the only site of malignant disease. The Society of Nuclear Medicine and Molecular Imaging recommends FDG-PET/CT for patients with an SPN to (1) detect potential malignant lesions early in the course of disease, (2) exclude malignancy in indeterminate lesions in low-risk patients, and (3) improve health care outcomes by avoiding futile surgery in low-risk patients and enabling curative surgery in high-risk patients.[11]

PET/CT plays a crucial role in lung cancer staging, particularly where there is curative treatment intent. Evaluation of disease extent is critical to determine appropriate therapy and prognosis of patients with lung cancer. Limited disease may be amenable to surgical resection, whereas delineation of tumor margins is needed for effective radiation treatment planning. Indeed, the 5-year overall survival for patients with lung cancer localized to a small pulmonary nodule postsurgery may be higher than 90%,[12,13] whereas survival is dismal for patients with distant metastases. CT is the preferred modality to evaluate lesion size, location, and invasion of adjacent structures, whereas PET provides complementary metabolic information.

The advent of hybrid PET/CT scanners has overcome many of the limitations of anatomic imaging alone.[14-17] For staging the site of primary disease (T status), PET/CT can help pinpoint metabolically active malignant disease and distinguish this from an adjacent benign process, such as atelectasis.[16] For evaluating spread of malignant disease to lymph nodes (N status), PET/CT is complementary to mediastinoscopy. The principal strengths of PET in this setting include detection of malignant cells within lymph nodes that appear morphologically normal, and evaluation of the entire mediastinum. Indeed, it is estimated that PET/CT changes N stage in up to 20% of cases compared with CT alone.[18,19] However, it is important to recall that PET may be falsely positive in patients with benign conditions, such as infection or inflammation. Furthermore, PET may be falsely negative in the setting of micrometastases or nodal disease spread when the avidity of the primary site of disease is low.[20–23] Thus, although PET/CT is suggested for staging patients who are surgical candidates, mediastinoscopy is recommended to confirm the results of a positive or negative PET/CT study.[24] One of the true strengths of PET/CT lies in its ability to detect distant metastases (M status). It is estimated that more than 60% of adenocarcinoma metastases are CT occult,[25] with an 8% incidence of occult metastases for clinical stage I disease, and up to 24% incidence for stage III disease.[26] The sensitivity, specificity, and accuracy of PET/CT for detecting systemic metastases exceed 90%.[27] PET/CT is superior to skeletal scintigraphy for the detection of osseous metastases and superior to CT for the detection of liver metastases.[28,29] Of note, tissue sampling confirmation should be considered if a false-positive PET/CT finding could have a deleterious effect on therapy.[20,30] Also, MR imaging is the imaging modality of choice to identify cerebral metastases. To date, hybrid PET/MR imaging versus PET/CT scanners have shown similar results for lung cancer staging.[31] Regardless of whether a PET/CT or PET/MR imaging scanner is used, PET plays an important role in staging patients with lung cancer with a significant impact on precision management including therapy intent (ie, cure vs palliation) and treatment selection (ie, surgery vs radiation).

PET-BASED MOLECULAR IMAGING AND PRECISION MEDICINE IN THE SUBSEQUENT TREATMENT STRATEGY OF THE PATIENT WITH LUNG CANCER

Precision medicine aims to classify patients into subgroups by integrating molecular pathobiology and genetic make-up of disease with clinical manifestations to diagnose, stage, predict treatment response, and suggest patient outcome.[32] Once those who will benefit are identified, tailored "preventive or therapeutic interventions" can be used to avoid the expense and toxicity of futile treatment given to those who will not respond. The ultimate goal is to offer the right treatment, to the right patient, at the right time. Thus, medical imaging in general, and molecular imaging in particular, contribute to precision medicine by helping select

the correct treatment based on the observed extent of disease, by monitoring response to the said treatment, and by prognosticating outcomes based on the presence of specific image signatures.

It is already well accepted that the role of PET-based molecular imaging in precision medicine of patients with lung cancer rests on its value as a predictive biomarker of early response to cytotoxic and cytostatic treatments, to radiotherapy, and to image-guided interventions. However, it is also a biomarker of prognosis of patients with lung cancer. These biomarker attributes contribute to precision medicine by influencing the decision to treat, and the type and intensity of treatment to be used. Being able to assess tumoral response to treatment early and accurately is a critical step in the precision medicine of the patient with lung cancer. This allows clinicians to discontinue treatment when it is not working, adjust the treatment algorithm, or consider second-line therapeutics options.

PET AS A PREDICTIVE BIOMARKER OF RESPONSE TO LUNG CANCER THERAPY

Limitations and pitfalls of morphologic imaging criteria (ie, World Health Organization, Response Evaluation Criteria in Solid Tumours [RECIST]) to assess tumor response or progression after therapy have become evident over the years. Some of these shortcomings are related to issues of reproducibility and that results do not correlate with patient outcomes in certain tumor types. Other limitations are therapy specific, because morphologic response criteria were designed to monitor the cytolytic effect of therapy, in which clinical efficacy for the most part translates into a reduction in tumor mass. Targeted therapy, however, is cytostatic, slowing and halting tumor cell proliferation. Thus, the clinical introduction of these targeted therapies has challenged the follow-up paradigm of patients with lung cancer, supporting the clinical need to personalize tumor response assessment to therapy.[33]

Wahl and colleagues[34] recently proposed a new hybrid, anatomomolecular imaging-based response criteria (ie, PET Response Criteria in Solid Tumors) that combines the tumoral morphologic phenotype of response (RECIST) with its metabolic appearance (PET) to monitor response to treatment. So far, the preliminary evidence arising from recently published reports is promising, and shows that this approach might be more appropriate and consistent to better predict response to cancer treatment in a variety of cancers types, including lung cancer. Further validation of these criteria is necessary for specific cancer types and treatment algorithms.

The reported clinical superiority of FDG-PET as a predictive biomarker of lung cancer response to cytotoxic chemotherapy and more recently to cytostatic targeted therapies is based in part on the fact that metabolic and pathophysiologic changes often precede alterations in lesion morphology.[35] Therefore, it is safe to say that PET-based molecular imaging tends to predict response to treatment earlier than do morphologic imaging modalities (ie, CT and MR imaging). In general, the data show that the earlier the response the better the progression-free and overall survival of the patient with cancer. In most cases the PET phenotype of response can predict patient outcome as early as after a couple courses of neoadjuvant chemotherapy.[36,37]

Assessment of Response to Cytotoxic Cancer Therapy and to Radiotherapy

The reliability of PET to assess response during and after cytotoxic chemotherapy and radiotherapy is well documented. Some of the seminal publications that constitute a good representative excerpt of today's literature on the topic are reviewed next. Although there is no consensus as to what is the optimal cutoff in reduction of FDG uptake to define response, the findings described in the literature concur with those observed in daily clinical practice when imaging patients with cancer with FDG-PET to monitor response to therapy.

In a study by Weber and colleagues[36] of 57 patients with stage IIIB and IV non–small cell lung cancer (NSCLC) that underwent FDG-PET before and after one cycle of platinum-based chemotherapy, a reduction in tumor FDG uptake of more than 20% was predictive of long-term survival (252 days for metabolic responders vs 151 days for nonresponders). Vansteenkiste and coworkers[35] published similar observations using FDG-PET to monitor response after three cycles of neoadjuvant chemotherapy in stage IIIA-N2 patients with NSCLC. Longer survival was observed in those patients whose primary tumor uptake decreased by more than 50%. Hoekstra and colleagues[38] confirmed the findings reported by the previous groups in a prospective study of 47 patients with NSCLC with stage IIIA-N2. In their study, prolonged overall survival correlated with a 35% reduction in tumor FDG uptake after one cycle of induction therapy. Eschmann and coworkers[39] studied 70 patients with stage III NSCLC before and at the conclusion of neoadjuvant radiochemotherapy.

The investigators reported a sensitivity of 94.5%, a specificity of 80%, and overall accuracy of 91% of FDG-PET for the detection of residual viable primary tumor following therapy; and a sensitivity, specificity, and accuracy of 77%, 68%, and 73%, respectively, for the detection of lymph node metastases. A negative PET scan or a reduction in the SUV of more than 80% at the end of therapy was consistent with better prognosis in their patient population. In a study of 30 patients with stage IIIA-N2 NSCLC, Dooms and colleagues[40] showed that after treatment completion, significantly longer 5-year overall survival (62%) and benefit from subsequent surgical intervention were achieved following a reduction of 60% in primary tumor uptake and persistent minor FDG avidity in mediastinal nodes. The authors underscored that persistent significant mediastinal uptake at the end of treatment was consistent with a poor 5-year overall survival rate (0%), indicating that these patients should not be considered for surgery.

FDG-PET has also been used to monitor response to radiotherapy in patients with lung cancer. Mac Manus and colleagues[41] showed that tumor metabolic response predicts outcome following radiation therapy. The investigators studied 88 patients treated with concurrent platinum-based radical chemoradiotherapy (n = 73) and radical radiotherapy alone (n = 15), who underwent baseline and posttreatment (median, 70 days) FDG-PET. Complete metabolic responders had a 1-year survival rate of 93% compared with 47% for nonresponders, and 2-year survival rate of 62% versus 30%, respectively.

The recommendation has always been to image patients 3 to 4 months after radiotherapy to minimize false-positive FDG uptake in radiation-induced inflammation. However, Hicks and coinvestigators showed that radiation-induced inflammation after radical radiotherapy does not interfere with the assessment of therapeutic response during FDG-PET if acquired at a median of 70 days after completion of treatment.[42]

Assessment of Response to Cytostatic Cancer Therapy

Twelve years ago, Paez and colleagues[43] and Lynch and coworkers[44] demonstrated that treatment of lung tumors expressing somatic mutations of the epidermal growth factor receptor gene with tyrosine kinase inhibitors (TKI) arrested tumor growth. These targeted therapies (eg, erlotinib, gefitinib, afatinib, and crizotinib) brought to the clinic a new armamentarium of biomarker-directed precision treatments for the patient with lung cancer.

This discovery raised new precision medicine–based challenges for the conventional and the molecular imaging communities when attempting to assess response to treatment in these patients. Reduction in tumor size is not always consistent with cytostatic treatment efficacy and therefore, the use of RECIST or World Health Organization criteria to monitor response may result in underestimation of the effectiveness of these drugs. Thus, the PET-based molecular imaging community anticipated that its imaging tool would be more appropriate to monitor the effect of targeted therapies in patients with lung cancer. However, new challenges had to be faced, such as defining the ideal timing of PET during and after targeted therapy, and what should be considered a significant reduction in radiopharmaceutical uptake to be consistent with successful response to therapy. Several studies have been carried out to answer these questions, and to evaluate the role of FDG- and FLT-PET as biomarkers of early lung cancer response to TKIs, such as erlotinib and gefitinib.[45–55]

The first FDG-PET studies showed that successful response to erlotinib and gefitinib can be predicted 2 days after the start of therapy.[45,46] Subsequent studies also demonstrated that early and accurate prediction of response is possible when imaging at 1, 2, and 3 weeks after treatment, as confirmed by conventional imaging and clinical evaluation 4 to 6 weeks later.[47–50]

Five different studies yielded similar results with FLT-PET. A reduction in primary lung tumor FLT uptake at 2 days, 1 week, and 3 weeks during treatment successfully predicted tumoral response after 6 weeks of TKI therapy.[51–55]

Although FDG and FLT uptake in the primary lung lesion tends to increase significantly in nonresponding patients, the most important message is that earlier and larger reductions in radiotracer uptake as a function of TKI treatment are consistent with longer survival and better quality of life for these patients.[45–55]

PET AS A BIOMARKER OF PROGNOSIS IN LUNG CANCER

Several studies have been conducted to determine the prognostic value of FDG-PET in lung cancer. Understanding the prognostic value of FDG metabolism in these lesions facilitates the identification of patients at high risk of early disease progression irrespective of their clinical stage at diagnosis. This information can then be used early during the clinical management of the patient with lung cancer to personalize postsurgical therapy in those with early stage disease, but highly metabolically active tumors.

The prognostic value of different PET signatures in lung cancer has been tested and similar results have been reported in the literature by different investigators. Examples of these image signatures are the intensity of tumor metabolic activity in terms of SUV, metabolically active tumor bulk as defined by indices of metabolic volumes and total lesion glycolysis (TLG), tumoral metabolic heterogeneity estimated through texture analysis, and the prognostic value of the reduction in FDG uptake during and at the completion of treatment (discussed previously).

Tumor Uptake

High intensity of FDG uptake is associated with tumor aggressiveness and is considered a prognostic imaging biomarker in lung cancer.[56] Despite the lack of agreement on optimal SUV cutoff, the evidence shows that a high tumor SUV is consistently associated with poor prognosis across different stages and histologic types of lung cancer.[56]

The role of FDG-PET as biomarker of patient outcomes centers on the early prediction of progression-free and overall survival. The hallmark of the PET image phenotype of metabolic aggressiveness in the personalized care of the patient with lung cancer rests on the accurate selection of those at high risk of disease progression, independent of the morphologic extent of disease at diagnosis. Furthermore, the metabolic patterns of aggressive lesions have been used to stratify patients with lung cancer into subpopulations with different prognoses. The latter is accomplished by correlating FDG patterns and intensities of tumor uptake with protein expression. In a radiogenomics validation study to understand tumor metabolism, Nair and colleagues[57] correlated tumor FDG avidity with nuclear factor kappa-light-chain-enhancer of activated B cells (NK-κBp65) expression and prognosis in patients with lung cancer. NK-κBp65 controls DNA transcription, cytokine production, and tumor cell survival. When NK-κB is deregulated in lung cancers, it becomes constitutively active, leading to tumor cell proliferation and inhibition of apoptosis. In 365 NSCLCs from 355 patients the investigators reported that when higher tumor SUV was coupled with high NK-κBp65 expression, patients had more extensive disease, tumor invasion, and worse prognosis.

Ahuja and colleagues[58] in 1998 showed that a primary lung tumor SUV greater than 10 was an independent predictor of overall survival. Since then many studies have confirmed a correlation between outcomes and the intensity of tumor FDG uptake in patients with early and advanced stage NSCLC.

Ohtsuka and colleagues[59] reported shorter progression-free survival and thus a higher rate of recurrence in patients with stage IA and IB, moderately or poorly differentiated lung adenocarcinomas, with a primary SUVmax greater than or equal to 3.3. Based on the results of their study in 98 patients, the authors recommended that in early stage disease the intensity of tumor uptake could be used to predict who will benefit from postsurgical adjuvant chemotherapy. Two years later, Goodgame and colleagues[60] reported similar results in a study of 136 patients with stage I NSCLC. The authors found significantly worse 5-year progression-free and overall survival rates in patients with a tumor SUV greater than 5.5 and indicated that the high intensity of tumor uptake was an independent predictor of recurrence in multivariate analysis. The same year, Hanin and coworkers[61] published their results of a study of 96 patients with stage I and II NSCLC interrogating the prognostic value of tumor FDG uptake in early stage disease. The median SUVmax in the study cohort was 7.8. Both, the overall and progression-free survival were significantly longer in patients with an SUVmax less than or equal to 7.8 (127 months vs 69 months [P = .001] and 96.1 months vs 87.7 months [P = .01], respectively).[61]

The findings of Cerfolio and colleagues[62] concurred with the results of the preceding studies, yet they took their analysis one step further. They analyzed progression-free survival within each stage (I through III) as a function of high and low SUV. They concluded that a higher primary tumor SUV within the same stage predicted progression of disease and a shorter overall survival. The 4-year survival for stage IB patients with low and high SUV was 80% and 66%, respectively; 64% versus 32% for stage II disease, and 64% versus 16% for stage IIIA patients, respectively.

Similar results have been published interrogating the association between tumor SUV and survival in high-stage disease. Decoster and coworkers[63] reported the results of a phase II study of 31 patients with nonsurgical stage III lung cancer treated with three cycles of neoadjuvant chemotherapy followed by radiotherapy. The patients underwent FDG-PET at baseline and after chemotherapy. PET noncomplete responders, defined as having a tumor SUV greater than 2.5 after therapy, had significantly shorter progression-free (9.8 months) and overall survival (14.4 months) than the PET complete responders (19.9 months and 49 months, respectively).[63]

A recent trial of the National Cancer Institute–funded American College of Radiology Imaging Network/Radiation Therapy Oncology Group cooperative group (ACRIN 6668/RTOG 0235) studied the relationship between tumor SUV and survival in 253 stage III patients with NSCLC.[64] FDG-PET was obtained before and at 14 weeks of concurrent platinum-based chemoradiotherapy. The study found higher posttreatment SUVpeak and SUVmax to be associated with poor survival (hazard ratio, 1.087; 95% confidence interval, 1.014–1.166; P = .02); however, the investigators could not find a specific prognostic SUV cutoff that could be recommended for daily clinical use.

Metabolically Active Tumor Bulk

Tumor bulk has been described as a prognostic indicator in different tumor types, including lung and pleural malignancies, and it is always taken into consideration by the clinical team when making treatment decisions.[65]

Two volumetric indices of metabolic activity may be derived from PET images. The first is the metabolic tumor volume (MTV), which corresponds to the metabolically active tumor mass, and is estimated by using semiautomatic tumor-contouring software with a predefined SUV as the threshold to segment metabolic tumor boundaries. The second index is the TLG, which is calculated by multiplying the tumor's mean SUV by the MTV. By summing the values for each lesion in the body, whole-body MTV and TLG are obtained. The rationale behind using the MTV and TLG are that they provide three-dimensional measurements of total tumor volume and metabolic activity, they reflect changes throughout the tumor, and may be more sensitive than a single-pixel-derived SUV.[65]

Recent preliminary data from patients with lung cancer imaged with FDG-PET suggest that pretreatment metabolically active tumor volumes may play a role as biomarkers of prognosis.[56,66–71] Specifically, these studies evaluated the primary lesion and the whole-body metabolic tumor burden, and found that these indices may be independent predictors of survival in patients with early and advanced-stage lung cancer.[56,69–71] Some studies suggested that SUVmax and SUVmean may be inferior to pretreatment MTV as predictors of overall and progression-free survival.[72] Large prospective multicenter studies are called for to confirm these findings, instruct clinicians on how they should be used in daily clinical practice, and elucidate their contribution to precision medicine for the patient with lung cancer.

Tumoral Metabolic Heterogeneity

Intratumoral heterogeneity is considered a driver of tumor aggressiveness, resistance to treatment, and poor progression-free and overall survival.[73]

Recent data in the PET literature introduced PET-derived measures of tumor heterogeneity estimated through image texture analysis.[74,75] Different FDG-PET-based texture parameters have been described and are being studied to characterize noninvasively intratumoral metabolic heterogeneity. So far our experience is showing that they may be better when applied to larger tumors, because of the inaccuracy of PET to characterize metabolic distribution in small lesions.[74,75]

There is also preliminary evidence that measures of metabolic intratumoral heterogeneity may play an important prognostic role in patients with lung cancer. This is certainly promising clinically speaking, because this noninvasively image-derived information may be used to personalize the selection of more aggressive therapy for these patients. Cook and coworkers[76] reported on the role of FDG-PET-derived tumor textural features as biomarkers of response and outcomes in patients with NSCLC treated with TKIs. Although only a single-center study of 47 patients, the results are certainly promising. The investigators found that a reduction in metabolic heterogeneity at Week 6 during treatment was consistent with good response to erlotinib confirmed by CT at 12 weeks. In addition, PET image-derived texture parameters were found to be independent predictors of survival in their patient cohort.[76]

These metabolic signatures of tumoral heterogeneity show good clinical and prognostic potential; however, these results have to be corroborated by prospective, randomized trials before they are included in daily clinical practice.

SUMMARY

PET/CT is a sensitive molecular imaging technique with a major role in the precision medicine algorithm of the patient with lung cancer. On one hand, it provides anatomofunctional insight during diagnosis, staging, and restaging. On the other hand, it is a biomarker of tumoral heterogeneity that directs the selection of the most appropriate treatment, and predicts response early and accurately during the course of cytotoxic and cytostatic therapies. Last but not least, it is a biomarker of prognosis in lung cancer.

REFERENCES

1. American Cancer Society. Key statistics for lung cancer. 2016. Available at: http://www.cancer.org/cancer/lungcancer-non-smallcell/detailedguide/non-small-cell-lung-cancer-key-statistics. Accessed July 9, 2016.

2. Mena E, Yanamadala A, Cheng G, et al. The current and evolving role of PET in personalized management of lung Cancer. PET Clin 2016;11(3):243–59.

3. Warburg O, Wind F, Negelein E. The metabolism of tumours in the body. J Gen Physiol 1927;8(6):519–30.

4. Warburg O. On respiratory impairment in cancer cells. Science 1956;124(3215):269–70.

5. Gerbaudo VH, Garcia CA. PET/CT of lung cancer. In: Schoepf UJ, Meinel F, editors. Multidetector-Row CT of the thorax, 2nd edition. Switzerland: Springer International Publishing; 2016.

6. Gould MK, Tang T, Liu IL, et al. Recent trends in the identification of incidental pulmonary nodules. Am J Respir Crit Care Med 2015;192(10):1208–14.

7. Gould MK, Maclean CC, Kuschner WG, et al. Accuracy of positron emission tomography for diagnosis of pulmonary nodules and mass lesions: a meta-analysis. JAMA 2001;287:914–24.

8. Gambhir SS, Czernin J, Schwimmer J, et al. A tabulated summary of the FDG PET literature. J Nucl Med 2001;42:1S–93S.

9. Cronin P, Dwamena B, Kelly AM, et al. Solitary pulmonary nodules: meta-analytic comparison of cross-sectional imaging modalities for diagnosis of malignancy. Radiology 2008;246:772–82.

10. Garcia-Velloso MJ, Bastarrika G, de-Torres JP, et al. Assessment of indeterminate pulmonary nodules detected in lung cancer screening: diagnostic accuracy of FDG PET/CT. Lung Cancer 2016;97:81–6.

11. Fletcher JW, Djulbegovic B, Soares HP, et al. Recommendations on the use of ^{18}F-FDG PET in oncology. J Nucl Med 2008;49(3):480–508.

12. Kodama K, Higashiyama M, Okami J, et al. Oncologic outcomes of segmentectomy versus lobectomy for clinical T1a N0 M0 non-small cell lung cancer. Ann Thorac Surg 2016;101(2):504–11.

13. Carr SR, Schuchert MJ, Pennathur A, et al. Impact of tumor size on outcomes after anatomic lung resection for stage 1A non-small cell lung cancer based on the current staging system. J Thorac Cardiovasc Surg 2012;143(2):390–7.

14. Lardinois D, Weder W, Hany TF, et al. Staging of non–small-cell lung cancer with integrated positron emission tomography and computed tomography. N Engl J Med 2003;348:2500–7.

15. Antoch G, Stattaus J, Nemat AT, et al. Non-small cell lung cancer: dual-modality PET/CT in preoperative staging. Radiology 2003;229(2):526–33.

16. Gerbaudo VH, Julius B. Anatomo-metabolic characteristics of atelectasis in F-18 FDG-PET/CT imaging. Eur J Radiol 2007;64(3):401–5.

17. Dizendorf EV, Baumert BG, von Schulthess GK, et al. Impact of whole-body ^{18}F-FDG PET on staging and managing patients for radiation therapy. J Nucl Med 2003;44:24–9.

18. Gould MK, Kuschner WG, Rydzak CE, et al. Test performance of positron emission tomography and

computed tomography for mediastinal staging in patients with non-small-cell lung cancer: a meta-analysis. Ann Intern Med 2003;139:879–92.

19. Toloza EM, Harpole L, McCrory DC. Noninvasive staging of non-small cell lung cancer: a review of the current evidence. Chest 2003;123(1 Suppl):137S–46S.

20. Reed CE, Harpole DH, Posther KE, et al. American College of Surgeons Oncology Group Z0050 trial. results of the American College of Surgeons Oncology Group Z0050 trial: the utility of positron emission tomography in staging potentially operable non-small cell lung cancer. J Thorac Cardiovasc Surg 2003;126(6):1943–51.

21. Kim BT, Lee KS, Shim SS, et al. Stage T1 non-small cell lung cancer: preoperative mediastinal nodal staging with integrated FDG PET/CT: a prospective study. Radiology 2006;241(2):501–9.

22. Vansteenkiste JF. FDG-PET for lymph node staging in NSCLC: a major step forward, but beware of the pitfalls. Lung Cancer 2005;47(2):151–3.

23. Kaseda K, Watanabe K, Asakura K, et al. Identification of false-negative and false-positive diagnoses of lymph node metastases in non-small cell lung cancer patients staged by integrated (18F-)fluorodeoxy-glucose-positron emission tomography/computed tomography: a retrospective cohort study. Thorac Cancer 2016;7(4):473–80.

24. Fischer BM, Mortensen J, Hansen H, et al. Multimodality approach to mediastinal staging in non-small cell lung cancer. faults and benefits of PET-CT: a randomised trial. Thorax 2011;66(4):294–300.

25. Sider L, Horejs D. Frequency of extrathoracic metastases from bronchogenic carcinoma in patients with normal-sized hilar and mediastinal lymph nodes on CT. AJR Am J Roentgenol 1988;151(5):893–5.

26. MacManus MP, Hicks RJ, Matthews JP, et al. High rate of detection of unsuspected distant metastases by PET in apparent stage III non-small-cell lung cancer: implications for radical radiation therapy. Int J Radiat Oncol Biol Phys 2001;50(2):287–93.

27. Hellwig D, Ukena D, Paulsen F, et al. Onko-PET der Deutschen gesellschaft fur nuklearmedizin. meta-analysis of the efficacy of positron emission tomography with F-18-fluorodeoxyglucose in lung tumors. basis for discussion of the German consensus conference on PET in oncology 2000. Pneumologie 2001;55(8):367–77.

28. Cook GJ, Houston S, Rubens R, et al. Detection of bone metastases in breast cancer by 18FDG PET: differing metabolic activity in osteoblastic and osteolytic lesions. J Clin Oncol 1998;16(10):3375–9.

29. Hustinx R, Paulus P, Jacquet N, et al. Clinical evaluation of whole-body ^{18}F-fluorodeoxyglucose positron emission tomography in the detection of liver metastases. Ann Oncol 1998;9(4):397–401.

30. Lardinois D, Weder W, Roudas M, et al. Etiology of solitary extrapulmonary positron emission tomography and computed tomography findings in patients with lung cancer. J Clin Oncol 2005;23:6846–53.

31. Schaarschmidt BM, Grueneisen J, Metzenmacher M, et al. Thoracic staging with ^{18}F-FDG PET/MR in non-small cell lung cancer: does it change therapeutic decisions in comparison to ^{18}F-FDG PET/CT? Eur Radiol 2016. [Epub ahead of print].

32. National Research Council (US) Committee on A Framework for Developing a New Taxonomy of Disease. Toward precision medicine: building a knowledge network for biomedical research and a new taxonomy of disease. Washington, DC: National Academies Press (US); 2011.

33. Erasmus JJ, Gladish GW, Broemeling L, et al. Interobserver and intraobserver variability in measurement of non-small-cell carcinoma lung lesions: implications for assessment of tumor response. J Clin Oncol 2003;21:2574–82.

34. Wahl RL, Jacene H, Kasamon Y, et al. From RECIST to PERCIST: evolving considerations for PET response criteria in solid tumors. J Nucl Med 2009;50(Suppl 1):122S–50S.

35. Vansteenkiste J, Fischer BM, Dooms C, et al. Positron-emission tomography in prognostic and therapeutic assessment of lung cancer: systematic review. Lancet Oncol 2004;5:531–40.

36. Weber WA, Petersen V, Schmidt B, et al. Positron emission tomography in non-small-cell lung cancer: prediction of response to chemotherapy by quantitative assessment of glucose use. J Clin Oncol 2003;21:2651–7.

37. Cerfolio RJ, Bryant AS, Winokur TS, et al. Repeat 18F-FDG-PET after neoadjuvant therapy is a predictor of pathologic response in patients with non-small cell lung cancer. Ann Thorac Surg 2004;78:1903–9.

38. Hoekstra CJ, Stroobants SG, Smit EF, et al. Prognostic relevance of response evaluation using [18F]-2-fluoro-2-deoxy-D-glucose positron emission tomography in patients with locally advanced non-small-cell lung cancer. J Clin Oncol 2005;23(33):8362–70.

39. Eschmann SM, Friedel G, Paulsen F, et al. 18F-FDG PET for assessment of therapy response and preoperative re-evaluation after neoadjuvant radiochemotherapy in stage III non-small cell lung cancer. Eur J Nucl Med Mol Imaging 2007;34(4):463–71.

40. Dooms C, Verbeken E, Stroobants S, et al. Prognostic stratification of stage IIIA-N2 non-small-cell lung cancer after induction chemotherapy: a model based on the combination of morphometric-pathologic response in mediastinal nodes and primary tumor response on serial 18-fluoro-2-deoxy-glucose positron emission tomography. J Clin Oncol 2008;26(7):1128–34.

41. Mac Manus MP, Hicks RJ, Matthews JP, et al. Metabolic (FDG-PET) response after radical radiotherapy/chemoradiotherapy for non-small cell

lung cancer correlates with patterns of failure. Lung Cancer 2005;49(1):95–108.

42. Hicks RJ, Mac Manus MP, Matthews JP, et al. Early FDG-PET imaging after radical radiotherapy for non-small-cell lung cancer: inflammatory changes in normal tissues correlate with tumor response and do not confound therapeutic response evaluation. Int J Radiat Oncol Biol Phys 2004;60(2):412–8.

43. Paez JG, Jänne PA, Lee JC, et al. EGFR mutations in lung cancer: correlation with clinical response to gefitinib therapy. Science 2004;304(5676):1497–500.

44. Lynch TJ, Bell DW, Sordella R, et al. Activating mutations in the epidermal growth factor receptor underlying responsiveness of non-small-cell lung cancer to gefitinib. N Engl J Med 2004;350(21):2129–39.

45. Sunaga N, Oriuchi N, Kaira K, et al. Usefulness of FDG-PET for early prediction of the response to gefitinib in non-small cell lung cancer. Lung Cancer 2008;59(2):203–10.

46. Takahashi R, Hirata H, Tachibana I, et al. Early [18F]fluorodeoxyglucose positron emission tomography at two days of gefitinib treatment predicts clinical outcome in patients with adenocarcinoma of the lung. Clin Cancer Res 2012;18(1):220–8.

47. van Gool MH, Aukema TS, Schaake EE, et al, NEL Study Group. Timing of metabolic response monitoring during erlotinib treatment in non-small cell lung cancer. J Nucl Med 2014;55(7):1081–6.

48. Benz MR, Herrmann K, Walter F, et al. (18)F-FDG PET/CT for monitoring treatment responses to the epidermal growth factor receptor inhibitor erlotinib. J Nucl Med 2011;52(11):1684–9.

49. Hachemi M, Couturier O, Vervueren L, et al. [18F]FDG positron emission tomography within two weeks of starting erlotinib therapy can predict response in non-small cell lung cancer patients. PLoS One 2014;9(2):e87629.

50. van Gool MH, Aukema TS, Schaake EE, et al. (18)F-fluorodeoxyglucose positron emission tomography versus computed tomography in predicting histopathological response to epidermal growth factor receptor-tyrosine kinase inhibitor treatment in resectable non-small cell lung cancer. Ann Surg Oncol 2014;21(9):2831–7.

51. Ullrich RT, Zander T, Neumaier B, et al. Early detection of erlotinib treatment response in NSCLC by 3'-deoxy-3'-[F]-fluoro-L-thymidine ([F]FLT) positron emission tomography (PET). PLoS One 2008;3(12):e3908.

52. Sohn HJ, Yang YJ, Ryu JS, et al. [18F]Fluorothymidine positron emission tomography before and 7 days after gefitinib treatment predicts response in patients with advanced adenocarcinoma of the lung. Clin Cancer Res 2008;14(22):7423–9.

53. Kahraman D, Scheffler M, Zander T, et al. Quantitative analysis of response to treatment with erlotinib in advanced non-small cell lung cancer using 18F-FDG and 3'-deoxy-3'-18F-fluorothymidine PET. J Nucl Med 2011;52(12):1871–7.

54. Zander T, Scheffler M, Nogova L, et al. Early prediction of nonprogression in advanced non-small-cell lung cancer treated with erlotinib by using [(18)F]fluorodeoxyglucose and [(18)F]fluorothymidine positron emission tomography. J Clin Oncol 2011;29(13):1701–8.

55. Bhoil A, Singh B, Singh N, et al. Can 3'-deoxy-3'-(18)F-fluorothymidine or 2'-deoxy-2'-(18)F-fluoro-d-glucose PET/CTbetter assess response after 3-weeks treatment by epidermal growth factor receptor kinase inhibitor, in non-small lung cancer patients? Preliminary results. Hell J Nucl Med 2014;17(2):90–6.

56. Paesmans M, Berghmans T, Dusart M, et al. Primary tumor standardized uptake value measured on fluorodeoxyglucose positron emission tomography is of prognostic value for survival in non-small cell lung cancer: update of a systematic review and meta-analysis by the European Lung Cancer Working Party for the International Association for the Study of Lung Cancer Staging Project. J Thorac Oncol 2010;5(5):612–9.

57. Nair VS, Gevaert O, Davidzon G, et al. NF-κB protein expression associates with (18)F-FDG PET tumor uptake in non-small cell lung cancer: a radiogenomics validation study to understand tumor metabolism. Lung Cancer 2014;83(2):189–96.

58. Ahuja V, Coleman RE, Herndon J, et al. The prognostic significance of fluorodeoxyglucose positron emission tomography imaging for patients with nonsmall cell lung carcinoma. Cancer 1998;83(5):918–24.

59. Ohtsuka T, Nomori H, Watanabe K, et al. Prognostic significance of [(18)F]fluorodeoxyglucose uptake on positron emission tomography in patients with pathologic stage I lung adenocarcinoma. Cancer 2006;107(10):2468–73.

60. Goodgame B, Pillot GA, Yang Z, et al. Prognostic value of preoperative positron emission tomography in resected stage I nonsmall cell lung cancer. J Thorac Oncol 2008;3(2):130–4.

61. Hanin FX, Lonneux M, Cornet J, et al. Prognostic value of FDG uptake in early stage non-small cell lung cancer. Eur J Cardiothorac Surg 2008;33(5):819–23.

62. Cerfolio RJ, Bryant AS, Ohja B, et al. The maximum standardized uptake values on positron emission tomography of a non-small cell lung cancer predict stage, recurrence, and survival. J Thorac Cardiovasc Surg 2005;130(1):151–9.

63. Decoster L, Schallier D, Everaert H, et al. Complete metabolic tumour response, assessed by 18-fluorodeoxyglucose positron emission tomography (18FDG-PET), after induction chemotherapy predicts a favourable outcome in patients with locally

advanced non-small cell lung cancer (NSCLC). Lung Cancer 2008;62(1):55–61.

64. Machtay M, Duan F, Siegel BA, et al. Prediction of survival by [18F]fluorodeoxyglucose positron emission tomography in patients with locally advanced non-small-cell lung cancer undergoing definitive chemoradiation therapy: results of the ACRIN 6668/RTOG 0235 trial. J Clin Oncol 2013;31(30): 3823–30.

65. Gerbaudo VH, Katz SI, Nowak AK, et al. Multimodality imaging review of malignant pleural mesothelioma diagnosis and staging. PET Clin 2011;6(3): 275–97.

66. Larson SM, Erdi Y, Akhurst T, et al. Tumor treatment response based on visual and quantitative changes in global tumor glycolysis using PET-FDG imaging. the visual response score and the change in total lesion glycolysis. Clin Positron Imaging 1999;2(3): 159–71.

67. Lee P, Weerasuriya DK, Lavori PW, et al. Metabolic tumor burden predicts for disease progression and death in lung cancer. Int J Radiat Oncol Biol Phys 2007;69(2):328–33.

68. Dehing-Oberije C, De Ruysscher D, van der Weide H, et al. Tumor volume combined with number of positive lymph node stations is a more important prognostic factor than TNM stage for survival of non-small-cell lung cancer patients treated with (chemo)radiotherapy. Int J Radiat Oncol Biol Phys 2008;70(4):1039–44.

69. Liao S, Penney BC, Zhang H, et al. Prognostic value of the quantitative metabolic volumetric measurement on 18F-FDG PET/CT in stage IV nonsurgical

small-cell lung cancer. Acad Radiol 2012;19(1): 69–77.

70. Zhang H, Wroblewski K, Liao S, et al. Prognostic value of metabolic tumor burden from (18)F-FDG PET in surgical patients with non-small-cell lung cancer. Acad Radiol 2013;20(1):32–40.

71. Park SY, Cho A, Yu WS, et al. Prognostic value of total lesion glycolysis by 18F-FDG PET/CT in surgically resected stage IA non-small cell lung cancer. J Nucl Med 2015;56(1):45–9.

72. Ohri N, Duan F, Machtay M, et al. Pretreatment FDG-PET metrics in stage III non-small cell lung cancer: ACRIN 6668/RTOG 0235. J Natl Cancer Inst 2015; 107(4) [pii:djv004].

73. Jamal-Hanjani M, Hackshaw A, Ngai Y, et al. Tracking genomic cancer evolution for precision medicine: the lung TRACERx Study. PLoS Biol 2014;12(7):e1001906.

74. Davnall F, Yip CS, Ljungqvist G, et al. Assessment of tumor heterogeneity: an emerging imaging tool for clinical practice? Insights Imaging 2012;3(6): 573–89.

75. van Gómez López O, García Vicente AM, Honguero Martínez AF, et al. Heterogeneity in [18F]fluorodeoxyglucose positron emission tomography/computed tomography of non-small cell lung carcinoma and its relationship to metabolic parameters and pathologic staging. Mol Imaging 2014;13:1–12.

76. Cook GJ, O'Brien ME, Siddique M, et al. Non-small cell lung cancer treated with erlotinib: heterogeneity of (18)F-FDG uptake at PET-association with treatment response and prognosis. Radiology 2015; 276(3):883–93.

Advancing Precision Nuclear Medicine and Molecular Imaging for Lymphoma

Chadwick L. Wright, MD, PhD[a], Joseph J. Maly, MD[b],
Jun Zhang, PhD[a], Michael V. Knopp, MD, PhD[a],*

KEYWORDS

- Lymphoma • Position emission tomography • Fluorodeoxyglucose • Biomarker
- Molecular imaging • Precision medicine

KEY POINTS

- Fluorodeoxyglucose F 18 (^{18}F FDG) is a PET imaging radiopharmaceutical that is evolving into an imaging biomarker for the detection and therapeutic response assessment of lymphomas.
- There are current challenges and opportunities for advancing the role and capabilities of ^{18}F FDG-PET in lymphoma.
- ^{18}F FDG-PET contributions will expand owing to new emerging technologies, clinical trial utilization, standardization, and its role in radiomics and big data analysis of lymphoma.
- Precision nuclear medicine and advanced molecular imaging approaches are poised to fundamentally adapt lymphoma management for the upcoming era of personalized medicine and precision medicine.

CLINICAL EVOLUTION OF PET WITH FLUORODEOXYGLUCOSE F 18 AS A BIOMARKER FOR LYMPHOMA

As our understanding of cancer expands, physicians are searching for new and improved tools to more precisely guide medical decision making as well as to accurately stratify each patient's risk at diagnosis and throughout the disease course. Many disciplines of medicine have contributed in this effort, but specifically regarding the diagnosis of lymphoma and its clinical management, PET with fluorodeoxyglucose F 18 (^{18}F FDG-PET) imaging has made a tremendous clinical impact. ^{18}F FDG-PET imaging is evolving into a standard of care modality for the majority of

Disclosure Statement: Dr C.L. Wright is supported by Grant no. IRG-67-003-50 from the American Cancer Society and the National Institutes of Health/National Cancer Institute, Clinical Loan Repayment Program. Dr J.J. Maly is supported by grant National Cancer Institute T32: CA165998. Drs C.L. Wright, J. Zhang and M.V. Knopp are also supported by the Wright Center of Innovation in Biomedical Imaging and ODSA TECH 09-028, TECH 10-012 and TECH 13-060. The authors declare that there is no conflict of interests regarding the publication of this paper.
[a] Wright Center of Innovation in Biomedical Imaging, Division of Imaging Science, Department of Radiology, The Ohio State University Wexner Medical Center, 395 West 12th Avenue, Room 430, Columbus, OH 43210, USA; [b] Division of Hematology, Department of Internal Medicine, The Ohio State University Wexner Medical Center, Starling Loving Hall 406C, 320 West 10th Avenue, Columbus, OH 43210, USA
* Corresponding author.
E-mail address: knopp.16@osu.edu

PET Clin 12 (2017) 63–82
http://dx.doi.org/10.1016/j.cpet.2016.08.005
1556-8598/17/© 2016 Elsevier Inc. All rights reserved.

lymphoma subtypes and its value in the molecular and functional characterization of lymphoma has overtaken more traditional anatomic imaging approaches. Additionally, in comparison to the nonimaging risk stratification tools (eg, molecular profile, International Prognostic Index [IPI], and International Prognostic Score) only ^{18}F FDG-PET has demonstrated real-time comprehensive disease evaluation, assessment of individual disease risk, likelihood of response to therapy, and survival, and therefore represents an emerging and important precision medicine tool to guide patient treatment.

Diagnostic Initial Staging

Initial diagnostic risk scoring systems for nearly every lymphoma subtype include Ann Arbor Stage[1] within its reference criteria: the IPI,[2,3] revised IPI (R-IPI),[4] Follicular Lymphoma IPI (FLIPI),[5] and International Prognostic Score.[6] In this regard, ^{18}F FDG-PET has been shown to improve diagnostic stage accuracy compared with other standard imaging modalities and staging tools and have, in some cases, led to change in therapeutic management in both Hodgkin lymphoma (HL) and non-Hodgkin lymphoma (NHL).[7–14] Interestingly, the improved salvage treatment options at relapse as well as the similarities in management of stage I versus stage II and stage III versus stage IV disease have probably limited this improved staging accuracy from contributing to an overall survival (OS) benefit. However, the improved staging accuracy of ^{18}F FDG-PET has led to the elimination of unnecessary consolidative radiation therapy and toxicity at diagnosis. For example, ^{18}F FDG-PET in follicular lymphoma (FL) has resulted in 11% to 31% upstaging from stage I and II (early stage) to stage III and IV (advanced stage).[15,16] The pretreatment ^{18}F FDG-PET also performed better than the FLIPI prognostic scoring system in identifying those patients who would have an incomplete therapeutic response or early relapse.[15] For the relatively common NHL subtype diffuse large B-cell lymphoma (DLBCL),[17] [18]F FDG-PET has demonstrated increased sensitivity for identifying both nodal[8,12,18–22] and extranodal[15,21] disease sites when compared with conventional computed tomography (CT) imaging at diagnosis and subsequently guides therapeutic management. [18]F FDG-PET is not only useful at complementing the assessment of the bone marrow involvement,[20,23] but is able to identify otherwise asymptomatic but high-risk/nonmarrow skeletal lesions,[24] providing an opportunity for involved field radiation therapy (IF-XRT) to improve event-free survival in such patients.

In addition to identifying disease sites at diagnosis, the semiquantitative assessment using standardized uptake value (SUV) with ^{18}F FDG-PET has also been shown to correlate with disease histology in lymphoma.[25] There are many instances in which this can be used to guide differentiation of indolent and aggressive lymphoma subtypes[26–28] and this diagnostic functionality becomes critically important when there is clinical suspicion for de novo or midtreatment transformation events. It is often the lesion with the highest ^{18}F FDG uptake (ie, highest SUV) on the ^{18}F FDG-PET that guides targeted biopsy for histopathologic confirmation.[29–31]

Interim Staging

The performance of ^{18}F FDG-PET during induction therapy has emerged as a treatment-defining diagnostic test for many lymphoma subtypes because its real-time insight into therapeutic response has improved the prognostic ability for ^{18}F FDG–avid lymphomas.[32,33] In particular, the subtype of lymphoma that has demonstrated the greatest usefulness from interim ^{18}F FDG-PET is HL. Studies have confirmed a negative interim ^{18}F FDG-PET scan after 1 to 3 cycles of induction chemotherapy[12,34,35] is a strong predictor of progression-free survival (PFS) and has also been shown to perform better than the International Prognostic Score for prediction of prognosis.[35] Conversely, a positive interim ^{18}F FDG-PET at the same treatment interval not only correlates with classically associated high-risk features of disease,[12,35] but has also been shown to predict either refractory disease or early disease relapse.[36] These data have driven the clinical use of interim ^{18}F FDG-PET to better evaluate, inform, and guide the course of treatment for HL patients. For example, the historical standard of care for patients with early stage HL has been IF-XRT at the completion of systemic induction chemotherapy. However, it was recently demonstrated that early stage HL patients with a negative ^{18}F FDG-PET scan after 4 systemic chemotherapy cycles of adriamycin, bleomycin, vinblastine, and dacarbazine (ABVD) regardless of risk factors had similar and in some cases better outcomes if they did not undergo the previously considered standard IF-XRT.[37] Conflicting data using this approach have been published in which an increased progression/relapse rate was observed after the preplanned 1-year interim analysis in the cohort of early stage favorable and unfavorable HL patients in which radiation was eliminated.[38] However, the relatively short period for this interim analysis, which led to it being discontinued per the experimental arm's inferiority, casts doubt unto the reliability of these conclusions. Subsequently, there have been data both published that continue to support the use of the interim ^{18}F FDG-PET scan to eliminate IF-XRT for early stage HL patients.[39] Specifically, IF-XRT toxicity can be eliminated in early stage good risk nonbulky HL patients if patients achieve a complete remission using ^{18}F FDG-PET after 3 cycles of ABVD.[39]

For advanced stage HL, bulky adenopathy has long been considered an indication for IF-XRT at the completion of 6 cycles of chemotherapy. However, recently published[40] and emerging data[41] suggest that a negative interim ^{18}F FDG-PET indicates that IF-XRT can be safely removed from the treatment regimen without compromising outcome. Similarly, systemic induction chemotherapy can be safely deescalated from more intensive chemotherapeutic regimen to the well-tolerated ABVD regimen if patients achieve complete response (CR) using ^{18}F FDG-PET after 2 cycles of chemotherapy.[42,43] In patients with relapsed/refractory HL treated with brentuximab vedotin as a bridge to autologous stem cell transplantation (ASCT), preliminary phase II data demonstrated that a negative interim ^{18}F FDG-PET after 2 cycles of brentuximab vedotin can eliminate the need for additional salvage chemotherapy (eg, augmented isophosphamide, cyclophosphamide, and etoposide) and can achieve an approximately 100% CR rate by proceeding directly to ASCT.[44] Interim ^{18}F FDG-PET has been used to intensify treatment as well. There is a PFS benefit to escalating systemic therapy from ABVD to bleomycin, etoposide, adriamycin, cyclophosphamide, oncovin, procarbazine, and prednisone (BEACOPP) or ASCT in advanced stage HL patients who remain ^{18}F FDG-PET positive after 2 cycles of therapy.[45–47] There has yet to be a proven OS benefit to this approach,[48] but as the landscape of systemic treatment options for such patients evolves, this concept will need to be revisited.

The role for interim ^{18}F FDG-PET to guide prognostic and therapeutic decision making in NHL has been less clear. Early data demonstrate a positive correlation between positive interim ^{18}F FDG-PET and other high-risk features[49] and evidence for its use in NHL is increasing. For example, the current standard of care as recommended by the British Columbia Cancer Agency for early stage DLBCL patients with a negative ^{18}F FDG-PET after 3 cycles of systemic chemotherapy using R-CHOP (rituximab, cyclophosphamide, doxorubicin, vincristine, and prednisone) is followed by 1 additional cycle and the elimination of the previously used IF-XRT.[50] These findings were supported in

early stage NHL patients in which IF-XRT was safely removed from the treatment regimen when CR by ^{18}F FDG-PET was achieved after 4 cycles of chemotherapy.[51] For advanced stage NHL, initial studies were encouraging; interim ^{18}F FDG-PET predicted CR rate, event-free survival, PFS, and OS (regardless of IPI risk group or rituximab therapy).[52–55] In addition, positive ^{18}F FDG-PET after 2 to 3 cycles of induction systemic chemotherapy was used to identify patients at greater risk who then proceeded to immediate ASCT and this provided a similar 2-year PFS when compared with patients with a negative interim ^{18}F FDG-PET scan.[56] Similarly, advanced stage DLBCL patients with a positive interim ^{18}F FDG-PET after 4 cycles of induction R-CHOP proceeded to ASCT and this resulted in similar PFS and OS to those patients with negative interim ^{18}F FDG-PET studies.[57]

In contrast, there are retrospective data[58,59] and prospective data[60,61] in patients with advanced stage NHL that indicate that interim ^{18}F FDG-PET may not serve as the best indicator of prognosis. An 87% false-positive rate in this population has been described as well as the observation that there is a similar PFS rate between those patients with a false-positive result and those with a negative ^{18}F FDG-PET.[62] It is possible that differences in the systemic therapeutic agents used for these patients may contribute to this observation.[63] Such considerations in conjunction with the biologic heterogeneity of NHL may confound the true usefulness of interim ^{18}F FDG-PET in NHL. Nevertheless, interim ^{18}F FDG-PET remains an integral diagnostic test within the context of related clinical trials and its usefulness for various NHL subtypes will be established. A complete list of the currently registered clinical trials at www.clinicaltrials.gov using this approach in lymphoma can be seen in **Table 1**.

Restaging at the Completion of Therapy

The use of ^{18}F FDG-PET after completing induction therapy serves to evaluate the patient's response to therapy and update the disease prognosis. In those patients who achieved CR by ^{18}F FDG-PET after completing therapy, 83% of NHL patients and 91% of HL patients maintained long-term CR as opposed to 0% of those patients who did not achieve CR.[64,65] Conversely, positive ^{18}F FDG-PET after completion of therapy portends disease progression in both NHL and HL.[66,67] In FL, median PFS was 48 months in the negative ^{18}F FDG-PET group compared with 17.2 months for the positive ^{18}F FDG-PET group with residual ^{18}F FDG uptake.[15] The poor prognostic implications of a positive ^{18}F FDG-PET after therapy

Table 1
Clinical trials using a ^{18}F FDG-PET–guided therapeutic decision model for lymphoma patients registered at www.clinicaltrials.gov and actively recruiting patients at the time of submission

Identifier	Phase	Population	[18]F FDG-PET Result–Based Intervention
NCT01659099	III	DLBCL CD20+	Patients with positive ^{18}F FDG-PET scan after 4 cycles of either experimental (GA101) or control (rituximab) arm will be taken to ASCT
NCT01359592	II	Limited stage DLBCL	Patients with positive ^{18}F FDG-PET + after 3 cycles of R-CHOP get IF-XRT followed by yttrium-90 ibritumomab tiuxetan and rituximab
NCT01118026	II	Bulky early stage cHL	Patients with positive ^{18}F FDG-PET after 2 cycles of ABVD escalated to BEACOPP + IF-XRT
NCT01390584	II	Early stage HL	Patients with positive ^{18}F FDG-PET after 2 cycles of ABVD escalated to BEACOPP + IF-XRT
NCT01804127	II	DLBCL	Identify number of cycles based on the interim ^{18}F FDG-PET result
NCT01478542	III	CD20+ aggressive B-cell lymphoma	Multiarm study using comparing investigational vincristine vs conventional vincristine in which patients could get up to 2 additional cycles of systemic chemotherapy and possibly IF-XRT based on result of ^{18}F FDG-PET after 4 cycles of chemotherapy
NCT01285765	III	Low-risk IPI DLBCL	Multiarm study using ^{18}F FDG-PET after 2 cycles of systemic chemotherapy to identify whether patients will complete 4 or 6 cycles of systemic chemotherapy
NCT02298283	II	Early stage HL	Patients with positive ^{18}F FDG-PET after 2 cycles of systemic chemotherapy will be transitioned to vedotin consolidation
NCT01356680	III	HL	Removal of IF-XRT from treatment regimen if negative ^{18}F FDG-PET after 4 total cycles of systemic chemotherapy
NCT02611323	I/II	NHL	CR, PR, or stable disease at the end of induction therapy per ^{18}F FDG-PET result will receive postinduction treatment with additional small molecule targeted therapy
NCT02624986	I/II	NHL	CR, PR, or stable disease at the end of induction therapy per ^{18}F FDG-PET result will receive postinduction treatment with additional small molecule targeted therapy
NCT02692248	II	DLBCL	Use of ^{18}F FDG-PET to identify patients in CR, PR, stable disease who will be eligible for additional cycles of systemic chemotherapy
NCT02405078	III	Relapsed/refractory DLBCL	Patients with response to systemic chemotherapy as assessed by ^{18}F FDG-PET will be eligible for standard maintenance systemic therapy vs further salvage treatment options if ^{18}F FDG-PET evidence of stable disease or PD
NCT02063685	III	FL	CR, PR, or stable disease at the end of induction therapy per ^{18}F FDG-PET result will receive postinduction treatment with additional small molecule targeted therapy
NCT01599559	III	Primary mediastinal B-cell lymphoma	Randomized assessment of consolidative IF-XRT to the mediastinum in patients with negative ^{18}F FDG-PET at the completion of induction chemotherapy

(continued on next page)

Table 1
(continued)

Identifier	Phase	Population	[18]F FDG-PET Result–Based Intervention
NCT01186978	II	DLBCL	Reduction of radiation dose from 30 to 20 Gy in addition to reduction of radiation field in patients achieving CR per ^{18}F FDG-PET after 4 or 6 cycles of systemic chemotherapy
NCT02244021	II	HL	Escalation to brentuximab vedotin salvage in patients who remain ^{18}F FDG-PET positive at the completion of systemic induction chemotherapy
NCT01858922	II	HL	Use of ^{18}F FDG-PET after 2 cycles of systemic chemotherapy to identify patient continues current therapy (experimental or control), undergoes IF-XRT, or taken off study
NCT02374424	II	DLBCL	Use of ^{18}F FDG-PET after 2 cycles of systemic chemotherapy to determine if patient eligible for immediate ASCT consolidation

Abbreviations: [18]F FDG-PET, PET with fluorodeoxyglucose F 18; ABVD, adriamycin, bleomycin, vinblastine, and dacarbazine; ASCT, autologous stem cell transplant; BEACOPP, bleomycin/etoposide/adriamycin/cyclophosphamide/oncovin/procarbazine/prednisone; cHL, classic Hodgkin lymphoma; CR, complete response; DLBCL, diffuse large B-cell lymphoma; FL, follicular lymphoma; HL, Hodgkin lymphoma; IF-XRT, involved field radiation therapy; IPI, International Prognostic Index; NHL, non-Hodgkin lymphoma; PR, partial response; PR, progressive disease; R-CHOP, rituximab/cyclophosphamide/doxorubicin/vincristine/prednisone.

also extends to the mantle cell lymphoma[68] subtype, and clinical trials using maintenance therapy in mantle cell lymphoma will ultimately determine whether ^{18}F FDG-PET can stratify which patients benefit from maintenance therapy.

[18]F FDG-PET also serves as the primary diagnostic modality to evaluate and characterize residual lymphoid masses (ie, distinguishing viable tumor from posttreatment fibrosis and necrosis).[8,9,66,69,70] In this way, restaging ^{18}F FDG-PET studies reduced the number of patients who were irradiated for residual tissue (and presumably residual disease) from 70% to 11%.[40] As such, restaging ^{18}F FDG-PET is now the determining factor for patients to receive consolidative radiotherapy as opposed to the initial presence of bulky nodes. There is no difference in the 5-year freedom from treatment failure for both bulky and nonbulky advanced stage HL without IF-XRT consolidation if a negative ^{18}F FDG-PET had been achieved after completing therapy.[41] Likewise for gray zone lymphoma, negative ^{18}F FDG-PET after completion of induction therapy improves PFS, and these data have largely eliminated IF-XRT (usually in the mediastinum).[71,72] In the unfortunate circumstance that the restaging ^{18}F FDG-PET results in an indeterminate lesion or node, a repeat ^{18}F FDG-PET study in 4 to 6 weeks can be helpful to confirm persistent or progressive disease because there is no survival advantage to treating asymptomatic patient in this situation.[73] It is when the second ^{18}F FDG-PET confirms a residual lesion that prompt pathologic confirmation and subsequent consolidative radiation therapy is needed to provide a 3-year PFS of 86% (compared with the 92% for negative restaging ^{18}F FDG-PET).[74]

PRECISION NUCLEAR MEDICINE AND THE EXISTING CHALLENGES

Although ^{18}F FDG-PET enables better clinical detection and management of lymphoma,[75–78] it has been recognized that the clinical effectiveness for ^{18}F FDG-PET in lymphoma for different patient populations as well as different lymphoma subtypes may still be improved.[79] Recently there has been the diagnostic trend to visually interpret and report ^{18}F FDG-PET assessment for lymphoma using the 5-point Deauville criteria[80] as opposed to more traditional quantitative approaches (eg, changes in SUV). Given the ability of PET to precisely and accurately quantify molecular processes, this latest trend should serve as a call for nuclear medicine physicians to actively engage in the development, refinement and validation of new analytical approaches to enable new precision medicine and personalized medicine practices demanded by our treating physicians and our patients. In particular, clinical nuclear medicine needs to transform into precision nuclear medicine. This paradigm of precision nuclear medicine seeks to advance existing and emerging tumor-specific targeting strategies to improve diagnostic imaging and quantification of disease burden while enhancing the multimodality therapeutic options for individual patients, reducing disease recurrence rates and minimizing treatment-related toxicities. In particular, precision nuclear medicine practices must enable better lesion detectability and assessment of whole body disease burden, more precise lesion characterization (eg, distinguishing benign vs malignant lymph nodes for lymphoma), and improved diagnostic confidence using existing and new imaging biomarkers.

At present, there are 3 challenges to address to advance precision nuclear medicine: (1) lesion detection, which is especially important in identifying disease at its earliest (and often smallest) stage as well as detection of reservoirs of disease which persist, (2) lesion characterization, which is important for distinguishing an otherwise indeterminate lesion (eg, lymph node) into either benign or malignant as well as describing the true heterogeneous nature of larger masses, and (3) diagnostic confidence, which is important both for nuclear medicine physicians to accurately describe the overall disease burden and for oncologists to determine which treatment modality or modalities are best suited to treat an individual's disease.

Lesion Detectability

One of the challenges for nuclear medicine physicians is lesion detection and this is especially true for small lesions or lesions within confounding tissues (eg, lesions near or involving tissues associated with high physiologic radiotracer uptake or excretion, lesions in regions of potential motion artifact like the diaphragm or extremities). In the initial staging of malignancy, intravascular contrast-enhanced CT or MR imaging provides excellent examples of improving lesion detectability owing to changes in vascular enhancement. This enhancement makes malignant/metastatic lesions more conspicuous within otherwise normal appearing tissues. For ^{18}F FDG-PET, lesion detectability can be influenced biologically by (1) ^{18}F FDG avidity of the lesion (ie, low-grade lymphoma tends to be less ^{18}F FDG avid than high-grade lymphoma and therefore can be more difficult to distinguish from background tissue uptake), (2) lesion size (smaller malignant lesions are more susceptible to partial volume effects with PET and therefore may falsely seem to be similar to background activity), and (3) patient body mass index.[81] In addition, lesion detectability can be influenced procedurally by the (1) dose of ^{18}F FDG administered, (2) injection-to-scan time, (3) image acquisition methodology, and (4) image reconstruction approach.[81–83]

Lesion Characterization

Although ^{18}F FDG-PET can aid in the characterization of indeterminate lesions detected on anatomic imaging as likely benign or likely malignant, there is another current unmet clinical need to better evaluate and characterize indeterminate lesions found on ^{18}F FDG-PET studies.[84,85] In the context of lesions with indeterminate ^{18}F FDG avidity, such lesions may relate to the underlying malignant/metastatic disease process, acute or chronic infection, acute or chronic inflammatory process, or even altered radiotracer biodistribution (eg, the presence of increased ^{18}F FDG in an axillary lymph node on the same side as a radiotracer that has been administered and extravasated, that is, lymphatic drainage and nodal accumulation of radiotracer, and lymph nodes in regions of increased physiologic ^{18}F FDG uptake corresponding with brown adipose tissue).[86] Clinical correlation with patient's symptomatology, history, physical examination, additional imaging, minimally invasive tissue sampling with fine needle aspiration or percutaneous biopsy, or more invasive tissue sampling with excisional biopsy is often needed. Depending on the patient's clinical context and physician's suspicion, such lesions may be closely monitored on follow-up imaging to document resolution and exclude any progressive/neoplastic process or direct tissue sampling may be pursued for more rapid and definitive assessment. Unfortunately, direct tissue sampling and histopathologic evaluation has associated nondiagnostic and complication rates as well. Therefore, the clinical dilemma of the indeterminate lymph node must be overcome with more precise lesion characterization by developing new imaging and analytical approaches with existing radiotracers (eg, ^{18}F FDG) or with new disease-specific imaging radiopharmaceuticals. In addition, there is need for better characterization of larger lesions and masses which may have heterogeneous appearance on CT or MR imaging. The presence and distribution of ^{18}F FDG uptake within such heterogeneous masses can help to distinguish areas of high versus low grade biology within a soft tissue lesion, areas of post-treatment change versus residual viable tumor within a treated lesion, and so on.

Diagnostic Confidence

Improved detection and localization of malignant lesions coupled with more precise characterization of such lesions will contribute to overall improved diagnostic confidence on the part of the reader and more consistent stratification of patients for therapy. In particular, new strategies and diagnostic/analytical tools that enable better intra-reader and interreader consistency for ^{18}F FDG-PET studies are needed.

PRECISION NUCLEAR MEDICINE: OPPORTUNITIES TO FUNDAMENTALLY ADVANCE MOLECULAR IMAGING
Emerging Technologies for PET with Fluorodeoxyglucose F 18

Given the role of ^{18}F FDG-PET in the detection and response assessment for lymphoma, its ability to further advance functional/molecular imaging when coupled with other anatomic imaging modalities depends on technical innovations, which then become integrated into new clinical PET systems and whose performance continues to improve with every system iteration.[87] There has been a recent technological revolution driven by the desire for PET/MR, which has led to the replacement of the conventional photomultiplier tubes in the PET gantry with solid state PET detectors, which are MR compatible but still rely on analog-to-digital signal conversion and Anger logic.[88,89] With the emergence of clinical PET/MR systems, there is now an opportunity for eliminating CT dose while maximizing soft tissue visualization with MR imaging and fusing this anatomic information with PET.[90,91] Such novel technical approaches may be useful for expanding functional/molecular PET imaging in pediatric oncology patients and potentially in pregnant patients.[92,93] At present, widespread use of PET/MR is limited by cost, less robust quantification of lesion activity owing to MR-based attenuation correction, patient compliance with MR imaging, and MR contraindications (eg, patients with incompatible implants). Such limitations ensure the continued role for ^{18}F FDG-PET/CT imaging in the foreseeable future.

Next-generation digital photon counting PET detectors have also been recently developed[94–98] and integrated into the first fully digital PET/CT system.[99] This digital photon counting PET detector technology has also been incorporated into PET/MR imaging devices for preclinical studies.[100–102] In general, digital PET detector technology improves overall PET image quality, quantitative accuracy, and diagnostic confidence when compared with conventional photomultiplier tube–based PET technology.[99] It is likely that PET vendors in the future will transition away from conventional photomultiplier tube–based PET systems to the solid state, digital PET detector systems.

Disruptive Innovations

Radiology and nuclear medicine are intricately dependent on technology and medical imagers are often the fastest adopters of new technologies. With each new innovation, there is potential disruption of the current standard of practice by either visualizing new lesions that are not appreciated using the older technology or the presence of pseudolesions that are now just better depicted regions of physiologic radiotracer distribution (eg, pituitary and adrenal glands). Likewise, the quantification of ^{18}F FDG-PET activity using SUV metrics can be significantly affected by new PET technology and image reconstruction methodologies.[103] With that said, potential disruptive innovations should not be avoided but rather adopted, optimized, translated, and validated for clinical use. Disruptive innovations are not only hardware innovations, but can also represent software innovations. For example, the measured tissue activity concentrations (ie, SUV) for lesions on ^{18}F FDG-PET studies can vary for the same image dataset when different methods of image reconstruction are used. Likewise, varying image reconstruction can affect the average and maximum SUVs of tumor lesions.[104] Time-of-flight (ToF)–based reconstruction improved quantitative accuracy and new approaches, which reduce the partial volume effects for SUV quantification (especially in small lesions) and will contribute to more accurate assessment of disease burden, response assessment, and prognosis.[105] The addition of advanced reconstruction approaches such as point-spread function in PET image reconstruction can qualitatively reduce image noise as well as improve signal to noise attributes when signal-to-noise ratios and activity recovery measures are evaluated.[106] Although this contributes to increased SUV values and tumor-to-background ratios, the use of point-spread function also improves the sensitivity of ^{18}F FDG-PET for the evaluation for smaller, nonenlarged but still malignant lymph nodes.[107] Furthermore, the incorporation of both point-spread function and ToF in ^{18}F FDG-PET image reconstruction results in even better image quality when the PET image reconstruction parameters are optimized.[108] These data suggest that parameter optimization of ^{18}F FDG-PET image reconstruction approaches that incorporate point-spread function and ToF has the potential to produce comparable image quality even if lower ^{18}F FDG dose is administered or if the total PET image acquisition time is reduced.[108,109] Recent work has suggested that these PET image reconstruction approaches may also be applicable and clinically useful in those patients with higher body mass indices.[109,110] Given the variability introduced by different/disruptive PET technologies in oncology clinical trials, it has become essential that consistent image acquisition parameters as well as consistent image reconstruction methodologies are used for serial ^{18}F FDG-PET assessments.[103,111]

New paradigms for dose reduction in PET with fluorodeoxyglucose F 18/computed tomography imaging

Another disruptive innovation for new PET technology is its ability to reduce the administered ^{18}F FDG dose to patients without significant impact in image quality or lesion quantification.[112] Such radiotracer dose reduction is consistent with ALARA (as low as reasonably achievable). It has been demonstrated that patient-specific ^{18}F FDG dosing can be based on the individual's body mass index to maximize PET image quality.[113] Although determining the lowest optimal ^{18}F FDG dose depends on multiple factors, one of the determinants is the underlying PET detector technology.[114–116] With the development of PET/MR technology, there has been renewed interest in the potential for radiotracer dose reduction in investigational and clinical PET studies.[92] In PET/MR, it has been demonstrated using phantoms that approximately 87% reduction of the ^{18}F FDG dose can be achieved while maintaining PET image quality, but this approach necessitates longer PET image acquisition time.[117] Likewise, preliminary PET/MR findings demonstrate that up to a 75% [18]F FDG dose reduction may be feasible in specific clinical applications.[118] New approaches for simulating ^{18}F FDG-PET dose reduction have been described using the fractional sampling of list-mode datasets obtained from PET/MR retrospectively. These simulated low-dose PET datasets demonstrate similar image characteristic (to a certain degree of relative dose reduction) when compared with the original full-dose PET dataset.[119] This type of approach will likely be tremendously enabling for future clinical trials to determine the lowest radiotracer dose necessary to maintain consistent clinical observations, quantification and outcomes in a large patient population. In the future, substantial ^{18}F FDG dose reductions for lymphoma patients undergoing serial imaging assessment may be realized without significant impact on clinical assessment.

Given that PET image reconstruction depends on attenuation correction (often with CT), there is interest in understanding the boundary conditions for ^{18}F FDG-PET in terms of lowering the CT dose while maintaining sufficient attenuation correction for quantitative PET image assessment as well as anatomic localization of PET findings.[120] Using model-based iterative reconstruction approaches in a simulation model, it appears feasible to use ultra-low CT doses to maintain consistent PET

attenuation correction and anatomic localization of PET findings when compared with-full dose CT.[120] Again, such CT dose reduction is consistent with ALARA. Dual-energy CT is an emerging technology that may also be useful in both attenuation correction and enhanced anatomic characterization of PET findings. In addition, optimized dual-energy CT approaches have the potential to improve quantitative PET assessment without increasing the overall CT dose.[121] Last, it has recently been noted that contrast-enhanced CT does not significantly affect the anatomic measurements of lymph node size for therapy response assessment when compared with non–contrast-enhanced/low-dose CT as a part of standard ^{18}F FDG-PET /CT assessment in lymphoma patients.[122] In terms of lymphoma, significant reductions in the doses of intravenous contrast, ^{18}F FDG, and CT radiation while maintaining diagnostic image quality and quantitative accuracy will be beneficial for patients.

New paradigms for faster and more precise PET with fluorodeoxyglucose F 18 imaging

One approach to achieve faster PET imaging is to incorporate more PET detectors rings into the z-axis of the PET gantry, which allows PET imaging using fewer PET bed positions.[123] Another approach is the use of ToF PET, which can also contribute to faster image acquisition times when compared with non-ToF PET while maintaining comparable image quality.[124,125] Over the last 4 decades, ToF PET image reconstruction has been demonstrated to be feasible[126,127] and clinically relevant.[128,129] The technical and clinical evolution of ToF PET has been previously reviewed in the literature.[130–134] Faster PET imaging helps to minimize patient motion artifacts caused by patient discomfort while lying on the imaging bed, and the need for imaging-related sedation or anesthesia. Faster PET imaging could also enable pseudodynamic imaging of specific lesions for better assessment of the lesion's pathophysiology to distinguish between benign and malignant disease. It should also be stated that ToF PET can also facilitate radiotracer dose reductions.[132] There are many other advantages with ToF PET capability and these include improved the lesion detectability, signal-to-noise ratio, image quality, precision, and accuracy of ^{18}F FDG uptake for quantification.[124,125,129,135–138] The use of ToF also contributes to significantly improved image quality in patients with higher body mass indices.[125,128,137] Again, innovations that enable faster PET imaging while maintaining comparable image quality and quantification will be beneficial for lymphoma patients.

New paradigms for higher definition PET with fluorodeoxyglucose F 18 imaging

PET imaging has been traditionally constrained to lower resolution image matrix sizes that are currently less than 200 × 200 (standard definition [SD]). For a 600-mm field of view, this size yields an axial voxel area of 3 × 3 mm^2, which is considerably lower than the default image matrix sizes used in CT of 512 × 512. Most detector geometries have an edge length of 4 mm, leading to the use of nonisotropic voxel sizes in some systems. Traditionally, smaller voxel volumes were considered not feasible in PET imaging owing to perceived higher count density requirements. This supposed constraint has been removed with the introduction of improved ToF timing resolution. A major leap forward was the introduction of solid state PET detectors and especially the ability for digital photon counting that facilitated the improvement of ToF from the 500 ps to the 300 ps range. Our team has been at the forefront to demonstrate the feasibility of high definition (HD) PET image reconstruction that, however, requires refined reconstruction approaches. Even with today's ToF PET photomultipler tube technology, HD 2 × 2 × 2 mm^3 voxel reconstruction is feasible, which substantially reduces partial volume effects in PET images and thus is highly relevant for PET imaging of malignant/metastatic lymph node disease (**Figs. 1** and **2**). Using the next-generation digital photon counting solid state PET detector technology, ultra-HD 1 × 1 × 1 mm^3 voxel volumes can be achieved enabling a highly precise visualization of small metabolically active disease with even further improved, excellent image quality (see **Figs. 1** and **2**). Thus, PET image detail is now approaching the level of CT and MR imaging that have been using higher resolving image matrices already for many years. Most important from an image quality perception, these HD reconstruction approaches substantially reduce partial volume effects and thus enable the true assessment of metabolic intensities even in small lesion and especially in heterogeneous masses. These improvements not only lead to better image quality, this more precise localization and quantification also advances the guidance for biopsy and therapy planning for radiation therapy. Most important, these advances have the opportunity to overcome the recognized limitations of current PET imaging with high quantitative variability that led to a relative disinterest of quantitative readout and the more common clinical adoption of visual referenced scores. PET imaging of lymphoma will readily benefit from HD ^{18}F FDG-PET imaging and it will not be a risky prediction that the imaging standards will rapidly change with the broader availability of the higher definition reconstructions even on current generation systems.

Image-Guided Biopsies and Interventions Using Fluorodeoxyglucose F 18

Although targeting anatomic lesions with ultrasound, CT, and MR imaging can facilitate prompt image-guided biopsy, whole body ^{18}F FDG-PET evaluation can confirm abnormal ^{18}F FDG uptake in the target lesion(s) of interest as well as excludes regions of disease involvement that might otherwise change the initial plan for tissue sampling. Given that ^{18}F FDG-PET can demonstrate malignancy in normal appearing tissues before anatomic changes as well as localize malignancy within heterogeneous tissue, the use of ^{18}F FDG-PET imaging as a guidance tool for direct tissue sampling can maximize the diagnostic accuracy of image-guided biopsies.[139–141] PET/CT has been used successfully for PET-guided targeted biopsy and tissue sampling of ^{18}F FDG–avid lymph nodes and lesions.[142,143] Furthermore, quantitative autoradiography of ^{18}F FDG–avid biopsy specimens is also feasible and may be a useful technique for verifying and localizing ^{18}F FDG uptake within the specimen.[144] [18]F FDG has also been used for the preoperative identification of malignant lymph nodes with PET imaging and subsequent radioguided resection of ^{18}F FDG–avid nodes using handheld gamma probes.[145–147] At present, there is no specific reimbursement for ^{18}F FDG-PET–guided tissue sampling in the United States.

Another approach for imaging lesions containing PET radioisotopes like ^{18}F FDG is the optical detection of Cerenkov radiation. Cerenkov radiation is produced during the process of positron emission and results in the production the visible and ultraviolet light photons.[148–150] In general, Cerenkov radiation is produced as the emitted positrons travel faster than the speed of light through the aqueous medium of the cells, tissues and organs containing ^{18}F FDG. As the positron travels through the aqueous medium, there is a disturbance of the local electromagnetic field of the water and atomic electrons within the water molecules become displaced. As the displaced electrons restore themselves to equilibrium, light photons are emitted, which can be detected using bioluminescence imaging technology. This optical detection of Cerenkov radiation is known as Cerenkov luminescence imaging[151] and detectable Cerenkov luminescence imaging has been described for medical positron-emitting radioisotopes and therapeutic beta-emitting radioisotopes.[152–154] Human Cerenkov luminescence imaging has been described using the therapeutic radioisotope iodine-131 and ^{18}F FDG[155,156] and

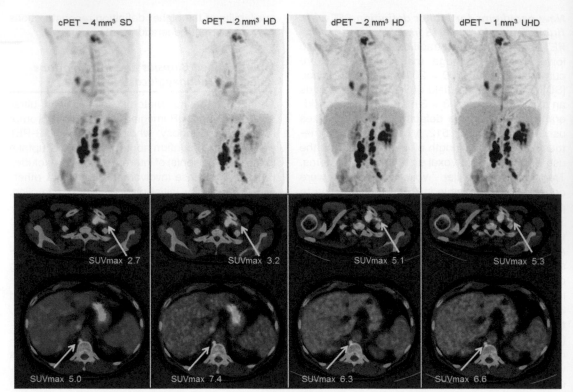

Fig. 1. Intraindividual comparison in a patient imaged using a conventional photomultiplier-tube based PET/CT (cPET; Gemini 64 ToF, Philips Healthcare, Stamford, CT) system and a precommercial release digital photon counting PET/CT (dPET; Vereos, Philips Healthcare) system with different reconstruction matrix/voxel volume sizes. The patient was intravenously administered a standard dose of 498 MBq of fluorodeoxyglucose F 18 (^{18}F FDG) and then underwent imaging on the dPET/CT system at 62 minutes and the cPET/CT system at 87 minutes after injection. Both cPET and dPET emission scans were acquired with 90 seconds per bed position. Although there are multiple ^{18}F FDG–avid lesions corresponding with enlarged lymph nodes noted in the chest and abdomen on both cPET and dPET images, there are subcentimeter nodes in the left supraclavicular and right retrocrural regions (*yellow arrows*) that are visually more apparent on dPET images and becomes more conspicuous (and more suspicious) with higher definition image reconstructions. (*Top*) Maximum intensity projection images from standard definition (SD) cPET (matrix size = 144 × 144; voxel volume = 4 × 4 × 4 mm³), high-definition (HD) cPET (matrix size = 288 × 288; voxel volume = 2 × 2 × 2 mm³), HD dPET (matrix size = 288 × 288; voxel volume = 2 × 2 × 2 mm³), and ultra-high definition (UHD) dPET (matrix size = 576 × 576; voxel volume = 1 × 1 × 1 mm³). Point spread function and Gaussian filtering was applied to both HD and UHD dPET reconstructed images but not to SD cPET or HD cPET images. (*Middle*: Axial images from SD cPET, HD cPET, HD dPET, and UHD dPET taken at the level of the node in the left supraclavicular region. (*Bottom*) Axial images from SD cPET, HD cPET, HD dPET, and UHD dPET taken at the level of the node in the right retrocrural region. This case illustrates the capability of higher definition cPET and dPET technology to radically improve lesion detectability, lesion characterization, and diagnostic confidence especially for subcentimeter lesions. SUV$_{max}$, maximum standardized uptake value.

this novel imaging approach will likely contribute to next-generation interventional/surgical imaging systems.

Big Data and the Role of PET with Fluorodeoxyglucose F 18 in the Future of Lymphoma

Routine medical imaging studies like ^{18}F FDG-PET require dedicated computational hardware and software as well as some computational time for image reconstruction of the acquired PET events into diagnostic images.[157] Despite expectations to the contrary, diagnostic ^{18}F FDG-PET images are not always immediately available for viewing and assessment when image acquisition ends. Today is the era of 'big data' and this simply refers to the continuous generation of large, complex datasets, often in different formats, which may not be easily amenable to conventional analysis or may require excessive computational time.[158] In addition, there are many scales to big data in medicine, which may range from (1) individual patient at one time point to (2) same patient at multiple time points

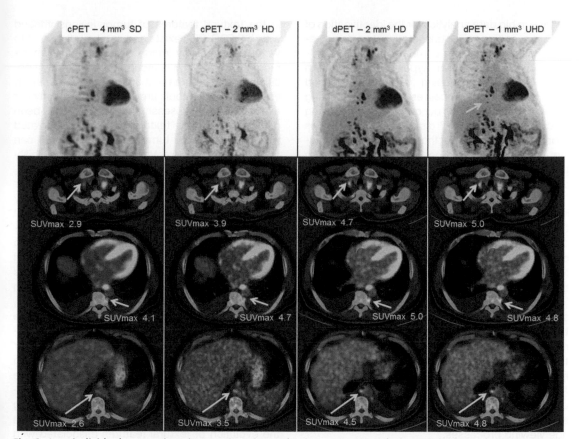

Fig. 2. Intraindividual comparison in a patient imaged using conventional photomultiplier-tube based PET/CT (cPET; Gemini 64 ToF) system and digital photon counting PET/CT (dPET; Vereos, both Philips Healthcare) system with different reconstruction matrix/voxel volume sizes. The patient was intravenously administered a standard dose of 478 MBq of fluorodeoxyglucose F 18 (^{18}F FDG) and then underwent imaging on the dPET/CT system at 53 minutes and the cPET/CT system at 81 minutes after injection. Both cPET and dPET emission scans were acquired with 90 seconds per bed position. Although there are multiple ^{18}F FDG-avid lesions corresponding with enlarged lymph nodes noted in the chest and abdomen on both cPET and dPET images, there are subcentimeter nodes in the right supraclavicular, paraaortic, and right retrocrural regions (*yellow arrows*) that are visually more conspicuous on high-definition (HD) cPET and dPET images. (*Top*) Maximum intensity projection images from standard definition (SD) cPET (matrix size = 144 × 144; voxel volume = 4 × 4 × 4 mm³), HD cPET (matrix size = 288 × 288; voxel volume = 2 × 2 × 2 mm³), HD dPET (matrix size = 288 × 288; voxel volume = 2 × 2 × 2 mm³), and ultra-high definition (UHD) dPET (matrix size =576 × 576; voxel volume = 1 × 1 × 1 mm³). Point spread function and Gaussian filtering was applied to both HD and UHD dPET reconstructed images but not to SD cPET or HD cPET images. (*Second from the top*) Axial images from SD cPET, HD cPET, HD dPET, and UHD dPET taken at the level of the node in the right supraclavicular region. (*Third from the top*) Axial images from SD cPET, HD cPET, HD dPET, and UHD dPET taken at the level of the node in the posterior paraaortic region. (*Bottom*) Axial images from SD cPET, HD cPET, HD dPET, and UHD dPET taken at the level of the node in the right retrocrural region. This case again illustrates the capability of higher definition cPET and dPET technology to improve lesion detectability, lesion characterization, and diagnostic confidence.

through his or her care to (3) subgroups of individual patients to (4) entire patient populations. With respect to medical imaging, this represents a large and ever-growing source of data as well as new opportunities for biomedical discovery.[159,160]

One challenge is that simple data searches within existing big data repositories may not even be possible without the development and support of information specialists using search or pattern recognition algorithms to identify the data of interest.[161] New methods for mining and analyzing large medical image dataset (eg, 19,000 CT images from >10,000 patients) to discover and characterize image features for specific diseases are now being described.[162] Given the existing registries and imaging data collections for various disease-specific clinical trials, there exists a tremendous opportunity for imagers to engage in big data analytics for the identification of new disease-specific quantitative imaging features, establishing new correlations between imaging and genetic phenotypes through pattern analysis, and developing new image-based models for disease processes. The use of existing trial registries to expand our current understanding of disease biology and disease management is promising, especially for those trials that are imaging intensive. Big data concepts will also inspire the development of new models for data registries and clinical trial design.[160,163,164]

To this end, the National Institutes of Health have launched the Big Data to Knowledge initiative to analyze, mine, and better understand the continuously increasing collection of biomedical data to further and generate new knowledge.[165] Many institutions and companies are embracing the future of big data in terms of local or remote 'cloud' data storage, data management, data sharing, and big data analytics and associated tool development. List-mode PET datasets may represent a very promising 'big data' source for the future advancement of our understanding of lymphoma within multiinstitutional clinical trials. At the very least, the list-mode dataset could be used to evaluate the impact of vendor-specific and vendor-neutral image reconstruction and image viewing processes.

Radiomics for PET with Fluorodeoxyglucose F 18 Assessment of Lymphoma: Challenges and Opportunities

It is notable that diagnostic images contain more information than may be used or even appreciated in routine clinical practice. When equipped with the necessary tools, this additional information can be extracted and can provide additional insight into the relevant disease process. The process of identifying, extracting and quantifying image features is known as radiomics. Radiomics promises to improve lesion characterization and perhaps even therapeutic response assessment.[166,167] In particular, textural features are used routinely for classifying images for the purposes of pattern analysis and pattern recognition. Texture analysis may someday serve as a precision nuclear medicine tool for PET in terms of segmenting tumor lesions, characterizing tumor lesions and measuring treatment response in tumor lesions. Although maximum SUV and mean SUV metrics are routinely reported for tumor lesions demonstrating ^{18}F FDG uptake, new radiomic approaches for quantitative assessment based on ^{18}F FDG-PET image features are also being investigated as potential biomarkers. It has been demonstrated that variability

in the textural features of tumor lesions imaged with ^{18}F FDG-PET exists and can be influenced to various degrees by image acquisition and image reconstruction.[168] It is incumbent to identify specific textural features that are most prone to error, especially if such tools are used for quantitative or even response assessment. It has also been demonstrated that textural features associated with heterogeneous tumors on ^{18}F FDG-PET can be consistently characterized with reproducibility better than standard SUV metrics for such tumors.[169–171] Likewise, some textural features for ^{18}F FDG-PET demonstrate high test–retest stability as well as high interobserver stability.[166] Given that image feature variability depends on image acquisition and image reconstruction, any attempt to assess ^{18}F FDG-PET image features as potential biomarkers within multiinstitutional clinical trials will necessitate appropriate standardization in terms of image acquisition, image reconstruction, and lesion analysis.[172–174] It also remains to be determined whether or not radiomic tools developed for ^{18}F FDG can be effectively used for different fluorine-18–labeled tumor-targeting agents or other PET-based imaging agents like carbon-11 and gallium-68.[175] It will be tremendously insightful for future preclinical studies using orthotopic tumor models to assess and describe the evolution of textural features associated with ^{18}F FDG–avid tumors throughout the natural progression of tumor development and subsequently during therapy. It is conceivable that radiomic evaluation of image features associated with different lymphoma subtypes on a very large scale may elucidate new biological processes and insights into disease management.

Continued Need for PET with Fluorodeoxyglucose F 18 Harmonization Within Clinical Trials

Quantitative assessment of ^{18}F FDG-PET studies using SUV depends on image acquisition, image reconstruction, and region of interest analysis, which can vary between institutions. For multiinstitutional clinical trials, standardization of acquisition, reconstruction, and analysis is essential to minimize differences in SUV quantification for the purposes of response assessment to various therapies.[176,177] In addition, standardized phantom-based imaging can also help to establish correction factors for SUV quantification between institutions[178] and such methods for multiinstitutional standardization for ^{18}F FDG-PET imaging have been successfully implemented.[179,180] Furthermore, new methodologies for ^{18}F FDG-PET standardization among institutions have been described to maximize the robustness of quantitative SUV metrics.[181] It should also be stressed that as new fluorine-18 or other PET-based tumor-targeting agents are developed, there remains a critical need to establish standardization methodologies for each of these agents for multi-institutional clinical trials.[182] It has also been demonstrated that new reconstruction approaches and methodologies (eg, ToF, point-spread function), which help to maximize lesion detectability for ^{18}F FDG-PET studies do not prevent subsequent standardization and harmonization for quantitative SUV assessment.[183–185]

SUMMARY

The treatment of lymphoma is complex and necessitates close collaboration among various medical specialties, including nuclear medicine, diagnostic and interventional radiology, medical oncology, radiation oncology, surgical oncology, and pathology. Over the last 4 decades, PET technology has rapidly advanced and evolved whereas the role of ^{18}F FDG as the primary PET radiotracer has not changed. There are current challenges and several opportunities to advance ^{18}F FDG-PET from a standard clinical nuclear medicine modality for lymphoma into a precision nuclear medicine platform. As new targeted therapeutic agents are developed and approved for clinical use in lymphoma, there will likely be a need for the concurrent development of companion diagnostic tests and imaging agents, which will help to identify and stratify which subgroup of patients will most likely respond to such therapies. Precision nuclear medicine can help to rapidly identify specific tumor targets in the body, quantify the overall burden of tumor disease, assess the pharmacokinetics of tumor and background tissue uptake, and assess for altered and unanticipated biodistribution while minimizing patient-related toxicities and radiation exposure.

REFERENCES

1. Lister TA, Crowther D, Sutcliffe SB, et al. Report of a committee convened to discuss the evaluation and staging of patients with Hodgkin's disease: Cotswolds meeting. J Clin Oncol 1989;7(11):1630–6.
2. Weisenburger DD, Savage KJ, Harris NL, et al. Peripheral T-cell lymphoma, not otherwise specified: a report of 340 cases from the International Peripheral T-cell Lymphoma Project. Blood 2011; 117(12):3402–8.
3. Mead GM, Sydes MR, Walewski J, et al. An international evaluation of CODOX-M and CODOX-M alternating with IVAC in adult Burkitt's lymphoma: results of United Kingdom Lymphoma Group LY06 study. Ann Oncol 2002;13(8):1264–74.
4. Sehn LH, Berry B, Chhanabhai M, et al. The revised International Prognostic Index (R-IPI) is a better predictor of outcome than the standard IPI for patients with diffuse large B-cell lymphoma treated with R-CHOP. Blood 2007;109(5):1857–61.
5. Solal-Celigny P, Roy P, Colombat P, et al. Follicular lymphoma International Prognostic Index. Blood 2004;104(5):1258–65.
6. Hasenclever D, Diehl V. A prognostic score for advanced Hodgkin's disease. International prognostic factors project on advanced Hodgkin's disease. N Engl J Med 1998;339(21):1506–14.
7. Bangerter M, Moog F, Buchmann I, et al. Whole-body 2-[18F]-fluoro-2-deoxy-D-glucose positron emission tomography (FDG-PET) for accurate staging of Hodgkin's disease. Ann Oncol 1998; 9(10):1117–22.
8. Buchmann I, Reinhardt M, Elsner K, et al. 2-(fluorine-18)fluoro-2-deoxy-D-glucose positron emission tomography in the detection and staging of malignant lymphoma. A bicenter trial. Cancer 2001;91(5):889–99.
9. Wirth A, Seymour JF, Hicks RJ, et al. Fluorine-18 fluorodeoxyglucose positron emission tomography, gallium-67 scintigraphy, and conventional staging for Hodgkin's disease and non-Hodgkin's lymphoma. Am J Med 2002;112(4):262–8.
10. Weihrauch MR, Re D, Bischoff S, et al. Whole-body positron emission tomography using 18F-fluorodeoxyglucose for initial staging of patients with Hodgkin's disease. Ann Hematol 2002;81(1):20–5.
11. Menzel C, Dobert N, Mitrou P, et al. Positron emission tomography for the staging of Hodgkin's lymphoma–increasing the body of evidence in favor of the method. Acta Oncol 2002;41(5):430–6.
12. Hutchings M, Loft A, Hansen M, et al. Position emission tomography with or without computed tomography in the primary staging of Hodgkin's lymphoma. Haematologica 2006;91(4):482–9.
13. Jerusalem G, Beguin Y, Fassotte MF, et al. Whole-body positron emission tomography using 18F-fluorodeoxyglucose compared to standard procedures for staging patients with Hodgkin's disease. Haematologica 2001;86(3):266–73.
14. Partridge S, Timothy A, O'Doherty MJ, et al. 2-Fluorine-18-fluoro-2-deoxy-D glucose positron emission tomography in the pretreatment staging of Hodgkin's disease: influence on patient management in a single institution. Ann Oncol 2000; 11(10):1273–9.
15. Le Dortz L, De Guibert S, Bayat S, et al. Diagnostic and prognostic impact of 18F-FDG PET/CT in follicular lymphoma. Eur J Nucl Med Mol Imaging 2010; 37(12):2307–14.

16. Wirth A, Foo M, Seymour JF, et al. Impact of [18f] fluorodeoxyglucose positron emission tomography on staging and management of early-stage follicular non-Hodgkin lymphoma. Int J Radiat Oncol Biol Phys 2008;71(1):213–9.

17. A clinical evaluation of the International Lymphoma Study Group classification of non-Hodgkin's lymphoma. The Non-Hodgkin's Lymphoma Classification Project. Blood 1997;89(11):3909–18.

18. Newman JS, Francis IR, Kaminski MS, et al. Imaging of lymphoma with PET with 2-[F-18]-fluoro-2-deoxy-D-glucose: correlation with CT. Radiology 1994;190(1):111–6.

19. Thill R, Neuerburg J, Fabry U, et al. Comparison of findings with 18-FDG PET and CT in pretherapeutic staging of malignant lymphoma. Nuklearmedizin 1997;36(7):234–9 [in German].

20. Jerusalem G, Beguin Y, Najjar F, et al. Positron emission tomography (PET) with 18F-fluorodeoxyglucose (18F-FDG) for the staging of low-grade non-Hodgkin's lymphoma (NHL). Ann Oncol 2001; 12(6):825–30.

21. Schaefer NG, Hany TF, Taverna C, et al. Non-Hodgkin lymphoma and Hodgkin disease: coregistered FDG PET and CT at staging and restaging–do we need contrast-enhanced CT? Radiology 2004; 232(3):823–9.

22. Pelosi E, Pregno P, Penna D, et al. Role of whole-body [18F] fluorodeoxyglucose positron emission tomography/computed tomography (FDG-PET/CT) and conventional techniques in the staging of patients with Hodgkin and aggressive non Hodgkin lymphoma. Radiol Med 2008;113(4):578–90.

23. Pakos EE, Fotopoulos AD, Ioannidis JP. 18F-FDG PET for evaluation of bone marrow infiltration in staging of lymphoma: a meta-analysis. J Nucl Med 2005;46(6):958–63.

24. Held G, Zeynalova S, Murawski N, et al. Impact of rituximab and radiotherapy on outcome of patients with aggressive B-cell lymphoma and skeletal involvement. J Clin Oncol 2013;31(32):4115–22.

25. Rodriguez M, Rehn S, Ahlstrom H, et al. Predicting malignancy grade with PET in non-Hodgkin's lymphoma. J Nucl Med 1995;36(10):1790–6.

26. Tsukamoto N, Kojima M, Hasegawa M, et al. The usefulness of (18)F-fluorodeoxyglucose positron emission tomography ((18)F-FDG-PET) and a comparison of (18)F-FDG-pet with (67)gallium scintigraphy in the evaluation of lymphoma: relation to histologic subtypes based on the World Health Organization classification. Cancer 2007; 110(3):652–9.

27. Schoder H, Noy A, Gonen M, et al. Intensity of 18fluorodeoxyglucose uptake in positron emission tomography distinguishes between indolent and aggressive non-Hodgkin's lymphoma. J Clin Oncol 2005;23(21):4643–51.

28. Watanabe R, Tomita N, Takeuchi K, et al. SUVmax in FDG-PET at the biopsy site correlates with the proliferation potential of tumor cells in non-Hodgkin lymphoma. Leuk Lymphoma 2010;51(2):279–83.

29. Noy A, Schoder H, Gonen M, et al. The majority of transformed lymphomas have high standardized uptake values (SUVs) on positron emission tomography (PET) scanning similar to diffuse large B-cell lymphoma (DLBCL). Ann Oncol 2009;20(3):508–12.

30. Uni M, Nakamura F, Yoshimi A, et al. Transformation of follicular lymphoma in the retroperitoneal muscles demonstrated by CT-guided needle biopsy of FDG-avid lesions; case series. Int J Clin Exp Pathol 2014;7(1):402–6.

31. Bodet-Milin C, Kraeber-Bodere F, Moreau P, et al. Investigation of FDG-PET/CT imaging to guide biopsies in the detection of histological transformation of indolent lymphoma. Haematologica 2008; 93(3):471–2.

32. Kostakoglu L, Coleman M, Leonard JP, et al. PET predicts prognosis after 1 cycle of chemotherapy in aggressive lymphoma and Hodgkin's disease. J Nucl Med 2002;43(8):1018–27.

33. Cahu X, Bodet-Milin C, Brissot E, et al. 18F-fluorodeoxyglucose-positron emission tomography before, during and after treatment in mature T/NK lymphomas: a study from the GOELAMS group. Ann Oncol 2011;22(3):705–11.

34. Friedberg JW, Fischman A, Neuberg D, et al. FDG-PET is superior to gallium scintigraphy in staging and more sensitive in the follow-up of patients with de novo Hodgkin lymphoma: a blinded comparison. Leuk Lymphoma 2004; 45(1):85–92.

35. Gallamini A, Barrington SF, Biggi A, et al. The predictive role of interim positron emission tomography for Hodgkin lymphoma treatment outcome is confirmed using the interpretation criteria of the Deauville five-point scale. Haematologica 2014; 99(6):1107–13.

36. Zinzani PL, Rigacci L, Stefoni V, et al. Early interim 18F-FDG PET in Hodgkin's lymphoma: evaluation on 304 patients. Eur J Nucl Med Mol Imaging 2012;39(1):4–12.

37. Meyer RM, Gospodarowicz MK, Connors JM, et al. ABVD alone versus radiation-based therapy in limited-stage Hodgkin's lymphoma. N Engl J Med 2012;366(5):399–408.

38. Raemaekers JM, Andre MP, Federico M, et al. Omitting radiotherapy in early positron emission tomography-negative stage I/II Hodgkin lymphoma is associated with an increased risk of early relapse: clinical results of the preplanned interim analysis of the randomized EORTC/LYSA/FIL H10 trial. J Clin Oncol 2014;32(12):1188–94.

39. Radford J, Illidge T, Counsell N, et al. Results of a trial of PET-directed therapy for early-stage Hodgkin's lymphoma. N Engl J Med 2015;372(17): 1598–607.

40. Engert A, Haverkamp H, Kobe C, et al. Reduced-intensity chemotherapy and PET-guided radiotherapy in patients with advanced stage Hodgkin's lymphoma (HD15 trial): a randomised, open-label, phase 3 non-inferiority trial. Lancet 2012; 379(9828):1791–9.

41. Savage KJ, Connors JM, Villa DR, et al. Advanced stage classical Hodgkin lymphoma patients with a negative PET-scan following treatment with ABVD have excellent outcomes without the need for consolidative radiotherapy regardless of disease bulk at presentation. Orlando (FL): American Society of Hematology; 2015.

42. Avigdor A, Bulvik S, Levi I, et al. Two cycles of escalated BEACOPP followed by four cycles of ABVD utilizing early-interim PET/CT scan is an effective regimen for advanced high-risk Hodgkin's lymphoma. Ann Oncol 2010;21(1):126–32.

43. Casasnovas O, Brice P, Bouabdallah R, et al. Randomized phase III study comparing an early PET driven treatment De-escalation to a Not PET-monitored strategy in patients with advanced stages Hodgkin lymphoma: interim analysis of the AHL2011 Lysa Study. Orlando (FL): American Society of Hematology; 2015.

44. Schoder H, Gerecitano JF, Hamlin P, et al. FDG-PET adapted sequential therapy with Brentuximab Vedotin and augmented ICE followed by autologous stem cell transplant for relapsed and refractory Hodgkin lymphoma. Blood 2013;122(21):2099.

45. Gallamini A, Rossi A, Patti C, et al. Early treatment intensification in advanced-stage high-risk Hodgkin lymphoma (HL) patients, with a positive FDG-PET scan after two ABVD courses – first interim analysis of the GITIL/FIL HD0607 clinical trial. Atlanta (GA): American Society of Hematology; 2012.

46. Straus DJ, Pitcher B, Kostakoglu L, et al. Initial results of US Intergroup trial of response-adapted chemotherapy or chemotherapy/radiation therapy based on PET for non-bulky stage I and II Hodgkin lymphoma (HL) (CALGB/Alliance 50604). Orlando (FL): American Society of Hematology; 2015.

47. Zinzani PL, Broccoli A, Gioia DM, et al. Interim positron emission tomography response-adapted therapy in advanced-stage Hodgkin lymphoma: final results of the phase II part of the HD0801 Study. J Clin Oncol 2016;34(12):1376–85.

48. Viviani S, Zinzani PL, Rambaldi A, et al. ABVD versus BEACOPP for Hodgkin's lymphoma when high-dose salvage is planned. N Engl J Med 2011;365(3):203–12.

49. Mikhaeel NG, Timothy AR, O'Doherty MJ, et al. 18-FDG-PET as a prognostic indicator in the treatment of aggressive Non-Hodgkin's lymphoma-comparison with CT. Leuk Lymphoma 2000;39(5–6):543–53.

50. Sehn LH, Savage KJ, Hoskins P, et al. Treatment of limited-stage DLBCL can be effectively tailored using a PET-based approach. Ann Oncol 2011;22: 90–1.

51. Lamy T, Damaj G, Gyan E, et al. R-CHOP with or without radiotherapy in non-bulky limited-stage diffuse large B cell lymphoma (DLBCL): preliminary results of the prospective randomized phase III 02–03 trial from the Lysa/Goelams Group. San Francisco (CA): American Society of Hematology; 2014.

52. Haioun C, Itti E, Rahmouni A, et al. [18F]fluoro-2-deoxy-D-glucose positron emission tomography (FDG-PET) in aggressive lymphoma: an early prognostic tool for predicting patient outcome. Blood 2005;106(4):1376–81.

53. Kostakoglu L, Goldsmith SJ, Leonard JP, et al. FDG-PET after 1 cycle of therapy predicts outcome in diffuse large cell lymphoma and classic Hodgkin disease. Cancer 2006;107(11):2678–87.

54. Spaepen K, Stroobants S, Dupont P, et al. Early restaging positron emission tomography with (18)F-fluorodeoxyglucose predicts outcome in patients with aggressive non-Hodgkin's lymphoma. Ann Oncol 2002;13(9):1356–63.

55. Safar V, Dupuis J, Itti E, et al. Interim [18F]fluorodeoxyglucose positron emission tomography scan in diffuse large B-cell lymphoma treated with anthracycline-based chemotherapy plus rituximab. J Clin Oncol 2012;30(2):184–90.

56. Kasamon YL, Wahl RL, Ziessman HA, et al. Phase II study of risk-adapted therapy of newly diagnosed, aggressive non-Hodgkin lymphoma based on midtreatment FDG-PET scanning. Biol Blood Marrow Transplant 2009;15(2):242–8.

57. Hertzberg MS, Gandhi MK, Butcher B, et al. Early treatment intensification with R-ICE chemotherapy followed by autologous stem cell transplantation (ASCT) using Zevalin-BEAM for patients with poor risk diffuse large B-cell lymphoma (DLBCL) as identified by interim PET/CT scan performed after four cycles of R-CHOP-14: a multicenter phase II study of the Australasian Leukaemia Lymphoma Study Group (ALLG). 57th Annual Meeting of the American Society of Hematology. Orlando, Florida, December 5–8, 2015.

58. Micallef IN, Maurer MJ, Wiseman GA, et al. Epratuzumab with rituximab, cyclophosphamide, doxorubicin, vincristine, and prednisone chemotherapy in patients with previously untreated diffuse large B-cell lymphoma. Blood 2011;118(15):4053–61.

59. Terasawa T, Lau J, Bardet S, et al. Fluorine-18-fluorodeoxyglucose positron emission tomography for interim response assessment of advanced-stage

Hodgkin's lymphoma and diffuse large B-cell lymphoma: a systematic review. J Clin Oncol 2009; 27(11):1906–14.

60. Cashen AF, Dehdashti F, Luo J, et al. 18F-FDG PET/CT for early response assessment in diffuse large B-cell lymphoma: poor predictive value of international harmonization project interpretation. J Nucl Med 2011;52(3):386–92.

61. Mamot C, Klingbiel D, Hitz F, et al. Final results of a prospective evaluation of the predictive value of interim positron emission tomography in patients with diffuse large B-cell lymphoma treated with R-CHOP-14 (SAKK 38/07). J Clin Oncol 2015; 33(23):2523–9.

62. Moskowitz CH, Schoder H, Teruya-Feldstein J, et al. Risk-adapted dose-dense immunochemotherapy determined by interim FDG-PET in advanced-stage diffuse large B-Cell lymphoma. J Clin Oncol 2010;28(11):1896–903.

63. Han HS, Escalon MP, Hsiao B, et al. High incidence of false-positive PET scans in patients with aggressive non-Hodgkin's lymphoma treated with rituximab-containing regimens. Ann Oncol 2009; 20(2):309–18.

64. Spaepen K, Stroobants S, Dupont P, et al. Prognostic value of positron emission tomography (PET) with fluorine-18 fluorodeoxyglucose ([18F]FDG) after first-line chemotherapy in non-Hodgkin's lymphoma: is [18F]FDG-PET a valid alternative to conventional diagnostic methods? J Clin Oncol 2001;19(2):414–9.

65. Spaepen K, Stroobants S, Dupont P, et al. Can positron emission tomography with [(18)F]-fluorodeoxyglucose after first-line treatment distinguish Hodgkin's disease patients who need additional therapy from others in whom additional therapy would mean avoidable toxicity? Br J Haematol 2001;115(2):272–8.

66. Jerusalem G, Beguin Y, Fassotte MF, et al. Whole-body positron emission tomography using 18F-fluorodeoxyglucose for posttreatment evaluation in Hodgkin's disease and non-Hodgkin's lymphoma has higher diagnostic and prognostic value than classical computed tomography scan imaging. Blood 1999;94(2):429–33.

67. Naumann R, Vaic A, Beuthien-Baumann B, et al. Prognostic value of positron emission tomography in the evaluation of post-treatment residual mass in patients with Hodgkin's disease and non-Hodgkin's lymphoma. Br J Haematol 2001; 115(4):793–800.

68. Visco C, Finotto S, Zambello R, et al. Combination of rituximab, bendamustine, and cytarabine for patients with mantle-cell non-Hodgkin lymphoma ineligible for intensive regimens or autologous transplantation. J Clin Oncol 2013;31(11): 1442–9.

69. Jerusalem G, Warland V, Najjar F, et al. Whole-body 18F-FDG PET for the evaluation of patients with Hodgkin's disease and non-Hodgkin's lymphoma. Nucl Med Commun 1999;20(1):13–20.

70. Stumpe KD, Urbinelli M, Steinert HC, et al. Whole-body positron emission tomography using fluorodeoxyglucose for staging of lymphoma: effectiveness and comparison with computed tomography. Eur J Nucl Med 1998;25(7):721–8.

71. Evens AM, Kanakry JA, Sehn LH, et al. Gray zone lymphoma with features intermediate between classical Hodgkin lymphoma and diffuse large B-cell lymphoma: characteristics, outcomes, and prognostication among a large multicenter cohort. Am J Hematol 2015;90(9):778–83.

72. Wilson WH, Pittaluga S, Nicolae A, et al. A prospective study of mediastinal gray-zone lymphoma. Blood 2014;124(10):1563–9.

73. Jerusalem G, Beguin Y, Fassotte MF, et al. Early detection of relapse by whole-body positron emission tomography in the follow-up of patients with Hodgkin's disease. Ann Oncol 2003;14(1): 123–30.

74. von Tresckow B, Plutschow A, Fuchs M, et al. Dose-intensification in early unfavorable Hodgkin's lymphoma: final analysis of the German Hodgkin Study Group HD14 trial. J Clin Oncol 2012;30(9): 907–13.

75. Allen-Auerbach M, de Vos S, Czernin J. The impact of fluorodeoxyglucose-positron emission tomography in primary staging and patient management in lymphoma patients. Radiol Clin North Am 2008; 46(2):199–211, vii.

76. Poeppel TD, Krause BJ, Heusner TA, et al. PET/CT for the staging and follow-up of patients with malignancies. Eur J Radiol 2009;70(3):382–92.

77. Baba S, Abe K, Isoda T, et al. Impact of FDG-PET/CT in the management of lymphoma. Ann Nucl Med 2011;25(10):701–16.

78. Cheson BD. Role of functional imaging in the management of lymphoma. J Clin Oncol 2011;29(14): 1844–54.

79. Facey K, Bradbury I, Laking G, et al. Overview of the clinical effectiveness of positron emission tomography imaging in selected cancers. Health Technol Assess 2007;11(44):iii–iv. xi-267.

80. Barrington SF, Kirkwood AA, Franceschetto A, et al. PET-CT for staging and early response: results from the response-adapted therapy in advanced Hodgkin lymphoma study. Blood 2016; 127(12):1531–8.

81. El Fakhri G, Santos PA, Badawi RD, et al. Impact of acquisition geometry, image processing, and patient size on lesion detection in whole-body 18F-FDG PET. J Nucl Med 2007;48(12):1951–60.

82. Lartizien C, Kinahan PE, Comtat C. A lesion detection observer study comparing 2-dimensional

versus fully 3-dimensional whole-body PET imaging protocols. J Nucl Med 2004;45(4):714–23.

83. Schaefferkoetter JD, Yan J, Townsend DW, et al. Initial assessment of image quality for low-dose PET: evaluation of lesion detectability. Phys Med Biol 2015;60(14):5543–56.

84. Liu Y, Ghesani NV, Zuckier LS. Physiology and pathophysiology of incidental findings detected on FDG-PET scintigraphy. Semin Nucl Med 2010; 40(4):294–315.

85. Metser U, Even-Sapir E. Increased (18)F-fluoro-deoxyglucose uptake in benign, nonphysiologic lesions found on whole-body positron emission tomography/computed tomography (PET/CT): accumulated data from four years of experience with PET/CT. Semin Nucl Med 2007;37(3):206–22.

86. Cohade C. Altered biodistribution on FDG-PET with emphasis on brown fat and insulin effect. Semin Nucl Med 2010;40(4):283–93.

87. Visvikis D, Ell PJ. Impact of technology on the utilisation of positron emission tomography in lymphoma: current and future perspectives. Eur J Nucl Med Mol Imaging 2003;30(Suppl 1):S106–16.

88. Pichler BJ, Judenhofer MS, Catana C, et al. Performance test of an LSO-APD detector in a 7-T MRI scanner for simultaneous PET/MRI. J Nucl Med 2006;47(4):639–47.

89. Solf T, Schulz V, Weissler B, et al. Solid-state detector stack for ToF-PET/MR. 2009 IEEE nuclear science symposium conference record, vols. 1-5. Orlando, FL, October 24 – November 1, 2009. p. 2798–99.

90. Judenhofer MS, Wehrl HF, Newport DF, et al. Simultaneous PET-MRI: a new approach for functional and morphological imaging. Nat Med 2008;14(4): 459–65.

91. Spick C, Herrmann K, Czernin J. 18F-FDG PET/CT and PET/MRI perform equally well in cancer: evidence from studies on more than 2,300 patients. J Nucl Med 2016;57(3):420–30.

92. Jones T, Budinger TF. The potential for low-dose functional studies in maternal-fetal medicine using PET/MR imaging. J Nucl Med 2013;54(11):2016–7.

93. Sher AC, Seghers V, Paldino MJ, et al. Assessment of sequential PET/MRI in comparison with PET/CT of pediatric lymphoma: a prospective study. AJR Am J Roentgenol 2016;206(3):623–31.

94. Degenhardt C, Rodrigues P, Trindade A, et al. Performance evaluation of a prototype positron emission tomography scanner using digital photon counters (DPC). 2012 IEEE Nuclear Science Symposium and Medical Imaging Conference Record (Nss/Mic). Anaheim, CA, October 27 – November 3, 2012. p. 2820–24.

95. Degenhardt C, Driessen H. Silicon photomultiplier technology goes fully digital. Laser Focus World 2011;47(1):83–5.

96. Degenhardt C, Zwaans B, Frach T, et al. Arrays of digital silicon photomultipliers - intrinsic performance and application to Scintillator Readout. 2010 IEEE Nuclear Science Symposium Conference Record (Nss/Mic). Knoxville, TN, October 30 – November 6, 2010. p. 1954–56.

97. Frach T, Prescher G, Degenhardt C, Zwaans B. The digital silicon photomultiplier - system architecture and performance evaluation. 2010 IEEE Nuclear Science Symposium Conference Record (Nss/ Mic). Knoxville, TN, October 30 – November 6, 2010. p. 1722–27.

98. Degenhardt C, Prescher G, Frach T, et al. The digital silicon photomultiplier - a novel sensor for the detection of scintillation light. 2009 IEEE Nuclear Science Symposium Conference Record, Vols. 1-5. Orlando, FL, October 24 – November 1, 2009. p. 2383–86.

99. Nguyen NC, Vercher-Conejero JL, Sattar A, et al. Image quality and diagnostic performance of a digital PET prototype in patients with oncologic diseases: initial experience and comparison with analog PET. J Nucl Med 2015;56(9):1378–85.

100. Schug D, Wehner J, Dueppenbecker PM, et al. PET performance and MRI compatibility evaluation of a digital, ToF-capable PET/MRI insert equipped with clinical scintillators. Phys Med Biol 2015;60(18): 7045–67.

101. Wehner J, Weissler B, Dueppenbecker PM, et al. MR-compatibility assessment of the first preclinical PET-MRI insert equipped with digital silicon photomultipliers. Phys Med Biol 2015;60(6):2231–55.

102. Weissler B, Gebhardt P, Dueppenbecker PM, et al. A digital preclinical PET/MRI insert and initial results. IEEE Trans Med Imaging 2015;34(11):2258–70.

103. Adams MC, Turkington TG, Wilson JM, et al. A systematic review of the factors affecting accuracy of SUV measurements. AJR Am J Roentgenol 2010;195(2):310–20.

104. Jaskowiak CJ, Bianco JA, Perlman SB, et al. Influence of reconstruction iterations on 18F-FDG PET/CT standardized uptake values. J Nucl Med 2005;46(3):424–8.

105. Basu S, Alavi A. Partial volume correction of standardized uptake values and the dual time point in FDG-PET imaging: should these be routinely employed in assessing patients with cancer? Eur J Nucl Med Mol Imaging 2007;34(10):1527–9.

106. Tong S, Alessio AM, Kinahan PE. Evaluation of noise properties in PSF-based PET image reconstruction. IEEE Nucl Sci Symp Conf Rec (1997) 2009; 2009(2009):3042–7.

107. Lasnon C, Hicks RJ, Beauregard JM, et al. Impact of point spread function reconstruction on thoracic lymph node staging with 18F-FDG PET/CT in non-small cell lung cancer. Clin Nucl Med 2012; 37(10):971–6.

108. Akamatsu G, Ishikawa K, Mitsumoto K, et al. Improvement in PET/CT image quality with a combination of point-spread function and time-of-flight in relation to reconstruction parameters. J Nucl Med 2012;53(11):1716–22.

109. Akamatsu G, Mitsumoto K, Ishikawa K, et al. Benefits of point-spread function and time of flight for PET/CT image quality in relation to the body mass index and injected dose. Clin Nucl Med 2013; 38(6):407–12.

110. Taniguchi T, Akamatsu G, Kasahara Y, et al. Improvement in PET/CT image quality in overweight patients with PSF and TOF. Ann Nucl Med 2015;29(1):71–7.

111. Schoder H, Erdi YE, Chao K, et al. Clinical implications of different image reconstruction parameters for interpretation of whole-body PET studies in cancer patients. J Nucl Med 2004;45(4):559–66.

112. Chen MK, Menard DH 3rd, Cheng DW. Determining the minimal required radioactivity of 18F-FDG for reliable semiquantification in PET/CT imaging: a Phantom study. J Nucl Med Technol 2016;44(1):26–30.

113. Lartizien C, Comtat C, Kinahan PE, et al. Optimization of injected dose based on noise equivalent count rates for 2- and 3-dimensional whole-body PET. J Nucl Med 2002;43(9):1268–78.

114. Freedenberg MI, Badawi RD, Tarantal AF, et al. Performance and limitations of positron emission tomography (PET) scanners for imaging very low activity sources. Phys Med 2014;30(1):104–10.

115. Nogueira SA, Dimenstein R, Cunha ML, et al. Low-dose radiation protocol using 3D mode in a BGO PET/CT. Radiol Med 2015;120(2):251–5.

116. Surti S, Karp JS. Impact of detector design on imaging performance of a long axial field-of-view, whole-body PET scanner. Phys Med Biol 2015; 60(13):5343–58.

117. Oehmigen M, Ziegler S, Jakoby BW, et al. Radiotracer dose reduction in integrated PET/MR: implications from national electrical manufacturers association phantom studies. J Nucl Med 2014; 55(8):1361–7.

118. Eldib M, Bini J, Lairez O, et al. Feasibility of (18)F-Fluorodeoxyglucose radiotracer dose reduction in simultaneous carotid PET/MR imaging. Am J Nucl Med Mol Imaging 2015;5(4):401–7.

119. Gatidis S, Wurslin C, Seith F, et al. Towards tracer dose reduction in PET studies: simulation of dose reduction by retrospective randomized undersampling of list-mode data. Hell J Nucl Med 2016;19(1):15–8.

120. Rui X, Cheng L, Long Y, et al. Ultra-low dose CT attenuation correction for PET/CT: analysis of sparse view data acquisition and reconstruction algorithms. Phys Med Biol 2015;60(19): 7437–60.

121. Xia T, Alessio AM, Kinahan PE. Dual energy CT for attenuation correction with PET/CT. Med Phys 2014;41(1):012501.

122. Simpson WL Jr, Lee KM, Sosa N, et al. Lymph nodes can accurately be measured on PET-CT for lymphoma staging/restaging without a concomitant contrast enhanced CT scan. Leuk Lymphoma 2016;57(5):1083–93.

123. Akamatsu G, Uba K, Taniguchi T, et al. Impact of time-of-flight PET/CT with a large axial field of view for reducing whole-body acquisition time. J Nucl Med Technol 2014;42(2):101–4.

124. Surti S, Karp JS, Popescu LM, et al. Investigation of time-of-flight benefit for fully 3-D PET. IEEE Trans Med Imaging 2006;25(5):529–38.

125. Surti S, Karp JS. Experimental evaluation of a simple lesion detection task with time-of-flight PET. Phys Med Biol 2009;54(2):373–84.

126. Mullani NA, Markham J, Ter-Pogossian MM. Feasibility of time-of-flight reconstruction in positron emission tomography. J Nucl Med 1980;21(11):1095–7.

127. Mallon A, Grangeat P. Three-dimensional PET reconstruction with time-of-flight measurement. Phys Med Biol 1992;37(3):717–29.

128. Surti S, Kuhn A, Werner ME, et al. Performance of Philips Gemini TF PET/CT scanner with special consideration for its time-of-flight imaging capabilities. J Nucl Med 2007;48(3):471–80.

129. Karp JS, Surti S, Daube-Witherspoon ME, et al. Benefit of time-of-flight in PET: experimental and clinical results. J Nucl Med 2008;49(3):462–70.

130. Lewellen TK. Time-of-flight PET. Semin Nucl Med 1998;28(3):268–75.

131. Conti M. State of the art and challenges of time-of-flight PET. Phys Med 2009;25(1):1–11.

132. Conti M. Focus on time-of-flight PET: the benefits of improved time resolution. Eur J Nucl Med Mol Imaging 2011;38(6):1147–57.

133. Surti S. Update on time-of-flight PET imaging. J Nucl Med 2015;56(1):98–105.

134. Surti S, Karp JS. Advances in time-of-flight PET. Phys Med 2016;32(1):12–22.

135. Daube-Witherspoon ME, Surti S, Perkins AE, et al. Determination of accuracy and precision of lesion uptake measurements in human subjects with time-of-flight PET. J Nucl Med 2014; 55(4):602–7.

136. Ter-Pogossian MM, Mullani NA, Ficke DC, et al. Photon time-of-flight-assisted positron emission tomography. J Comput Assist Tomogr 1981;5(2):227–39.

137. Surti S, Scheuermann J, El Fakhri G, et al. Impact of time-of-flight PET on whole-body oncologic studies: a human observer lesion detection and localization study. J Nucl Med 2011;52(5):712–9.

138. El Fakhri G, Surti S, Trott CM, et al. Improvement in lesion detection with whole-body oncologic time-of-flight PET. J Nucl Med 2011;52(3):347–53.

139. Kobayashi K, Bhargava P, Raja S, et al. Image-guided biopsy: what the interventional radiologist needs to know about PET/CT. Radiographics 2012;32(5):1483–501.

140. Nguyen ML, Gervais DA, Blake MA, et al. Imaging-guided biopsy of (18)F-FDG-avid extrapulmonary lesions: do lesion location and morphologic features on CT affect the positive predictive value for malignancy? AJR Am J Roentgenol 2013;201(2): 433–8.

141. Paparo F, Piccazzo R, Cevasco L, et al. Advantages of percutaneous abdominal biopsy under PET-CT/ultrasound fusion imaging guidance: a pictorial essay. Abdom Imaging 2014;39(5):1102–13.

142. Tatli S, Gerbaudo VH, Feeley CM, et al. PET/CT-guided percutaneous biopsy of abdominal masses: initial experience. J Vasc Interv Radiol 2011;22(4):507–14.

143. Solomon SB, Cornelis F. Interventional molecular imaging. J Nucl Med 2016;57(4):493–6.

144. Fanchon LM, Dogan S, Moreira AL, et al. Feasibility of in situ, high-resolution correlation of tracer uptake with histopathology by quantitative autoradiography of biopsy specimens obtained under 18F-FDG PET/CT guidance. J Nucl Med 2015; 56(4):538–44.

145. Cohn DE, Hall NC, Povoski SP, et al. Novel perioperative imaging with 18F-FDG PET/CT and intraoperative 18F-FDG detection using a handheld gamma probe in recurrent ovarian cancer. Gynecol Oncol 2008;110(2):152–7.

146. Povoski SP, Hall NC, Murrey DA Jr, et al. Multimodal imaging and detection approach to 18F-FDG-directed surgery for patients with known or suspected malignancies: a comprehensive description of the specific methodology utilized in a single-institution cumulative retrospective experience. World J Surg Oncol 2011;9:152.

147. Povoski SP, Hall NC, Murrey DA Jr, et al. Feasibility of a multimodal (18)F-FDG-directed lymph node surgical excisional biopsy approach for appropriate diagnostic tissue sampling in patients with suspected lymphoma. BMC Cancer 2015;15:378.

148. Holland JP, Normand G, Ruggiero A, et al. Intraoperative imaging of positron emission tomographic radiotracers using Cerenkov luminescence emissions. Mol Imaging 2011;10(3):177–86, 1–3.

149. Robertson R, Germanos MS, Li C, et al. Optical imaging of Cerenkov light generation from positron-emitting radiotracers. Phys Med Biol 2009;54(16):N355–65.

150. Spinelli AE, D'Ambrosio D, Calderan L, et al. Cerenkov radiation allows in vivo optical imaging of positron emitting radiotracers. Phys Med Biol 2010;55(2):483–95.

151. Thorek D, Robertson R, Bacchus WA, et al. Cerenkov imaging - a new modality for molecular imaging. Am J Nucl Med Mol Imaging 2012;2(2): 163–73.

152. Liu H, Ren G, Miao Z, et al. Molecular optical imaging with radioactive probes. PLoS One 2010;5(3): e9470.

153. Ruggiero A, Holland JP, Lewis JS, et al. Cerenkov luminescence imaging of medical isotopes. J Nucl Med 2010;51(7):1123–30.

154. Xu Y, Liu H, Cheng Z. Harnessing the power of radionuclides for optical imaging: Cerenkov luminescence imaging. J Nucl Med 2011;52(12): 2009–18.

155. Spinelli AE, Ferdeghini M, Cavedon C, et al. First human Cerenkography. J Biomed Opt 2013;18(2): 20502.

156. Thorek DL, Riedl CC, Grimm J. Clinical Cerenkov luminescence imaging of (18)F-FDG. J Nucl Med 2014;55(1):95–8.

157. Lee JH, Yao Y, Shrestha U, et al. Handling big data in medical imaging: iterative reconstruction with large-scale automated parallel computation. IEEE Nucl Sci Symp Conf Rec (1997) 2014;2014.

158. Toga AW, Foster I, Kesselman C, et al. Big biomedical data as the key resource for discovery science. J Am Med Inform Assoc 2015;22(6):1126 31.

159. Pentecost MJ. Big data. J Am Coll Radiol 2015; 12(2):129.

160. Kansagra AP, Yu JP, Chatterjee AR, et al. Big data and the future of radiology informatics. Acad Radiol 2016;23(1):30–42.

161. Kohli M, Dreyer KJ, Geis JR. Rethinking radiology informatics. AJR Am J Roentgenol 2015;204(4): 716–20.

162. Toews M, Wachinger C, Estepar RS, et al. A feature-based approach to big data analysis of medical images. Inf Process Med Imaging 2015; 24:339–50.

163. Liebeskind DS. Innovative interventional and imaging registries: precision medicine in cerebrovascular disorders. Interv Neurol 2015;4(1–2):5–17.

164. Margolies LR, Pandey G, Horowitz ER, et al. Breast imaging in the era of big data: structured reporting and data mining. AJR Am J Roentgenol 2016; 206(2):259–64.

165. Margolis R, Derr L, Dunn M, et al. The National Institutes of Health's Big Data to Knowledge (BD2K) initiative: capitalizing on biomedical big data. J Am Med Inform Assoc 2014;21(6):957–8.

166. Leijenaar RT, Carvalho S, Velazquez ER, et al. Stability of FDG-PET radiomics features: an integrated analysis of test-retest and inter-observer variability. Acta Oncol 2013;52(7):1391–7.

167. Tixier F, Le Rest CC, Hatt M, et al. Intratumor heterogeneity characterized by textural features on baseline 18F-FDG PET images predicts response to concomitant radiochemotherapy in esophageal cancer. J Nucl Med 2011;52(3):369–78.

168. Galavis PE, Hollensen C, Jallow N, et al. Variability of textural features in FDG PET images due to different acquisition modes and reconstruction parameters. Acta Oncol 2010;49(7):1012–6.

169. Tixier F, Hatt M, Le Rest CC, et al. Reproducibility of tumor uptake heterogeneity characterization through textural feature analysis in 18F-FDG PET. J Nucl Med 2012;53(5):693–700.

170. Bagci U, Yao J, Miller-Jaster K, et al. Predicting future morphological changes of lesions from radiotracer uptake in 18F-FDG-PET images. PLoS One 2013;8(2):e57105.

171. van Velden FH, Kramer GM, Frings V, et al. Repeatability of radiomic features in non-small-cell lung cancer [F]FDG-PET/CT studies: impact of reconstruction and delineation. Mol Imaging Biol 2016; 18(5):788–95.

172. Nyflot MJ, Yang F, Byrd D, et al. Quantitative radiomics: impact of stochastic effects on textural feature analysis implies the need for standards. J Med Imaging (Bellingham) 2015;2(4):041002.

173. Yan J, Chu-Shern JL, Loi HY, et al. Impact of image reconstruction settings on texture features in 18F-FDG PET. J Nucl Med 2015;56(11):1667–73.

174. Leijenaar RT, Nalbantov G, Carvalho S, et al. The effect of SUV discretization in quantitative FDG-PET radiomics: the need for standardized methodology in tumor texture analysis. Sci Rep 2015;5: 11075.

175. Chicklore S, Goh V, Siddique M, et al. Quantifying tumour heterogeneity in 18F-FDG PET/CT imaging by texture analysis. Eur J Nucl Med Mol Imaging 2013;40(1):133–40.

176. Zijlstra JM, Boellaard R, Hoekstra OS. Interim positron emission tomography scan in multi-center studies: optimization of visual and quantitative assessments. Leuk Lymphoma 2009;50(11): 1748–9.

177. Boellaard R. Need for standardization of 18F-FDG PET/CT for treatment response assessments. J Nucl Med 2011;52(Suppl 2):93S–100S.

178. Westerterp M, Pruim J, Oyen W, et al. Quantification of FDG PET studies using standardised uptake values in multi-centre trials: effects of image reconstruction, resolution and ROI definition parameters. Eur J Nucl Med Mol Imaging 2007;34(3):392–404.

179. Boellaard R, Oyen WJ, Hoekstra CJ, et al. The Netherlands protocol for standardisation and quantification of FDG whole body PET studies in multicentre trials. Eur J Nucl Med Mol Imaging 2008; 35(12):2320–33.

180. Boellaard R. Standards for PET image acquisition and quantitative data analysis. J Nucl Med 2009; 50(Suppl 1):11S–20S.

181. Makris NE, Huisman MC, Kinahan PE, et al. Evaluation of strategies towards harmonization of FDG PET/CT studies in multicentre trials: comparison of scanner validation phantoms and data analysis procedures. Eur J Nucl Med Mol Imaging 2013; 40(10):1507–15.

182. Makris NE, Boellaard R, Visser EP, et al. Multicenter harmonization of 89Zr PET/CT performance. J Nucl Med 2014;55(2):264–7.

183. Quak E, Le Roux PY, Hofman MS, et al. Harmonizing FDG PET quantification while maintaining optimal lesion detection: prospective multicentre validation in 517 oncology patients. Eur J Nucl Med Mol Imaging 2015;42(13):2072–82.

184. Boellaard R. The engagement of FDG PET/CT image quality and harmonized quantification: from competitive to complementary. Eur J Nucl Med Mol Imaging 2016;43(1):1–4.

185. Sunderland JJ, Christian PE. Quantitative PET/CT scanner performance characterization based upon the society of nuclear medicine and molecular imaging clinical trials network oncology clinical simulator phantom. J Nucl Med 2015;56(1):145–52.

Molecular Imaging and Precision Medicine in Prostate Cancer

Francesco Ceci, MD, PhD[a],*, Michelangelo Fiorentino, MD[b],
Paolo Castellucci, MD[a], Stefano Fanti, MD[a]

KEYWORDS

- 68Ga-PSMA PET/CT • Prostate cancer • Biochemical relapse • Castrate resistant prostate cancer
- Androgen receptor

KEY POINTS

- PET/computed tomography (CT) with prostate-specific membrane antigen gallium 68 (68Ga-PSMA PET/CT) is valuable diagnostic tool with promising performance to detect the site of relapse in prostate cancer patients.
- 68Ga-PSMA, as theranostics agent, will be effective in delivering high doses for systemic radionuclide therapy, offering a new therapeutic approach to patients with resistance to castration in PCa (CRPC).
- Molecular biomarkers are expected to become in the future robust test to predict appropriateness of the new second-generation antiandrogen agents in CRPC patients.

INTRODUCTION

Prostate cancer (PCa) is the most common solid neoplasm and the third leading cause of cancer-related death in men in Europe and the United States.[1,2] Although primary treatment of clinically localized PCa is associated with excellent oncologic results, up to 50% of the patients treated with radical prostatectomy or external-beam radiotherapy (EBRT) experience biochemical recurrence (BCR) during follow-up.[3–7] Nowadays, several tools evaluating clinical and pathologic parameters (prostate-specific antigen [PSA], PSA doubling time [PSAdt], PSA velocity, pathologic Gleason score [GS], pathologic T, lymph node [LN] invasion, and distant metastases) are available to assess the probability of harboring local versus systemic recurrence after radical prostatectomy or EBRT.[8–10] Although these models are characterized by a relatively good accuracy in distinguishing between local and distant relapse, they are not able to provide precise and individual information about the site of relapse (visceral vs bone metastases, pelvic vs extrapelvic lesions) and/or the number of metastases.

As a consequence, clinicians are currently not able to target individualized and precise salvage therapies according to the information provided by these tools only. Thus, individuals experiencing BCR are generally referred for salvage radiotherapy (S-RT) to the prostate bed versus systemic androgen deprivation therapy (ADT) when a local versus systemic relapse is suspected, respectively. In this context, patients are generally treated without any efforts to detect the real sites of the disease. Metastases-directed therapy might play a role in the management of these patients[11,12] if

The authors have nothing to disclose.

[a] Service of Nuclear Medicine, S. Orsola-Malpighi University Hospital, University of Bologna, Via Massarenti 9, Bologna 40138, Italy; [b] Department of Pathology, S. Orsola-Malpighi University Hospital, University of Bologna, Via Massarenti 9, Bologna 40138, Italy
* Corresponding author. Servizio di Medicina Nucleare, PAD.30, Azienda Ospedaliero-Universitaria S. Orsola-Malpighi, Università di Bologna, Via Massarenti, 9, Bologna 40138, Italy.
E-mail address: francesco.ceci@studio.unibo.it

PET Clin 12 (2017) 83–92
http://dx.doi.org/10.1016/j.cpet.2016.08.004
1556-8598/17/© 2016 Elsevier Inc. All rights reserved.

an imaging modality that accurately identifies number and site(s) of metastases were available.

Conventional imaging techniques, including computed tomography (CT), bone scintigraphy, and MR imaging, are characterized by low sensitivity for detecting the sites of PCa recurrence.[10] Functional imaging, in particular PET, demonstrated to be a useful imaging procedure showing molecular function and metabolic activity information not available with other diagnostic modalities, in a single-step examination.[13] Over the last decade, PET/CT with ^{11}C-choline and/or ^{18}F-choline has proven its role for investigating PCa.[10,14] Particularly, choline PET/CT proved to be a better diagnostic tool for restaging PCa patients presenting BCR, as compared with conventional imaging.[10,14] This modality allows for differentiating between an early relapse limited to the pelvis and a systemic progression[14] and already proved its impact on the management of patients with recurrent PCa.[15]

Moreover, despite some limitations including the presence of nodal micrometastases, functional molecular imaging could provide valuable information also for staging PCa, in selected cases, before primary therapies (radical prostatectomy or EBRT).[16] In patients with high risk of extraprostatic involvement (high PSA values and/or high GS), PET/CT imaging could show the presence of nodal metastases in uncommon sites (eg, presacral and retroperitoneal LNs). Thus, an image-guided treatment strategy including PET-positive findings, such as an extended pelvic lymph-node dissection or an EBRT performed with an enlarged planned target volume, could be performed. In contrast, choline-PET/CT may lead to exclude the patient from a radical therapy owing to the assessment of a systemic metastatic spread–diffusion.[16] Nevertheless, the main application of PET imaging in PCa remain the restaging of the disease, with the detection of the site(s) of relapse in case of BCR as the main purpose. In this context, choline-PET/CT still holds relatively low sensitivity, especially in patients with low PSA levels at the time of imaging.[14] Unfortunately, the optimal timing for salvage treatments to obtain the best chance of cure in case of PCa recurrence would be when the PSA level is low, which reflect a still limited cancer burden.[17–19]

Several efforts have been made over the last years to develop new probes able to provide better performances when compared with the choline-PET/CT, particularly in case of low PSA levels during BCR.[20] The development of radiotracers designed to specifically target the extracellular domains of substrates overexpressed in PCa cells, could lead to the development of theranostics tracers, valuable both for diagnostic and therapeutic purposes.[21] Finally, understanding the molecular mechanisms underlying resistance to castration in PCa (CRPC) and the maintenance of active androgen receptor (AR) would be of interest, because they may represent predictive biomarkers for response to antiandrogen therapy.

PROSTATE-SPECIFIC MEMBRANE ANTIGEN–BASED PET AND COMPUTED TOMOGRAPHY IMAGING

A new molecular probe targeting the prostate-specific membrane antigen (PSMA) has been developed recently.[22] PSMA, the glutamate carboxypeptidase II (GCPII), is a membrane-bound metallopeptidase expressed in several tissues, including the prostate, brain, small intestine, and kidney. Although the function of GCPII in prostate remains unclear, it is well-known that this protein is overexpressed in PCa. Hence, GCPII is a putative target for PCa diagnosis and treatment.[23] The precise localization of the catalytic site of PSMA in the extracellular domain allowed for the development of small, highly specific inhibitors that are internalized inside the cell after ligand binding.[24] Molecular imaging, precisely targeting the GCPII, has seen an unprecedentedly rapid adoption in PCa imaging in the last few years.[25,26] There is a broad range of GCPII enzyme activities as represented by the biodistribution of gallium 68 (^{68}Ga-PSMA).[27] In normal organs, high uptake of ^{68}Ga-PSMA was demonstrated in the kidney cortex and the duodenum, as well as in the lachrymal and salivary glands. The liver and spleen showed moderate uptake. Regarding the prostate, it was observed a significantly higher median uptake in primary prostate tumors as compared with the normal prostate stroma. Considering metastatic tumor lesions, LNs and bone metastases were easily detectable owing to their high tracer uptake.[27] The agent mostly used in clinical studies (Glu-NH-CO-NH-Lys-(Ahx)-[68Ga(HBED-CC)]) is labeled with [68]Ga (^{68}Ga-PSMA).[28] However, it is important to mention that the different available probes, including ^{68}Ga-PSMA-I&T, ^{18}F-DCFBC, and ^{18}F-DCFPyL, seem to show equivalent efficacy for evaluating PCa. Although no direct comparisons have been performed yet, advantages of ^{18}F over ^{68}Ga are mostly owing to a higher feasibility of these compounds and possibly to higher quality standards of fluorinated isotopes.[28]

The first investigations reported a higher tumor to background ratio for ^{68}Ga-PSMA PET/CT for the detection of suspected PCa metastases when compared with ^{18}F-choline PET/CT[29] and very promising performances also at very low PSA levels.[25,26] Morigi and colleagues[30] performed a prospective comparative study between

[18]F-fluoromethylcholine and ^{68}Ga-PSMA PET/CT on a cohort of 38 patients. The study specifically addressed patients in the low and very low PSA area (mean PSA, 1.72 ng/mL; range 0,04–12), also remarking possible changes in clinical management of these patients. The study confirmed a major detection rate for PSMA over ^{18}F-fluoromethylcholine regardless of the PSA level. More in detail, when PSA was 0.5 to 2.0 ng/mL, the positivity rate was 69% for ^{68}Ga-PSMA PET/CT versus 31% for ^{18}F-fluoromethylcholine and when PSA was greater than 2.0, the positivity rate was 86% for ^{68}Ga-PSMA versus 57% for ^{18}F-fluoromethylcholine. The TBR in positive scans was higher for ^{68}Ga-PSMA than for ^{18}F-fluoromethylcholine (28.6 for ^{68}Ga-PSMA vs 9.4 for ^{18}F-fluoromethylcholine; $P<.001$). It was also observed a change in clinical management in 63% (24 of 38 patients) of the overall population, with 54% (13 of 24 patients) being owing to ^{68}Ga-PSMA PET/CT alone. These results were later confirmed by Bluemel and colleagues[31] in a population of 139 recurrent PCa patients, in which ^{68}Ga-PSMA PET/CT was offered in case of negative choline PET/CT. The sequential imaging approach designed to limit ^{68}Ga-PSMA PET/CT imaging to patients with negative choline scans (32 ^{68}Ga-PSMA PET/CT scan performed in this patient series) resulted in high detection rates. ^{68}Ga-PSMA PET/CT identified sites of recurrent disease in 43.8% of the patients with negative choline PET/CT scans. In the largest patient series published so far, Afshar-Oromieh and colleagues[25] evaluated the diagnostic accuracy of ^{68}Ga-PSMA PET/CT in a cohort of 319 patients with recurrent PCa. Despite inhomogeneous characteristics in the population (mean, PSA 161 ng/mL; median, PSA 4.59; 28 of 319 patients not treated with radical therapies) the investigators assessed an overall positivity rate of 82.8%. In particular, a total of 901 lesions were assessed by ^{68}Ga-PSMA PET/CT and considered suspicious for malignancy, with a mean per-lesion maximum standardized uptake value of 13.4 ± 14.6. This study confirmed the high tumor to background ratio for ^{68}Ga-PSMA PET/CT allowing a proper visualization of the suspected lesions, together with the assessment of the high specificity for PCa cells in a clinical investigation. Histology, as a reference standard of validation, was available in 42 patients with an overall amount of 416 lesions evaluated. In all the 98 PET-positive lesions, the presence of PCa cells was confirmed in all cases. Eiber and colleagues[26] later confirmed these promising results. Their results were obtained in a cohort of 248 patients with recurrent PCa (median PSA, 1.99 ng/mL; range 0.2–59.4). The authors observed a promising

overall positivity rate of 89.5% for ^{68}Ga-PSMA PET/CT. More in detail, the authors observed a considerably high positivity rate with low PSA levels with positivity rate of 93.0% (67 of 72) for a PSA value between 1 and 2 ng/mL, 72.7% (24 of 33) between 0.5 and 1 ng/mL, and 57.9% (11 of 19) for a PSA value between 0.2 and 0.5 ng/m. Recently, Ceci and colleagues[32] investigated the role of ^{68}Ga-PSMA PET/CT for restaging PCa patients and evaluated which clinical and pathologic features were associated with PET/CT positivity rate. In their patient series (70 PCa patients; mean PSA, 3.5 ng/mL; median, 1.7), it was described a positivity rate of 74.2%. A PSA level of 0.83 ng/mL and a PSAdt of 6.5 months were found to be valuable cutoff values for predicting with high probability a positive or negative scan result. Moreover, PSA at the time of the scan and PSAdt were associated significantly ($P<.05$) with an increased probability of a positive ^{68}Ga-PSMA PET/CT result. These results were later confirmed in the retrospective analysis published by Verburg and colleagues[33] on 151 patients. The investigators specifically inquired about the extent of disease in recurrent PCa determined by ^{68}Ga-PSMA PET/CT in relation to PSA levels, PSAdt, and Gleason score. The authors demonstrated that high PSA levels and fast PSA kinetics are more likely to relate to a positive PSMA scan. No association was observed for Gleason score; this finding confirmed other data suggesting that PSMA overexpression is not directly related to the tumor grading. Two examples of recurrent PCa patients investigated with ^{68}Ga-PSMA PET/CT are reported in **Figs. 1** and **2**.

Despite these promising results, the results obtained by ^{68}Ga-PSMA PET/CT in recurrent PCa have not been validated extensively with either histology (namely, biopsy of the suspicious metastatic site) or with lesion-directed imaging provided with high specificity.[34] This is important, because the performance characteristics of any novel imaging methodology should be validated and its performance characteristics supported by confirmatory assessments. Lack of this information may have contributed to an artificial inflation of the sensitivity and specificity of ^{68}Ga-PSMA PET/CT reported in the literature. However, this novel approach proved its promising performance for investigating PCa, confirming the importance of this imaging modality for the precise individualization of the site of recurrence.[25,26,32] As a consequence, lesion-targeted therapy performed with curative intent and in accordance with this highly specific imaging procedure could impact on patient management. In addition, the assessment of those parameters more likely to relate to a positive

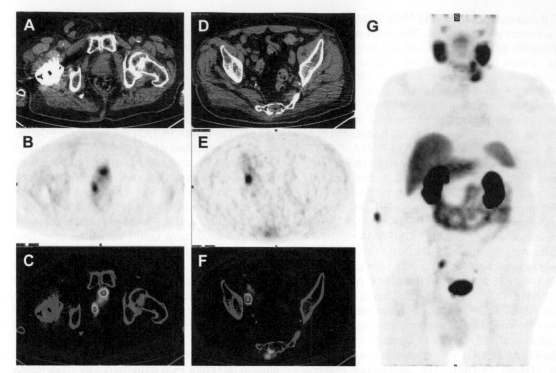

Fig. 1. Z.S. is a 73-year-old man treated in October 2010 with external beam radiation therapy as primary treatment for prostate cancer (GS 4 + 3; cT2cNxMx) with a prostate-specific antigen (PSA) nadir of 0.07 ng/mL. Biochemical recurrence (BCR) occurred in September 2013 with a PSA of 0.29 ng/mL. PSA constantly increased up to 2.03 ng/mL on March 2016. No androgen deprivation therapy was administrated during BCR. The patient subsequently underwent PET/computed tomography (CT) with gallium 68 (68Ga- prostate-specific membrane antigen [PSMA] PET/CT; [G] maximum intensity projection) revealing the presence of local relapse in prostate bed ([A] CT, [B] 68Ga-PSMA PET, [C] fused images), right iliac lymph node (LN; [D] CT, [E] 68Ga-PSMA PET, [F] fused images) and left iliac LN (not shown). These findings were later confirmed at conventional imaging (MR imaging).

scan may lead to a better patient selection with an improvement in sensitivity, thus decreasing the number of false negative findings. This would help in optimizing the use of lesion-targeted approach in PCa recurrent disease.

LESION-TARGETED RADIOTHERAPY AND RADIONUCLIDE THERAPY

The efficacy of EBRT for treating recurrent PCa patients with BCR and suspected for local relapse is already established in literature.[34,35] The optimal timing for S-RT to obtain the best chance of cure would be when the tumor burden is low, that is, when PSA first reaches detectable levels during BCR.[34,35] It was reported in literature a disease-free survival at 6 years after S-RT of 40% for patients presenting with a PSA of less than 0.5 ng/mL before the treatment and of 18% for patients with a PSA of greater than 1.5 ng/mL.[35] Despite this therapeutic approach, the majority of patients treated with S-RT will experience disease progression after treatment.[34,35] For this reason,

all efforts should be made to exclude the presence of metastasis not included in the planned target volume. In this context, functional imaging with PET/CT, particularly with choline PET/CT, proved its role selecting patient with a low tumor burden (oligometastatic disease) and addressing a lesion target therapy instead of a palliative treatment, with benefit in terms of biochemical-free survival and ADT-free survival.[34,35]

Recently, Sterzing and colleagues[36] evaluated the impact of 68Ga-PSMA-PET/CT on a cohort of 57 patients with PCa who were candidates for radiotherapy, evaluating the changes in the radiotherapeutic management. 68Ga-PSMA-PET/CT detected 85 lesions characteristic for PCa in 34 of the 57 patients (59.6%), 25 with BCR and 9 (26.5%) at initial diagnosis; conventional CT was positive only in 12 of 57 patients (21.1%). The TNM staging of 29 of 57 (50.8%) patients was changed after 68Ga-PSMA-PET/CT, leading to a subsequent alteration in the radiotherapeutic management. Based on 68Ga-PSMA-PET/CT, lesion target radiotherapy was performed: 29 of the 57

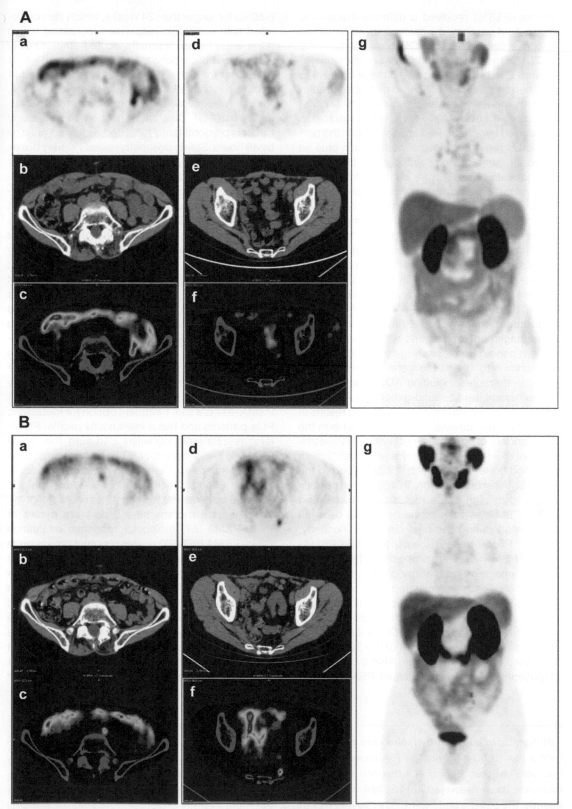

Fig. 2. A.C. is a 68-year-old man treated in February 2012 with radical prostatectomy plus pelvic lymph node dissection for prostate cancer GS 4 + 4; pT23aN0(0/22)Mx with a prostate-specific antigen (PSA) nadir of

patients (50.8%) received a different therapeutic approach, if compared with the initial plan based on conventional staging. Of these 29 patients, 18 (62.1%) received an additional simultaneous integrated LNs boost owing to a change from N0 to N1, whereas the extent of pelvic lymphatic irradiation remained the same. Eight patients (27.5%) were changed from M0 to M1a, which resulted in an enlarged lymphatic field irradiation with the paraaortic LN region or inguinal node region plus an additional simultaneous integrated LN boost. Four patients (13.8%) were changed from M0 to M1b and radiotherapy was canceled and systemic therapy was given. These preliminary results suggest that a sensitive and specific imaging procedures helps to exclude stage IV patients from IMRT and enables individualized dose escalation to LNs metastases or subvolumes of the prostate. Despite the consequences in terms of changes for disease-free survival and overall survival remain to be investigated, ^{68}Ga-PSMA-PET/CT lesion-target therapy could have an impact on the management of patients with recurrent PCa who are candidates for salvage therapies.[37]

Patients with CRPC are generally treated with palliative therapies including ADT, taxane-based chemotherapy, and second-generation ADT (abiraterone, enzaluatamide). Recently, good results in terms of overall survival, when compared with the best standard of care, were obtained with the combination of [223]Ra and steroids in patients with advanced bone involvement.[38] With regard to the high PSMA expression on PCa cells, especially increased in high-grade metastatic disease and CRPC, PSMA as therapeutic target has been an investigated during the past decade.[39] Recently, different PSMA-based agents, including PSMA-617 and PSMA I&T, were proposed as theranostics agent in imaging and therapy of PCa. Kratochwil and colleagues[40] investigated the efficacy of ^{177}Lu-PSMA-617–targeted radionuclide therapy in a case series of 30 patients with metastatic CRPC resistant to other treatments. Of the 30 patients, 21 had a PSA response; in 13 of the 30, the PSA decreased by more than 50%. After 3 cycles, 8 of 11 patients achieved a sustained PSA response

(>50%) for longer than 24 weeks, which also correlated with radiologic response (decreased lesion number and size). Normally, acute hematotoxicity was mild. Diffuse bone marrow involvement was a risk factor for higher grade myelosuppression, but could be identified by PSMA imaging in advance. Xerostomia, nausea, and fatigue occurred sporadically (<10%). Clearance of non–tumor-bound tracer is predominantly renal and widely completed by 48 hours. Safety dosimetry reveals kidney doses of approximately 0.75 Gy/GBq, red marrow 0.03 Gy/GBq, and salivary glands 1.4 Gy/GBq, irrespective of tumor burden and consistent on subsequent cycles. Mean tumor absorbed dose ranged from 6 to 22 Gy/GBq during cycle 1. These results were subsequently confirmed by Ahmadzadehfar and colleagues[41] in a cohort of 24 CRPC, refractory to chemotherapy and treated with a mean dose of mean of 6.0 GBq and 2 scheduled cycles of ^{177}Lu-PSMA-617. Eight weeks after the first cycle of ^{177}Lu-PSMA-617 therapy, 79.1% experienced a decline in PSA level. Eight weeks after the second cycle of ^{177}Lu-PSMA-617 therapy, 68.2% experienced a decline in PSA relative to the baseline value. Apart from 2 cases of grade 3 anemia, there was no relevant hematotoxicity or nephrotoxicity (grade 3 or 4). These results confirmed that ^{177}Lu-PSMA-617 is a safe treatment option for metastatic PCa patients and has a low toxicity profile. Promising results were obtained also with the ^{177}Lu-PSMA-I&T in a cohort of 56 CRPC patients.[42] All patients tolerated the therapy without any acute adverse effects. Decreases in PSA was noted in 45 of 56 patients (80.3%). In 25 patients, followed up at least 6 months after 2 or more cycles of ^{177}Lu-PSMA-I&T, molecular response evaluation (^{68}Ga-PSMA PET/CT) revealed partial remission in 14, stable disease in 2, and progressive disease in 9 patients. The severity of pain significantly reduced in 2 of 6 patients (33.33%). The median progression-free survival was 13.7 months, and the median overall survival was not reached at a follow-up of 28 months. Except for mild reversible xerostomia in 2 patients, no long-term side effect was observed. There was a small, but significant reduction in erythrocyte and leukocyte counts, of

---

0.01 ng/mL. No adjuvant therapies were performed. Biochemical recurrence (BCR) occurred in November 2015 with a PSA of 0.21 ng/mL. The PSA increased to 0.83 ng/mL in April 2016. No androgen deprivation therapy was administrated during BCR. Patient was addressed to ^{11}C-choline PET/computed tomography (CT; [A] g, maximum intensity projection) resulted negative ([a, d] ^{11}C-choline PET, [b, e] CT, [c, f] fused images). Subsequently, the patient underwent ^{68}Ga-PSMA PET/CT ([B] g, maximum intensity projection) revealing the presence of 2 subcentiemtric lymph nodes in left common iliac and presacral region, respectively ([a, d] ^{68}Ga-PSMA PET, [b, e] CT, [c, f] fused images).

which only the erythrocytes decreased slightly below the normal range. No thrombocytopenia occurred.

^{177}Lu-PSMA radionuclide therapy confirmed in the preliminary results its promising role as a new treatment option for CRPC, demonstrating substantial antitumor activity with few side effects. Therefore, this agent merits further attention in larger prospective trials.

BIOMARKERS IN CASTRATION-RESISTANT PROSTATE CANCER

Lethal PCa is typically a metastatic disease resistant to castration, where the AR is still active. The recently developed second-generation antiandrogens are expected to improve the survival of these patients, alone or in combination with taxane-based chemotherapeutic regimens. Second generation antiandrogens effectively reduce the effects of circulating androgens by either blocking their synthesis (abiraterone) or preventing the binding with the AR (enzalutamide). However, most patients with CRPC eventually develop resistance in the late phase of the disease, even to second-generation agents. Molecular mechanisms underlying resistance to castration and the maintenance of active AR have been in part elucidated and may represent predictive biomarkers for response to antiandrogens.[43,44]

The first of these mechanisms involves the constitutive expression within the CRPC tumor cells of splicing variants of the AR gene. The expression of such variants influences protein translation, leading to the synthesis of truncated AR proteins where the ligand-binding domain of the receptor is lost or is highly reduced. These truncated receptors lose the binding properties but still maintain the portion of the AR with transcriptional activity (N-terminal domain) that is therefore able to function independently of the androgen binding. This mechanism mimics at the cell level the clinical syndrome of androgen resistance. In fact, several lines of evidence showed that these AR variants are enriched in CRPC patients when compared with still androgen-sensitive tumors. In addition, the presence of these variants in CRPC patients is associated with resistance to second-generation antiandrogens and poorer outcomes. In fact, the expression of truncated receptors lacking the ligand binding domain of the AR makes ineffective drugs such as the enzalutamide that prevents the binding of the androgen with its receptor. Similarly, this mechanism is associated with poor response to the inhibitor of the androgen synthesis, such as abiraterone because the reduction of circulating androgen ligands caused by these agents is ineffective owing to the peripheral absence of the receptor. Among the 18 splicing variant of the AR, the most frequently encountered in CRPC is that named AR-V7. Recent clinical reports evidenced that the presence of the AR-V7 variant in circulating tumor cells of CRPC patients was associated with resistance to abiraterone and enzalutamide but not to a decrease sensitivity chemotherapies based on taxanes (docetaxel, cabazitaxel).[45] Therefore, taxanes might be more effective in patients harboring truncated AR proteins compared with second-generation antiandrogens targeting the androgen and its receptor.[46] If these data will be confirmed in prospective randomized trials designed specifically on patients with or without AR-V7 and other AR variants, this will become the first predictive biomarker in CRPC patients. Unfortunately, there are currently technical and scientific limitations to the clinical implementation of a test based on the AR variants. First, reports published so far have investigated just the AR-V7 variant from circulating tumor cells in the blood of CRPC patients using an immunomagnetic enrichment method followed by a real-time polymerase chain reaction quantification. This method is not currently certified for in vitro diagnostics.[47] Second, there are several other known variants of the AR that might be an alternative or coexist with the AR-V7 in the same tumor cells. These other variants are often associated with full-length or variably truncated receptors whose biological function is currently unknown. Third, there are no large epidemiologic data on the prevalence of the AR variants in cohorts of CRPC patients.

Another important mechanism of resistance to antiandrogens in CRPC involves the aberrations in the exon 8 of the AR gene. This part of the gene encodes for the ligand binding domain of the AR and there are more than 100 known point mutations in exon 8, leading to variable changes in the steric conformation of the receptor. These aberrations are known to change in experimental models the affinity of the receptor to peripheral antiandrogens such as bicalutamide and enzalutamide.[48,49] In particular, the occurrence of the F876L and the H874Y and T877A variants in the circulating DNA of patients with CRPC seem able to confer resistance to enzalutamide and to abiraterone respectively.[50] All these achievements in the knowledge of the biology behind advanced PCa have been corroborated by the data published from the Cancer Genome Atlas Consortium and disclose the opportunity of new adjunctive predictive biomarkers in advanced PCa.[51]

The landscape on the predictive biomarkers in advanced PCa has changed significantly in the last few years. At least we have now putative molecular biomarkers that are expected to become in the future robust test to predict appropriateness of the new second-generation antiandrogen agents. This would help to save money for the health services and avoid unnecessary side effects to the patients.

SUMMARY

Considering the wide diffusion of PCa in the Europe and the United States, the presence of diagnostic techniques able to detect the site of relapse with high sensitivity and specificity could have an impact on the management of recurrent patients. As a consequence, PET/CT imaging targeting the external domain of the GCPII (PSMA PET/CT) could be considered as imaging modality able to guide lesion target therapies with curative intent (eg, salvage EBRT) in patients who experienced BCR after primary therapies. Furthermore, the inhibitors of the PSMA could be bound also to an high-energy beta emitter (eg, ^{177}Lu). Thus, it seems promising that a radioactive PSMA-ligand, which is directly internalized into tumor cells, will be effective in delivering high doses for systemic radionuclide therapy, offering a new therapeutic approach to CRPC patients. Finally, the landscape on the predictive biomarkers in CRPC has changed significantly in the last few years. At least we have now putative molecular biomarkers that are expected to become in the future robust test to predict appropriateness of the new second-generation antiandrogen agents in CRPC patients.

REFERENCES

1. Siegel RL, Miller KD, Jemal A, et al. Cancer statistics. CA Cancer J Clin 2015;2015(65):5–29.
2. Heidenreich A, Bastian PJ, Bellmunt J, et al. EAU guidelines on prostate cancer. part 1: screening, diagnosis, and local treatment with curative intent-update 2013. Eur Urol 2014;65:124–37.
3. Briganti A, Karnes RJ, Gandaglia G, et al. Natural history of surgically treated high-risk prostate cancer. Urol Oncol 2015;33(163):e7–13.
4. Punnen S, Cooperberg MR, D'Amico AV, et al. Management of biochemical recurrence after primary treatment of prostate cancer: a systematic review of the literature. Eur Urol 2013;64:905–15.
5. Freedland SJ, Presti JC Jr, Amling CL, et al. Time trends in biochemical recurrence after radical prostatectomy: results of the SEARCH database. Urology 2003;61:736–41.
6. Boorjian SA, Eastham JA, Graefen M, et al. A critical analysis of the long-term impact of radical

7. prostatectomy on cancer control and function outcomes. Eur Urol 2012;61:664–75.
7. Khuntia D, Reddy CA, Mahadevan A, et al. Recurrence-free survival rates after external-beam radiotherapy for patients with clinical T1-T3 prostate carcinoma in the prostate-specific antigen era: what should we expect? Cancer 2004;100:1283–92.
8. Heidenreich A, Bastian PJ, Bellmunt J, et al. EAU guidelines on prostate cancer. Part II: treatment of advanced, relapsing, and castration-resistant prostate cancer. Eur Urol 2014;65:467–79.
9. Kattan MW, Wheeler TM, Scardino PT, et al. Postoperative nomogram for disease recurrence after radical prostatectomy for prostate cancer. J Clin 1999;17:1499–507.
10. Choueiri TK, Dreicer R, Paciorek A, et al. A model that predicts the probability of positive imaging in prostate cancer cases with biochemical failure after initial definitive local therapy. J Urol 2008;179:906–10 [discussion: 10].
11. Suardi N, Gandaglia G, Gallina A, et al. Long-term outcomes of salvage lymph node dissection for clinically recurrent prostate cancer: results of a single-institution series with a minimum follow-up of 5 years. Eur Urol 2015;67:299–309.
12. Ost P, Bossi A, Decaestecker K, et al. Metastasis-directed therapy of regional and distant recurrences after curative treatment of prostate cancer: a systematic review of the literature. Eur Urol 2015;67:852–63.
13. Phelps ME. Inaugural article: positron emission tomography provides molecular imaging of biological processes. Proc Natl Acad Sci U S A 2000;97:9226–33.
14. Castellucci P, Ceci F, Graziani T, et al. Early biochemical relapse after radical prostatectomy: which prostate cancer patients may benefit from a restaging 11C-Choline PET/CT scan before salvage radiation therapy? J Nucl Med 2014;55:1424–9.
15. Ceci F, Herrmann K, Castellucci P, et al. Impact of 11C-choline PET/CT on clinical decision making in recurrent prostate cancer: results from a retrospective two-centre trial. Eur J Nucl Med Mol Imaging 2014;41(12):2222–31.
16. Evangelista L, Guttilla A, Zattoni F, et al. Utility of choline positron emission tomography/computed tomography for lymph node involvement identification in intermediate- to high-risk prostate cancer: a systematic literature review and meta-analysis. Eur Urol 2013;63(6):1040–8.
17. Briganti A, Karnes RJ, Joniau S, et al. Prediction of outcome following early salvage radiotherapy among patients with biochemical recurrence after radical prostatectomy. Eur Urol 2014;66:479–86.
18. Fossati N, Karnes RJ, Cozzarini C, et al. Assessing the optimal timing for early salvage radiation therapy in patients with prostate-specific antigen rise after radical prostatectomy. Eur Urol 2015;69(4):728–33.

19. Stephenson AJ, Scardino PT, Kattan MW, et al. Predicting the outcome of salvage radiation therapy for recurrent prostate cancer after radical prostatectomy. J Clin Oncol 2007;25:2035–41.

20. Afshar-Oromieh A, Malcher A, Eder M, et al. PET imaging with a [68Ga]gallium-labelled PSMA ligand for the diagnosis of prostate cancer: biodistribution in humans and first evaluation of tumour lesions. Eur J Nucl Med Mol Imaging 2013;40(4):486–95.

21. Afshar-Oromieh A, Hetzheim H, Kratochwil C, et al. The theranostic PSMA Ligand PSMA-617 in the diagnosis of prostate Cancer by PET/CT: biodistribution in humans, radiation dosimetry, and first evaluation of tumor lesions. J Nucl Med 2015;56(11): 1697–705.

22. Ghosh A, Heston WD. Tumor target prostate specific membrane antigen (PSMA) and its regulation in prostate cancer. J Cell Biochem 2004;91:528–39.

23. Barinka C, Rojas C, Slusher B, et al. Glutamate carboxypeptidase II in diagnosis and treatment of neurologic disorders and prostate cancer. Curr Med Chem 2012;19:856–70.

24. Foss CA, Mease RC, Fan H, et al. Radiolabeled small-molecule ligands for prostate-specific membrane antigen: in vivo imaging in experimental models of prostate cancer. Clin Cancer Res 2005; 11:4022–8.

25. Afshar-Oromieh A, Avtzi E, Giesel FL, et al. The diagnostic value of PET/CT imaging with the (68)Ga-labelled PSMA ligand HBED-CC in the diagnosis of recurrent prostate cancer. Eur J Nucl Med Mol Imaging 2015;42:197–209.

26. Eiber M, Maurer T, Souvatzoglou M, et al. Evaluation of hybrid 68Ga-PSMA Ligand PET/CT in 248 patients with biochemical recurrence after radical prostatectomy. J Nucl Med 2015;56:668–74.

27. Prasad V, Steffen IG, Diederichs G, et al. Biodistribution of [(68)Ga]PSMA-HBED-CC in patients with prostate Cancer: Characterization of uptake in normal organs and tumour lesions. Mol Imaging Biol 2016;18(3):428–36.

28. McBride WJ, Sharkey RM, Karacay H, et al. A novel method of 18F radiolabeling for PET. J Nucl Med 2009;50:991–8.

29. Afshar-Oromieh A, Zechmann CM, Malcher A, et al. Comparison of PET imaging with a (68)Ga-labelled PSMA ligand and (18)F-choline-based PET/CT for the diagnosis of recurrent prostate cancer. Eur J Nucl Med Mol Imaging 2014;41:11–20.

30. Morigi JJ, Stricker PD, van Leeuwen PJ, et al. Prospective comparison of 18F-Fluoromethylcholine versus 68Ga-PSMA PET/CT in prostate Cancer patients who have rising PSA after curative treatment and are being considered for targeted therapy. J Nucl Med 2015;56:1185–90.

31. Bluemel C, Krebs M, Polat B, et al. 68Ga-PSMA-PET/CT in patients with biochemical prostate cancer recurrence and negative 18F-choline-PET/CT. Clin Nucl Med 2016;41(7):515–21.

32. Ceci F, Uprimny C, Nilica B, et al. (68)Ga-PSMA PET/CT for restaging recurrent prostate cancer: which factors are associated with PET/CT detection rate? Eur J Nucl Med Mol Imaging 2015;42:1284–94.

33. Verburg FA, Pfister D, Heidenreich A, et al. Extent of disease in recurrent prostate cancer determined by [(68)Ga]PSMA-HBED-CC PET/CT in relation to PSA levels, PSA doubling time and Gleason score. Eur J Nucl Med Mol Imaging 2016;43(3):397–403.

34. Bolla M, Van Tienhoven G, Warde P, et al. External irradiation with or without long-term androgen suppression for prostate cancer with high metastatic risk: 10-year results of an EORTC randomised study. Lancet Oncol 2010;11:1066–73.

35. Stephenson AJ, Bolla M, Briganti A, et al. Postoperative radiation therapy for pathologically advanced prostate cancer after radical prostatectomy. Eur Urol 2012;61(3):443–51.

36. Sterzing F, Kratochwil C, Fiedler H, et al. 68Ga-PSMA-11 PET/CT: a new technique with high potential for the radiotherapeutic management of prostate cancer patients. Eur J Nucl Med Mol Imaging 2016; 43:34–41.

37. Schiavina R, Ceci F, Romagnoli D, et al. (68)Ga-PSMA-PET/CT-guided salvage retroperitoneal lymph node dissection for disease relapse after radical prostatectomy for prostate cancer. Clin Genitourin Cancer 2015;13(6):e415–7.

38. Parker C, Nilsson S, Heinrich D. Alpha emitter radium-223 and survival in metastatic prostate cancer. N Engl J Med 2013;369:213–23.

39. Deb N, Goris M, Trisler K, et al. Treatment of hormone-refractory prostate cancer with 90Y-CYT-356 monoclonal antibody. Clin Cancer Res 1996;2: 1289–97.

40. Kratochwil C, Giesel FL, Stefanova M, et al. PSMA-targeted radionuclide therapy of metastatic castration-resistant prostate cancer with Lu-177 labeled PSMA-617. J Nucl Med 2016;57(8): 1170–6.

41. Ahmadzadehfar H, Eppard E, Kurpig S, et al. Therapeutic response and side effects of repeated radioligand therapy with 177Lu-PSMA-DKFZ-617 of castrate-resistant metastatic prostate cancer. Oncotarget 2016;7(11):12477–88.

42. Baum RP, Kulkarni HR, Schuchardt C, et al. Lutetium-177 PSMA radioligand therapy of metastatic castration-resistant prostate cancer: safety and efficacy. J Nucl Med 2016;57(7):1006–13.

43. Robinson D, Van Allen EM, Wu YM, et al. Integrative clinical genomics of advanced prostate cancer. Cell 2015;161(5):1215–28.

44. Nakazawa M, Antonarakis ES, Luo J. Androgen receptor splice variants in the era of enzalutamide and abiraterone. Horm Cancer 2014;5(5):265–73.

45. Antonarakis ES, Lu C, Wang H, et al. AR-V7 and resistance to enzalutamide and abiraterone in prostate cancer. N Engl J Med 2014;371(11): 1028–38.

46. Antonarakis ES, Lu C, Luber B, et al. Androgen receptor splice variant 7 and efficacy of taxane chemotherapy in patients with metastatic castration-resistant prostate cancer. JAMA Oncol 2015;1(5):582–91.

47. Nakazawa M, Lu C, Chen Y, et al. Serial blood-based analysis of AR-V7 in men with advanced prostate cancer. Ann Oncol 2015;26(9):1859–65.

48. Joseph JD, Lu N, Qian J, et al. A clinically relevant androgen receptor mutation confers resistance to second-generation antiandrogens enzalutamide and ARN-509. Cancer Discov 2013;3(9):1020–9.

49. Korpal M, Korn JM, Gao X, et al. An F876L mutation in androgen receptor confers genetic and phenotypic resistance to MDV3100 (enzalutamide). Cancer Discov 2013;3(9):1030–43.

50. Azad AA, Volik SV, Wyatt AW, et al. Androgen receptor gene aberrations in circulating cell-free DNA: biomarkers of therapeutic resistance in castration-resistant prostate cancer. Clin Cancer Res 2015; 21(10):2315–24.

51. Cancer Genome Atlas Research Network. The molecular taxonomy of primary prostate Cancer. Cell 2015;163(4):1011–25.

Radionuclide Therapies in Molecular Imaging and Precision Medicine

A. Tuba Kendi, MD[a],*, Valeria M. Moncayo, MD[a],
Jonathon A. Nye, PhD[b], James R. Galt, PhD[b],
Raghuveer Halkar, MD[a], David M. Schuster, MD[a]

KEYWORDS

- PET/CT • SPECT/CT • [131]I MIBG • [131]I therapy • [90]Y microspheres
- Peptide radionuclide receptor therapy

KEY POINTS

- Individualized treatment, also known as precision medicine, aims to target tumor cells to the maximum extent while minimizing the toxicity to the organs at risk.
- Determination of radionuclide therapy doses according to patient-specific data, such as age, weight, height, kidney function, and other generic information, is not sufficient to provide precision medicine.
- For each patient, an individualized dosimetry workup should be determined not only using patient-specific data demographics but also according to the patient-specific radionuclide distribution.
- Recent introduction of single-photon emission computed tomography (SPECT)-based and PET-based dosimetry in routine clinical use has improved applications of precision medicine in radionuclide therapy.

INTRODUCTION

With recent advances in molecular imaging and cancer therapy, a rapid growth in radionuclide therapy as part of precision medicine is expected. Dual-purpose therapeutic and diagnostic ("theragnostic") radiopharmaceuticals permit low-dose imaging with one radionuclide to assess biodistribution kinetics for tumor dosimetry, as well as radionuclide therapy at high doses using a different radionuclide but the same uptake pattern. Recent developments in the imaging modalities, including PET/computed tomography (CT), PET/ MR imaging and SPECT/CT contribute to the more precise localization of radiopharmaceuticals and thus dosimetry calculations. The ability to predict precisely the radiation dose before delivery of the therapy is an important component of personalized medicine. In this article, we focused on use of [131]MIBG, [131]NaI therapy, peptide radionuclide receptor therapy, and targeted delivery of radionuclides with embolizing ^{90}Y microspheres.

METAIODOBENZYLGUANIDINE

Metaiodobenzylguanidine (MIBG) is an analog of guanethidine that shares structural features of norepinephrine, developed in 1979 as a diagnostic agent for imaging of the adrenal medulla.[1] Cellular MIBG uptake occurs by 2 different pathways. The

The authors have nothing to disclose.
[a] Division of Nuclear Medicine and Molecular Imaging, Department of Radiology and Imaging Sciences, Emory University School of Medicine, 1364 Clifton Road Northeast, Atlanta, GA 30322, USA; [b] Division of Research, Department of Radiology and Imaging Sciences, Emory University School of Medicine, 1364 Clifton Road Northeast, Atlanta, GA 30322, USA
* Corresponding author.
E-mail address: drtubakendi@yahoo.com

PET Clin 12 (2017) 93–103
http://dx.doi.org/10.1016/j.cpet.2016.08.006
1556-8598/17/© 2016 Elsevier Inc. All rights reserved.

dominant means of uptake is mediated by the noradrenaline (NA) transporter as an active ATPase-dependent, saturable system.[1–3] The second pathway is nonspecific, low-level diffusion. As most tumors of neural crest origin have high levels of NA transporter, radiolabeled MIBG has been used successfully for imaging of a variety of neuroendocrine tumors (NETs), with higher sensitivities for pheochromocytoma (PHEO), paraganglioma (PGL), and neuroblastoma (NB) than other NETs.[4]

Demonstration of adequate targeting by using either ^{131}I MIBG or ^{123}I MIBG is a prerequisite for successful ^{131}I MIBG treatment. ^{131}I-labeled MIBG decays by beta radiation, releasing energy to tumor cells. Beta particles are responsible for most cell damage and deposit their energy within a localized tissue region of a few millimeters from the decay origin.[4]

A variety of drugs may interfere with MIBG uptake by tumor cells; hence, they should be discontinued before therapy. A full list of interfering agents and suggested cessation times has been published.[2–5] Patients using antihypertensive medications can be prescribed phenoxybenzamine (alpha blockade), atenolol, or nifedipine.[4] Patient selection criteria include adequate bone marrow reserve (hemoglobin ≥ 9 g/dL, white blood cell count $\geq 3.0 \times 10^9$/L, platelets $\geq 100 \times 10^9$/L) and renal function (glomerular filtration rate ≥ 30 mL/min). Therapy is contraindicated for patients who are pregnant or breastfeeding. Female patients of reproductive age must agree to birth control for 6 months after therapy. Patients should be able to follow radiation safety instructions. Acute spinal cord compression and hemodynamic/neurologic instability are also contraindications. Patients should have a reasonable performance status (Karnofsky >60) and a life expectancy of at least 3 months.[2–5]

Free radioactive iodine in the administered dose may accumulate in the thyroid gland and may result in hypothyroidism.[2–5] To prevent this side effect, administration of agents that block the radioactive iodine uptake in the thyroid gland are necessary. These agents include potassium iodine (KI), saturated solution of potassium iodine (SSKI), or Lugol solution.[4,5] The recommendation is to start thyroid blockade 24 to 48 hours before therapy and continue for 10 to 15 days after therapy.

Although diagnostic MIBG is approved by the Food and Drug Administration (FDA), ^{131}I MIBG treatment in the United States is not FDA approved. [131]I MIBG treatment is performed either under the practice of medicine or with an investigational new drug grant[4] (**Figs. 1** and **2**).

Data regarding use of ^{131}I MIBG in PHEO and PGL are limited to a few prospective studies. There is currently no consensus on an optimal

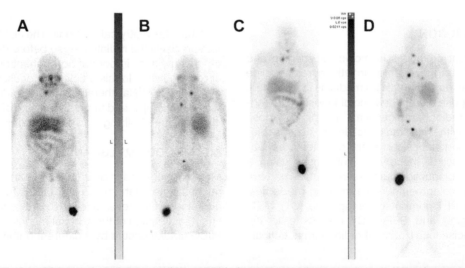

Fig. 1. A 58-year-old woman presenting with intractable hypertension 5 years ago. Patient underwent abdomen MR imaging and ^{123}I MIBG studies. There was a large left adrenal mass with local invasion, which was avid in the MIBG study. Patient underwent left adrenalectomy and left nephrectomy. Pathology was PHEO. Patient presented with distal femoral fracture after 3 years. Fracture was fixed with intramedullary rod placement. Pathology result of the femoral fracture was positive for metastatic PHEO. Patient underwent whole body ^{123}I MIBG study. (*A*) Anterior and (*B*) Posterior show multiple foci of radiotracer uptake in the chest, abdomen/pelvis, and distal left femoral region, corresponding to bone and intrathoracic metastasis from PHEO. Patient underwent 419 mCi of ^{131}I MIBG therapy. Posttherapy imaging (*C, D*) showed foci of radiotracer uptake with more conspicuous uptake compared with before therapy.

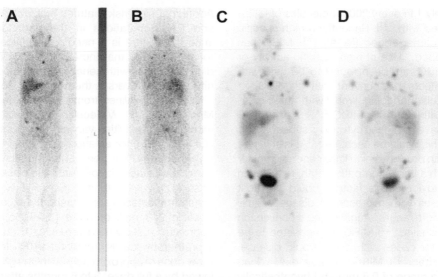

Fig. 2. A 68-year-old man with metastatic PGL. Patient initially presented with flank pain, with suspicion for kidney stones. Further workup revealed a large retroperitoneal mass, consistent with PGL. Patient underwent resection of the primary. [123]I MIBG study showed multiple bone metastases (*A, B*). Patient underwent 380 mCi ^{131}I MIBG therapy. The 1-year follow-up ^{123}I MIBG showed progression with worsening bone metastasis and new hepatic metastasis. Patient underwent a second MIBG therapy with 422 mCi. Posttherapy MIBG imaging showed multiple bone and hepatic metastases (*C, D*). The 1-year follow-up after second MIBG therapy showed stable metastatic disease.

dose strategy. There is some evidence that high doses (>500 mCi) or myeloablative regiments maybe associated with better response. There are, however, no direct comparisons to determine if smaller doses result in improved survival. A recent meta-analysis of MIBG therapy of PGL and PHEO suggested that stable disease and partial response could be achieved in more than 50% and 40% of patients, respectively.[6] Recently, Zhou and colleagues[7] showed that soft tissue disease responded better than bone lesions to MIBG therapy.

Limited data are available for the use of MIBG as first-line therapy in presurgical NB. One study showed a response rate of 66% in presurgical high-risk patients with NB.[2] In refractory NB, a response rate of 36% with additional 34% cases with stable disease has been reported.[2] Zhou and colleagues[7] compared the outcomes of MIBG therapy for relapsed versus refractory NB. This study showed that patients with relapse had higher rates of progressive disease and had lower 2-year survival compared with patients with refractory disease.[7]

Doses could be given empirically as fixed dose amounts with limited toxicity or in fixed activity/body weight (GBq/kg).[4] Most centers administer a fixed dose of 7.4 to 11.2 GBq (100–300 mCi).[3] Doses also can be given based on dosimetric estimations as well to deliver less than 2 to 4 Gy to blood or whole body.[4] Although the initial approach in the 1980s was to deliver palliation therapy with low doses, increasing experience has led most centers to administer high-activity therapy with frequent intervals. Administration of a relatively high first dose is preferred, as MIBG uptake is optimal during the first treatment cycle, and may decrease in the subsequent cycles. Mathematical modeling supports high-activity therapy for microscopic disease. The frequency of therapies is usually between 3 and 6 months, based on recovery from toxicity. Fast-growing tumors are usually treated in 3-month intervals and slow-growing tumors are treated every 6 months.[2–4]

[124]I is an emerging radionuclide for imaging with PET/CT.[8] Currently, [124]I MIBG PET/CT offers the best alternative for pretherapy dosimetry, as it has advantages of image quantification and better spatial resolution compared with ^{131}I MIBG. However, the number of reports is still limited and more investigation is necessary for effective use of [124]I MIBG for patient-specific dosimetry. A recent study by Huang and colleagues[9] also found that patient-specific dosimetry by using [124]I MIBG PET/CT provides better dose estimates to organs and tumors with more realistic simulation geometry and may improve therapy planning for MIBG.

Currently, the specific activity of ^{131}I MIBG ranges from 30 to 50 mCi/mg,[4] hence approximately 1 in every 2000 molecules of MIBG will be labeled with [131]I. Recently, a high specific activity, no-carrier-added (NCA), ^{131}I MIBG has been developed.[4] Use of high specific activity or NCA ^{131}I MIBG has been found to be safe with fewer side effects than conventional ^{131}I MIBG.[4,10]

There is also ongoing work with the alpha-emitter astatine ([211]At)-MIBG.[2,4] [211]At MIBG proved to have a higher cytotoxic superiority to ^{131}I MIBG. This could be because [211]At is an alpha emitter, which produces high linear energy transfer radiation with a very short path length, resulting in potent cytotoxicity. This feature could be most useful in cases with microscopic disease. Similarly, a short-range Auger and conversion electron-producing ^{125}I MIBG is suggested to be best suited for cases with microscopic disease, as beta emitter ^{131}I MIBG therapy has a long average beta range of 0.8 mm and hypothetically fails to deliver an adequate tumoricidal radiation dose to small tumors.[3,5]

NA I-131 FOR WELL-DIFFERENTIATED THYROID CANCER

The incidence of differentiated thyroid cancer (DTC) is increasing worldwide.[11] This is partly due to increasing diagnosis, mostly by widespread use of high-quality anatomic cross-sectional imaging. In comparison with most adult cancers, DTC is typically diagnosed at a younger age. On average, 2.3% of cases are found in people younger than 55 years and 2% of cases occur in children and teenagers.[12] Thyroid cancer, as well as other thyroid diseases, are approximately 3 to 5 times higher in incidence in female compared with male patients.[13] Although cumulative radiation exposure is always a concern in a young population, it is of even greater concern in young female patients.

Tailored radioiodine therapies for patients with thyroid cancer represent an opportunity to put into practice the concept of precision medicine. A recent article by Ladenson[14] describes the many applications of the concept of precision medicine in thyroidology, including benign and malignant disease.

More specific for nuclear medicine, radioiodine ablation and therapy for DTC are based on the principle of iodine-symporter expression and the necessity to eliminate residual tissue for follow-up with serum thyroglobulin levels. Several factors are taken into consideration when deciding a dose of radioiodine for a patient, ranging from the risk stratification based on patient age, gender, and micro and macroscopic characteristics of the tumor, lymph node status, and metastatic disease.

Additional high-risk features include BRAF, RAS, and PAX8 mutations in the pathologic specimen.[15,16] There is a need for additional studies to demonstrate that increased doses of radioiodine in patients with genetic mutations offer a significant benefit versus the traditional doses.

Current guidelines from the Society of Nuclear Medicine and Molecular Imaging (SNMMI) recommend activities varying from 30 to 100 mCi (1.11–3.7 GBq) for ablation of residual tissue after thyroidectomy.[16] If cervical or mediastinal lymph node metastasis is present, the recommended dose is 150 to 200 mCi (5.55–7.4 GBq), and if distant metastases are present, the recommended dose is 200 mCi or more (7.4 GBq). A 2-step approach is used when the residual tissue identified in pretherapy scan is greater than 10%. In that case, a low dose of approximately 30 mCi is given first followed by a full dose, 3 to 6 months after.[16]

New guidelines by the American Thyroid Association (ATA), released in late 2015, recommend lower doses of radioiodine depending on the risk stratification.[15] For low-risk patients, post thyroidectomy ablation is not recommended. The ATA guidelines recommend the use of a lower dose of radioiodine for remnant ablation in intermediate-risk patients (approximately 30 mCi), with use of up to 150 mCi for adjuvant therapy. If structural disease is known, then empiric doses are recommended (100–200 mCi).[15]

Dosimetry is frequently applied in thyroid cancer treatment, when there is evidence of progressing disease and the patient has received previous radioiodine therapies. SNMMI guidelines and ATA guidelines recommend dosimetry in older patients, and/or patients with renal function impairment. The objective is to keep the radiation dose to the bone marrow in safe ranges.[15,16]

In dosimetry, after a low dose of NaI-131, typically 4 mCi, serial imaging is acquired, immediately after dosing, and subsequently at 24 and 48 hours. From the serial image data, an effective clearance rate is calculated for the thyroid that represents the combination of biological and physical decay. The total committed absorbed dose to the thyroid is the product of the administered activity, the time-integrated activity of the thyroid, and the specific absorption factor. Dose committed to the thyroid from peripheral sources is negligible. The absorbed dose can be adjusted for the patient-specific thyroid mass if it can be accurately delineated from a CT or MR image. Simpler methodologies of absorbed dose calculation may assume a population-based effective clearance rate and a single image time point to determine the fraction of administered activity in the thyroid.[17]

An alternative for planar NaI-131 dosimetry is [124]I PET-based, patient-specific 3-dimensional (3D) dosimetry with sequential PET to obtain cumulated activity images.[16,18] This technique also has been used for dosimetry of ^{131}I MIBG.[9]

The dose-limiting organ in radioactive iodine therapy is the bone marrow. This limit has been set as the dose administered that delivers 2 Gy (200 rad) to the blood.[19]

Second primary malignancies in patients with thyroid cancer represent a concern in patients receiving radioactive iodine therapy. This risk is increased in patients treated with large cumulative doses (higher than 600 mCi).[20] No clear evidence exists to suggest that there is increased risk of a secondary malignancy after a single administration of 30 to 100 mCi.[15,20] Gilabert and Prebet[21] addressed the issue of secondary myeloid neoplasms after exposure to radioiodine, and they found 10 cases of acute leukemia in a period of 19 years. Patients need to be informed of this potential risk.

Imaging is another role of nuclear medicine in thyroid cancer treatment. Pretherapy scans, with ^{123}I or ^{131}I after thyroidectomy can reveal the presence of significant residual tissue, where a smaller dose of radioiodine would be indicated for initial ablation versus a second surgery if the amount is significant. Also, a larger dose could be indicated if the patient is upstaged based on the imaging findings (ie, neck uptake corresponding to a lymph node in previously node-negative patients). Posttherapy planar and SPECT or SPECT/CT scans illustrate the radioiodine distribution, often revealing the extent of metastatic disease, and sometimes may show new areas not seen on pretherapy scans. Readers should be aware of false-positive uptake that relates to sodium iodine-symporter activity (Fig. 3).

PET with fludeoxyglucose F 18 (^{18}F-FDG-PET)/CT is valuable in the evaluation of non–iodine-avid dedifferentiated thyroid cancer, particularly high-risk patients with elevated thyroglobulin (Tg) (generally >10 ng/mL), in patients with Tg antibodies, and in patients with aggressive pathology, like poorly differentiated, tall cell, and Hurthle cell thyroid cancer. ^{18}F-FDG-PET/CT scans are useful for evaluation of recurrent and/or metastatic disease and are complementary to ^{131}I whole body scans (WBS).[15] ^{18}F-FDG-PET/CT scans may be able to detect foci of metastatic disease, which are noniodine avid[22,23] (Fig. 4).

Because survival rates at 10 years among patients with radioiodine-avid metastatic thyroid cancer is approximately 60% compared with approximately 10% if the disease is non–radioiodine avid, has prompted the development of strategies to "redifferentiate" thyroid disease. One approach is the use of the current investigational drug selumetinib, which has shown to produce a clinically meaningful increase in iodine uptake and retention in patients with non–iodine-avid DTC.[24]

Patients with thyroid cancer and candidates for ^{131}I MIBG therapy in our institution undergo a personalized checklist-based pretherapy consultation with the nuclear medicine therapy provider to address radiation safety instructions, patient preparation, and answer patients' questions. With this approach, the delivery of precision medicine is more feasible and a physician–patient relationship is established providing more value to the encounter and increasing patient satisfaction.[25]

PEPTIDE-RECEPTOR RADIONUCLIDE THERAPY

NETs are epithelial neoplasms with neuroendocrine differentiation. The annual incidence is approximately 3.65 per 100,000 and rising.[26] Some are truly functional and patients may present with symptoms related to secretion of various peptides or amines, whereas some are not functional (nonsecretory). The patients with nonfunctional tumors may remain asymptomatic for years.

The aim of therapy for unresectable tumors is to control the symptoms and tumor growth. Systemic therapy includes somatostatin (SST) analogs (SSAs), molecularly targeted, cytotoxic chemotherapies, surgery, and regional therapies (hepatic arterial embolization, ablative procedures).

SST has antiproliferative functions that are mediated by its inhibitory effects by binding to 5 high-affinity G-protein–coupled receptors (SSTR1-5).[26] NETs of small bowel and pancreas exhibit high density of SSTRs, predominantly SSTR2. Because SSTs are very short-lived, long-acting and short-acting synthetic analogs (SSAs) have been under use since the early 1980s. Routine follow-up of patients on SSA treatment is usually performed every 3 months. Response to therapy is usually assessed by CT, MR imaging, or ultrasonography. SSTR scintigraphy, or ^{111}In pentetreotide (OctreoScan), is usually performed initially to localize primary and metastatic SST-positive tumors, but scintigraphy usually is not used during follow-up. Peptides labeled with ^{68}Ga include DOTAtate, DOTAtoc, and DOTAnoc. PET/CT with these tracers outperforms ^{111}In pentetrotide whole body and SPECT and is expected to replace ^{111}In pentetrotide where they are available.[26,27] FDG-PET/CT can be used for SSTR imaging negative cases and for assessment of aggressiveness of the tumor.[27]

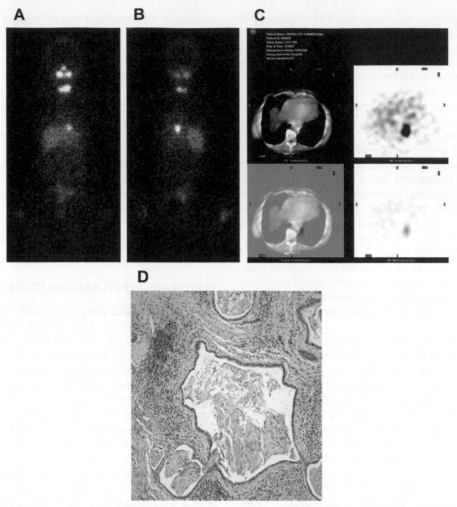

Fig. 3. Postablation scan on a 62-year-old woman with Hurthle cell cancer s/p thyroidectomy (*A*). Ablation with 150 mCi of NaI-131 was performed and demonstrates a focus of tracer uptake in the upper abdomen or inferior thorax near midline on planar anterior (*A*) and posterior (*B*) views. SPECT/CT localizes the area of abnormal NaI 1 to 131 uptake to a left pleural-based soft tissue density, worrisome for malignancy (*C*). Pathology slide after wedge resection of the mass shows bronchiectasis and surrounding acute and chronic inflammation (*D*) (hematoxylin-eosin, original magnification ×20).

Peptide-receptor radionuclide therapy (PRRT) for NETs is a relatively new and promising treatment modality that has been applied for more than 10 years. It is an effective treatment with tumor response in 20% and tumor stabilization in 60%.[27] In reported objective responses in terms of overall survival (OS) and progression-free survival (PFS), PRRT compared favorably with other therapies.[28] PRRT uses radionuclide-labeled SSAs to target the SSTRs (mostly SSTR2) on the surface of NET cells.[29] The first radionuclide used was ^{111}In-DTPA-octreotide, which is an Auger emitter. Although this therapy was effective in relief of symptoms, the tumor response was none or was very modest.[27,28] Recently Beta emitter [90]Yttrium as ^{90}Y-DOTATOC (Y-PRRT) or both beta and gamma emitter [177]Lutetium as ^{177}Lu-DOTATATE (Lu-PRRT) have much better results with objective response rates ranging from 15% to 35%.[28]

[90]Y has maximal tissue penetration of 12 mm and half-life of 2.7 days, whereas ^{177}Lu has 2-mm tissue penetration and 6.7 days of half-life. Because of the deeper penetration of ^{90}Y, it is better suited for larger tumors and ^{177}Lu is considered better suited for smaller tumors. Because of different sizes of multifocal metastatic disease, combination therapy, known as the duo or "cocktail approach," [90]Y and ^{177}Lu may be more effective than individual treatment with either ^{90}Y or [177]Lu.

Other attempts to improve the antitumoral efficacy of PRRT include combining PRRT with radiosensitizing chemotherapeutic agents or

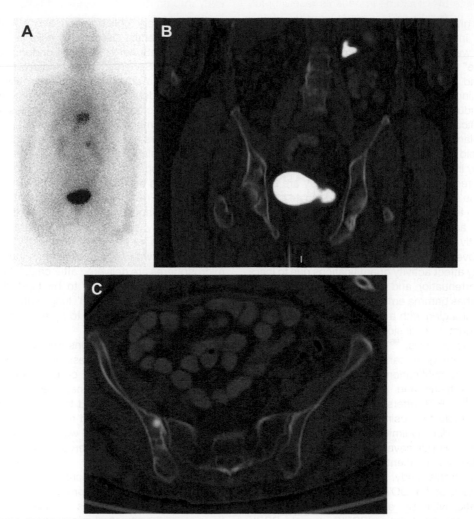

Fig. 4. An 85-year-old woman diagnosed with papillary thyroid carcinoma. After total thyroidectomy and neck dissection, she underwent NaI-131 therapy. During follow-up, Tg level started to rise. Patient underwent Tg-stimulated NaI-131 imaging followed with a whole body FDG-PET/CT. I-131 whole body image (*A*) showed no evidence of iodine-avid disease. FDG-PET/CT performed 2 days after NaI-131 image showed multiple foci of bone metastases, mainly in the pelvic bones (*B, C*). Patient underwent external-beam radiation therapy, however progressed in follow-up.

intra-arterial administration of PRRT in patients with hepatic metastases.

Prerequisites for PRRT include uptake in tumor and metastases higher than liver at SSTR imaging, normal kidney function, normal bone marrow, limited bone metastases, and high performance status.[28,30,31]

PRRT is usually well tolerated.[27,28,31] Early side effects include nausea and vomiting, mostly caused by concomitant infusion of amino acids for kidney protection. Abdominal pain and fatigue can be seen but are rare. In a few cases, mild carcinoid crisis was observed. This could be treated with small dose of octreotide. Temporary hair loss is also one of the side effects that is reported in 60% of cases treated with Lu-PRRT.[28,31] Late side effects include bone marrow and renal toxicities.[27] Treatment with ^{90}Y more frequently was associated with renal toxicity compared with [177]Lu. This could be related to deeper tissue penetration of [90]Y. Risk factors for kidney damage include hypertension, diabetes, previous chemotherapy, and hemoglobin toxicity.[27] Co-infusion of positively charged amino acids is performed to protect against renal toxicity.[27,28,31] Bone marrow toxicity is generally mild and temporary, and mostly presents with reduction in platelets, leukocytes, or hemoglobin. Again, bone marrow toxicity is mostly associated with ^{90}Y therapy than [177]Lu. Development of myelodysplastic syndrome and leukemia is reported but extremely rare.[27,28,31]

^{90}Y is given usually in 2 or 3 cycles with 6-week to 8-week intervals, and ^{177}Lu is given in 4 cycles every 8 weeks. More cycles can be considered as "salvage" therapy depending on toxicity to the kidneys and bone marrow. Most centers have been performing standardized doses as therapy instead of individualized doses. However, to improve patient efficacy and reduce toxicity, individualized PRRT planning should be considered. This concept may avoid severe hematologic and/or renal toxicity, and may improve the quality of life.[27,28,30,31]

Data required as input for dosimetry are blood and urine samples and WBSs at adequate interval times up to at least 3 days after PRRT. Regions of interest are drawn on planar images to obtain time-activity curves.[31] However, background and organ overlay are a problem in planar images that may affect activity quantifications due to inaccurate attenuation and scatter corrections.[29]

^{177}Lu has gamma emission, which makes it suitable for imaging with a gamma camera. Although lack of gamma emission of ^{90}Y is a drawback for dosimetric analysis, ^{86}Y and ^{90}Y PET or bremsstrahlung imaging can be used for dosimetry. However, quantification using bremsstrahlung images is difficult and requires complex corrections.[31] ^{86}Y PET offers better quantification and more suitable for dosimetry. However, high cost and low availability limit its routine use.

Recently, Hardiansyah and colleagues[29] investigated the role of patient-based treatment planning in PRRT. In this study, they performed individualized dosing of ^{90}Y-DOTATOC of 15 patients with metastatic NET by applying a physiologically based pharmacokinetic (PBPK) model. PBPK modeling is shown to be a powerful method to simulate the biodistribution of radiopharmaceuticals in PRRT. The prediction of biodistribution to kidneys and bone marrow is extremely important, as these are dose-limiting organs at PRRT.[29] Hardiyanshah and colleagues[29] also implemented 3D imaging data from ^{68}Ga-DOTA-peptide PET/CT to calculate individualized therapy. As a conclusion, they strongly recommended use of 3D data during individualized treatment planning. However, the short half-life of ^{68}Ga limits its use for pretherapeutic dosimetry. ^{44}Sc or ^{64}Cu PET/CT could enable pretherapeutic organ and tumor dosimetry.[31]

SELECTIVE INTERNAL RADIATION THERAPY

Selective internal radiation therapy with ^{90}Y-labeled microspheres is another example in which the concept of precision medicine is applied in nuclear medicine therapeutics. Patients with unresectable liver tumors are carefully selected, given the complexity of the entire procedure, the multidisciplinary collaboration and coordination, and the potential associated risks. ^{90}Y-labeled glass (TheraSphere; BTG, London, England) or resin (SIR-Spheres; Sirtex Medical, North Sydney, Australia) microspheres are delivered via intra-arterial deposition to treat liver primary hepatocellular carcinoma and metastatic lesions from colorectal primary, respectively.[32] Other metastatic liver tumors are treated as an "off-label" application. Calculations for dosing are made based on patient-specific parameters. Individualized therapy plans are coordinated with interventional radiology. Previous imaging, patient-specific anatomic variants, hepatic function tests, previous chemotherapy, or radiation therapy are taken into consideration for treatment planning.[32,33]

In patients with hepatocellular carcinoma, glass microspheres are delivered after calculation of volume of liver parenchyma to be treated (usually lobar or segmental) and lung shunt fraction. Ideally, a dose of 120 Gy to a segment is calculated for tumor treatment.

Hepatic metastatic lesions from colorectal carcinoma are treated with resin microspheres after calculation of dose based on body surface area, relative hepatic lobe volume, specific tumor load percent on each lobe, and the factors described previously. A standardized method of calculation has been developed and widely used, in which the specific data are entered on a spreadsheet for dose calculation.

Preprocedural ^{99m}Tc–microaggregated albumin (MAA) imaging and postprocedural ^{90}Y bremsstrahlung SPECT/CT scans are useful to evaluate the potential and actual microsphere distribution, respectively, and to identify radiotracer activity outside the tumoral coverage areas.[32,34]

Imaging at each step of the procedure allows treatment planning to be tailored to the specific patient, verification that the treatment dose has been delivered to the tumor, and follow-up that allows remaining tumor to be correlated with the treatment dose. Use of the ^{99m}Tc-MAA SPECT/CT as a predictor of the ^{90}Y radiation dose has proven to be problematic.[35–37]

Although ^{90}Y bremsstrahlung SPECT/CT has to be considered semiquantitative at best, it is possible to use these scans to estimate the delivered radiation dose.[32,38] ^{90}Y has a very low occurrence of positron emission that allows much more accurate posttreatment imaging.[39,40]

Sirtex and theraspheres are alternatives for targeted therapy for primary and secondary liver malignancies, in which patient-specific variables are taken into consideration for individualized therapy. Pretreatment and posttreatment imaging are essential tools for the delivery of precision medicine. **Fig. 5**

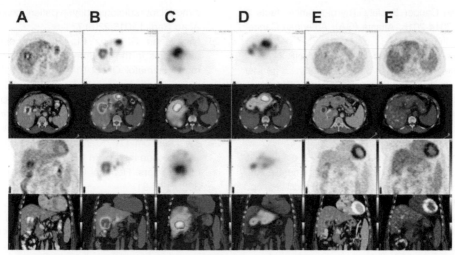

Fig. 5. PET/CT and SPECT/CT transaxial (*upper row*) and coronal (*lower row*) slices demonstrating changes before and after treatment with ^{90}Y-labeled resin microspheres, for metastatic liver cancer from a pancreatic neuroendocrine primary tumor. (*A*) FDG-PET/CT 13 days before the first treatment showing a necrotic liver lesion in the right hepatic lobe with peripheral metabolic activity and a less prominent lesion in the left hepatic lobe. (*B*) ^{99m}Tc MAA SPECT/CT 12 days before the first treatment demonstrates MAA uptake in the right and left hepatic lobes corresponding to the lesion seen in FDG-PET/CT. MAA was administered to both lobes of the liver. Although the primary purpose of the MAA scan is to determine if there is a shunt that would allow microspheres to enter and give an unacceptable radiation dose to the lung, SPECT/CT demonstrates uptake in tumor (as shown here) and evaluation of extrahepatic uptake in the abdomen if present. (*C*) Bremsstrahlung SPECT/CT after ^{90}Y treatment of the right lobe of the liver demonstrating microsphere localization in the tumor intended to be treated. (*D*) Bremsstrahlung SPECT/CT after repeat ^{90}Y treatment, now to the left lobe of the liver 42 days after the first treatment. (*E*) FDG-PET/CT 145 days after the first treatment showing markedly less tumor uptake. (*F*) FDG-PET/CT 220 days after the first treatment with tumor uptake reduced to nearly normal background liver activity.

illustrates an example of the evolution of imaging before and after therapy with ^{90}Y microspheres.

REFERENCES

1. Wieland DM, Brown LE, Tobes MC, et al. Imaging the primate adrenal medulla with [123I] and [131I] meta-iodobenzylguanidine: concise communication. J Nucl Med 1981;22(4):358–64.

2. Sharp SE, Trout AT, Weiss BD, et al. MIBG in neuroblastoma diagnostic imaging and therapy. Radiographics 2016;36(1):258–78.

3. Val Lewington. I-131 Metaiodobenzylguanidine therapy. In: Baum PR, editor. Therapeuctic nuclear medicine. Berlin, Heidelberg: Springer; 2014. p. 571–81.

4. Carrasquillo JA, Pandit-Taskar N, Chen CC. Radionuclide therapy of adrenal tumors. J Surg Oncol 2012;106(5):632–42.

5. Bombardieri E, Giammarile F, Aktolun C, et al. 131I/123I-metaiodobenzylguanidine (mIBG) scintigraphy: procedure guidelines for tumour imaging. Eur J Nucl Med Mol Imaging 2010;37(12):2436–46.

6. van Hulsteijn LT, Niemeijer ND, Dekkers OM, et al. (131)I-MIBG therapy for malignant paraganglioma and phaeochromocytoma: systematic review and meta-analysis. Clin Endocrinol 2014;80(4):487–501.

7. Zhou MJ, Doral MY, DuBois SG, et al. Different outcomes for relapsed versus refractory neuroblastoma after therapy with (131)I-metaiodobenzylguanidine ((131)I-MIBG). Eur J Cancer 2015;51(16):2465–72.

8. Lopci E, Chiti A, Castellani MR, et al. Matched pairs dosimetry: 124I/131I metaiodobenzylguanidine and 124I/131I and 86Y/90Y antibodies. Eur J Nucl Med Mol Imaging 2011;38(Suppl 1):S28–40.

9. Huang SY, Bolch WE, Lee C, et al. Patient-specific dosimetry using pretherapy [(1)(2)(4)I]m-iodobenzylguanidine ([(1)(2)(4)I]mIBG) dynamic PET/CT imaging before [(1)(3)(1)I]mIBG targeted radionuclide therapy for neuroblastoma. Mol Imaging Biol 2015;17(2):284–94.

10. Kayano D, Kinuya S. Iodine-131 metaiodobenzylguanidine therapy for neuroblastoma: reports so far and future perspective. ScientificWorldJournal 2015;2015:189135.

11. Pellegriti G, Frasca F, Regalbuto C, et al. Worldwide increasing incidence of thyroid cancer: update on epidemiology and risk factors. J Cancer Epidemiol 2013;2013:965212.

12. American Cancer Society. Thyroid cancer facts & figures 2014-2015. Atlanta (GA): American Cancer Society, Inc.

13. Moncayo VM, Aarsvold JN, Alazraki NP. Nuclear medicine imaging and therapy: gender biases in disease. Semin Nucl Med 2014;44(6): 413–22.

14. Ladenson PW. Precision medicine comes to thyroidology. J Clin Endocrinol Metab 2016;101(3):799–803.

15. Haugen BR, Alexander EK, Bible KC, et al. 2015 American Thyroid Association management guidelines for adult patients with thyroid nodules and differentiated thyroid cancer: the American Thyroid Association guidelines task force on thyroid nodules and differentiated thyroid cancer. Thyroid 2016; 26(1):1–133.

16. Silberstein EB, Alavi A, Balon HR, et al. The SNMMI practice guideline for therapy of thyroid disease with 131I 3.0. J Nucl Med 2012;53(10):1633–51.

17. Sgouros G, Song H, Ladenson PW, et al. Lung toxicity in radioiodine therapy of thyroid carcinoma: development of a dose-rate method and dosimetric implications of the 80-mCi rule. J Nucl Med 2006; 47(12):1977–84.

18. Sgouros G, Kolbert KS, Sheikh A, et al. Patient-specific dosimetry for 131I thyroid cancer therapy using 124I PET and 3-dimensional-internal dosimetry (3D-ID) software. J Nucl Med 2004;45(8): 1366–72.

19. Dorn R, Kopp J, Vogt H, et al. Dosimetry-guided radioactive iodine treatment in patients with metastatic differentiated thyroid cancer: largest safe dose using a risk-adapted approach. J Nucl Med 2003;44(3):451–6.

20. Rubino C, de Vathaire F, Dottorini ME, et al. Second primary malignancies in thyroid cancer patients. Br J Cancer 2003;89(9):1638–44.

21. Gilabert M, Prebet T. Acute leukemia arising after radioiodine treatment for thyroid cancer. Haematologica 2012;97(8):e28–9 [author reply: e30].

22. Leboulleux S, Schroeder PR, Schlumberger M, et al. The role of PET in follow-up of patients treated for differentiated epithelial thyroid cancers. Nat Clin Pract Endocrinol Metab 2007;3(2): 112–21.

23. Robbins RJ, Wan Q, Grewal RK, et al. Real-time prognosis for metastatic thyroid carcinoma based on 2-[18F]fluoro-2-deoxy-D-glucose-positron emission tomography scanning. J Clin Endocrinol Metab 2006;91(2):498–505.

24. Ho AL, Grewal RK, Leboeuf R, et al. Selumetinib-enhanced radioiodine uptake in advanced thyroid cancer. N Engl J Med 2013;368(7):623–32.

25. Moncayo VM, Applegate KE, Duszak R Jr, et al. The nuclear medicine therapy care coordination service: a model for radiologist-driven patient-centered care. Acad Radiol 2015;22(6):771–8.

26. Narayanan S, Kunz PL. Role of somatostatin analogues in the treatment of neuroendocrine tumors. Hematol Oncol Clin North Am 2016;30(1): 163–77.

27. Kjaer A, Knigge U. Use of radioactive substances in diagnosis and treatment of neuroendocrine tumors. Scand J Gastroenterol 2015;50(6):740–7.

28. Kwekkeboom DJ, Krenning EP. Peptide receptor radionuclide therapy in the treatment of neuroendocrine tumors. Hematol Oncol Clin North Am 2016; 30(1):179–91.

29. Hardiansyah D, Maass C, Attarwala AA, et al. The role of patient-based treatment planning in peptide receptor radionuclide therapy. Eur J Nucl Med Mol Imaging 2016;43(5):871–80.

30. Sabet A, Biersack HJ, Ezziddin S. Advances in peptide receptor radionuclide therapy. Semin Nucl Med 2016;46(1):40–6.

31. Baum PRKH. Peptide receptor radionuclide therapy of neuroendocrine tumors expressing somatostatin receptors. In: Baum PR, editor. Therapeutic nuclear medicine. Berlin, Heidelberg: Springer; 2014. p. 583–603.

32. Camacho JC, Moncayo V, Kokabi N, et al. (90)Y Radioembolization: multimodality imaging pattern approach with angiographic correlation for optimized target therapy delivery. Radiographics 2015; 35(5):1602–18.

33. Murthy R, Nunez R, Szklaruk J, et al. Yttrium-90 microsphere therapy for hepatic malignancy: devices, indications, technical considerations, and potential complications. Radiographics 2005;25(Suppl 1):S41–55.

34. Ahmadzadehfar H, Sabet A, Muckle M, et al. 99mTc-MAA/90Y-Bremsstrahlung SPECT/CT after simultaneous Tc-MAA/90Y-microsphere injection for immediate treatment monitoring and further therapy planning for radioembolization. Eur J Nucl Med Mol Imaging 2011;38(7): 1281–8.

35. Wondergem M, Smits ML, Elschot M, et al. 99mTc-macroaggregated albumin poorly predicts the intrahepatic distribution of 90Y resin microspheres in hepatic radioembolization. J Nucl Med 2013;54(8): 1294–301.

36. Ulrich G, Dudeck O, Furth C, et al. Predictive value of intratumoral 99mTc-macroaggregated albumin uptake in patients with colorectal liver metastases scheduled for radioembolization with 90Y-microspheres. J Nucl Med 2013;54(4): 516–22.

37. Kao YH, Hock Tan AE, Burgmans MC, et al. Image-guided personalized predictive dosimetry by artery-specific SPECT/CT partition modeling for safe and effective 90Y radioembolization. J Nucl Med 2012; 53(4):559–66.

38. Eaton BR, Kim HS, Schreibmann E, et al. Quantitative dosimetry for yttrium-90 radionuclide therapy: tumor dose predicts fluorodeoxyglucose positron emission tomography response in hepatic metastatic melanoma. J Vasc Interv Radiol 2014;25(2):288–95.

39. Willowson KP, Tapner M, Team QI, et al. A multicentre comparison of quantitative (90)Y PET/CT for dosimetric purposes after radioembolization with resin microspheres: the QUEST phantom study. Eur J Nucl Med Mol Imaging 2015;42(8):1202–22.

40. Lhommel R, van Elmbt L, Goffette P, et al. Feasibility of 90Y TOF PET-based dosimetry in liver metastasis therapy using SIR-Spheres. Eur J Nucl Med Mol Imaging 2010;37(9):1654–62.

Molecular Imaging and Precision Medicine
PET/Computed Tomography and Therapy Response Assessment in Oncology

Sara Sheikhbahaei, MD, MPH[a], Esther Mena, MD[a],
Puskar Pattanayak, MD[a], Mehdi Taghipour, MD[a], Lilja B. Solnes, MD[a],
Rathan M. Subramaniam, MD, PhD, MPH[a,b,c,d,e,*]

KEYWORDS

- Molecular imaging • Precision medicine • PET/computed tomography • Therapy response
- Oncology

KEY POINTS

- A variety of methods have been developed to assess the tumor response to therapy.
- Standardized qualitative criteria based on ^{18}F-fluoro-deoxyglucose PET/computed tomography have been proposed to evaluate the treatment effectiveness in specific cancers and these allow more accurate therapy response assessment and survival prognostication.
- Multiple studies have addressed the utility of the volumetric PET biomarkers, including metabolic tumor volume and total lesion glycolysis, as prognostic indicators in several malignancies; however, there is still no consensus about the preferred segmentation methodology for these metrics.
- Tumor heterogeneity (heterogeneous intratumoral uptake) was proposed as a novel PET metric for therapy response assessment.
- Advanced and novel PET imaging techniques will be used to study the specific biological behavior of cancer during therapy.

INTRODUCTION

Cancer is the second leading cause of death worldwide and has emerged as a major public health problem.[1] In 2013, there were 14.9 million new cancer cases and more than 8 million cancer-related deaths worldwide. The top 3 most commonly diagnosed cancers are breast, tracheobronchial-lung, and colorectal cancer, which accounted for 34.6% of all cancers in 2013.[1,2] Overall, the prognosis has improved for the most prevalent cancers in both developing and more developed countries, resulting in a steady decrease in mortalities (1% annually).[3] Recent advances in molecular biology, targeted

Disclosure: Dr E. Mena is supported by NIBI/NIH under the award number T32EB006351. Drs S. Sheikhbahaei, P. Pattanayak, M. Taghipour, L.B. Solnes, and R.M. Subramaniam have nothing to disclose.

[a] Russell H. Morgan Department of Radiology and Radiological Sciences, Johns Hopkins School of Medicine, Johns Hopkins University, 601 North Caroline Street, Baltimore, MD 21287, USA; [b] Department of Radiology, University of Texas Southwestern Medical Center, 5323 Harry Hines Boulevard, Dallas, TX 75390, USA; [c] Department of Clinical Sciences, University of Texas Southwestern Medical Center, 5323 Harry Hines Boulevard, Dallas, TX 75390, USA; [d] Department of Biomedical Engineering, University of Texas Southwestern Medical Center, 5323 Harry Hines Boulevard, Dallas, TX 75390, USA; [e] Advanced Imaging Research Center, University of Texas Southwestern Medical Center, 5323 Harry Hines Boulevard, Dallas, TX 75390, USA
* Corresponding author. Department of Radiology, University of Texas Southwestern Medical Center, 5323 Harry Hines Boulevard, Dallas, TX 75390.
E-mail address: rathan.subramaniam@UTsouthwestern.edu

PET Clin 12 (2017) 105–118
http://dx.doi.org/10.1016/j.cpet.2016.08.002

therapies, and molecular imaging result in early diagnosis and improved survival of oncologic patients.[4] One of the most relevant advances was the introduction of ^{18}F-fluoro-deoxyglucose (FDG) PET combined with computed tomography (CT) in the diagnosis and management of oncologic patients. FDG-PET/CT has rapidly become an important imaging tool for the initial tumor staging and the assessment of cancer recurrence, and has also gained increased acceptance in the setting of tumor response assessment.[5]

The traditional approach to treatment monitoring through imaging has relied on anatomic changes assessing tumor size before and after therapy, using anatomic imaging modalities such as CT and MR imaging that mainly depend on tumor morphology and size, whereas FDG-PET has the ability to provide functional information by identifying metabolically active lesions and monitoring changes after therapy. Thus, FDG-PET/CT imaging has become a promising technique for monitoring therapy response and tumor heterogeneity, and for the early identification of patients who are likely to fail targeted or standard therapies. Furthermore, FDG-PET imaging has proved to be a successful tool with high diagnostic performance in the restaging of oncologic patients during and after completion of treatment, especially in lung cancer, head and neck cancer, breast cancer, and lymphoma, because of its ability to distinguish scar tissue and fibrosis from residual viable tumors.[6–9] To facilitate the assessment of treatment response using FDG-PET/CT imaging, several PET-based visual, semiquantitative, and absolute quantitative criteria have been developed.[4,7,8,10,11] Furthermore, the role of imaging as a determinant of therapeutic decisions in patients with cancer has become increasingly important in the era of genomic medicine, in which genomically defined subsets of patients are treated with anticancer therapy targeting. These targeted therapies vary significantly from the traditional cytotoxic effects of standard chemotherapy, thus response assessment should evolve in parallel with the advances in cancer treatment.

This article reviews and illustrates the commonly used PET/CT-based therapy assessment criteria and future directions for therapy response assessment in oncology.

QUANTITATIVE PET THERAPY RESPONSE ASSESSMENT CRITERIA

Postchemotherapy assessment is a necessary step in the overall treatment algorithm to determine the efficacy and the necessity of continuing treatment. Historically, a variety of methods were introduced and have been developed to assess tumor response to therapy.[4,10] Specifically, they were all designed to quantify therapy effectiveness by assessing tumor shrinkage, which has been shown to correlate with survival.[10]

The first anatomic tumor response criterion was the World Health Organization (WHO) method (1976), which was introduced before the widespread use of CT in the standard practice and the posttherapy follow-up of oncology patients.[10] The original WHO criteria included bidimensional measurements of the tumors, and tumor response was defined as a decrease of the product of these 2 perpendicular diameters of the tumor sites, in order to categorize the amount of shrinkage into 4 categories: complete response, partial response, no response, or progressive disease.[5,10] The WHO criteria did not fully standardize response assessment because of its limitation in specifying critical factors, such as the total number of tumor foci needed to be measured and the minimum measurable tumor size.[10]

With the growing use of CT as a standard for care, the WHO criteria were reevaluated by the National Cancer Institute (NCI) and the European Association for Research and Treatment of Cancer (EORTC) in order to enhance their sensitivity in the assessment of the posttherapy response. In 2000, following a series of clinical trials, the Response Evaluation Criteria in Solid Tumors (RECIST 1.0) provided a new set of CT-based guidelines that assessed tumor response from unidimensional measurements made on CT along the tumor's longest axis, rendering the process more reproducible and applicable to the clinical practice.[12] RECIST 1.0 also defined parameters such as a maximum of 10 lesions, with a maximum of 5 per organ, and the minimum measurable lesion size of 1 cm. The RECIST 1.0 criteria divide intrinsically continuous data (tumor size) into 4 distinct outcome categories by defining the percentage reduction in target lesion size for each category (Table 1). RECIST 1.0 underwent further reevaluation and was modified as RECIST 1.1 in 2008.[10] The current RECIST 1.1 has a few key changes from the WHO criteria and the original RECIST that have contributed to its dominance in tumor response assessment. RECIST 1.1 simplifies the number of lesions required to assess the tumor burden, to a maximum of 5 tumors, and 2 per organ. It also specifies that the longest node diameter measurement is sufficient for assessing therapy response, rather than the product of the 2 longest perpendiculars.[5,10] In addition, the new criteria provided recalculated quantitative values for lymph node tumor response in which total response did not imply complete tumor shrinkage. The RECIST

Table 1
Summary of RECIST 1.1, EORTC, PERCIST 1.0, and IrRC therapy assessment criteria

	RECIST 1.1	EORTC	PERCIST 1.0	IrRC
CMR	No target lesions, Reduction of all pathologic nodes to <10 mm	Complete resolution of FDG uptake within all lesions	Complete resolution of FDG uptake within measurable target lesion, so that it is less than liver activity and indistinguishable from surrounding background blood-pool levels	Disappearance of all lesions in 2 consecutive observations ≥4 wk apart
PMR	Reduction of at least 30% in target lesions from baseline	Reduction of at least 25% in SUV of target lesion	Reduction of at least 30% in target measurable tumor SUL peak. Absolute decrease in SUL ≥0.8	Reduction of at least 50% in tumors in 2 observations ≥4 wk apart
SMD	Not meeting criteria for CMR, PMR, in absence of PD	Increase in SUV of <25% or decrease in SUV of <15% with no increase in extend of uptake	Not meeting criteria for CMR, PMR, in absence of PD	Not meeting criteria for IrCMR or IrPMR, in absence of IrPD
PD	Increase of at least 20% in target lesions or 5-mm increase in lesion size. One or more new visible lesions	Decline in SUV of more than 15% after 1 cycle or more than 25% after two or more cycles	Increase of at least 30% in SUL peak, with >0.8 SUL unit increase in tumor SUV peak from baseline scan. Visible increase in uptake. New FDG-avid lesions	Increase of at least 25% in tumor burden compared with nadir in 2 consecutive observations ≥4 wk apart

Abbreviations: CMR, complete metabolic response; IrRC, immune-related response criteria; PERCIST, PET Response Criteria in Solid Tumors; PD, progressive disease; PMR, partial metabolic response; SMD, stable metabolic disease; SUL, SUV normalized to body mass; SUV, standardized uptake value.

1.1 criteria are the standard CT-based criteria for clinical trials with therapies for solid tumor because of their applicability to a broad range of cancers.

Despite its superiority to the older criteria, RECIST 1.1 has been shown to be inconsistent when multiple reviewers provide the measurements. For example, when multiple reviewers measured lesions of identical diameters, there was disagreement about size, ranging from 25% to 50% in 31.8% of cases.[13] Although this type of classification is simple and allows clear categorization of data, it only takes into consideration tumor size, which is not always an accurate indication of a tumor's functional state. Furthermore, a discontinuous organization of data may exclude potentially valuable information. Incorrect categorization of lesions occurs in cases in which a residual mass is present. In cancers such as sarcoma, hepatoma, and lymphoma, the percentage of tumor shrinkage is not an appropriate indicator of

survival.[10] These patients still have residual masses after treatment, which may either represent treated disease or persistent neoplastic process.[14]

The incorporation of functional imaging modalities helped to address the issue of residual masses detected after therapy, which frequently comprise inflammatory, necrotic, and fibrotic tissue rather than residual viable tumor. The first attempt to apply guidelines to a functional imaging modality was released by the EORTC in 1999, defining tumor response as a 25% reduction in the target lesion FDG maximum standardized uptake value (SUV_{max}); and recommending a normalization of SUV values from the body surface area (see **Table 1**).

In 2009, Wahl and colleagues[10] proposed the PET Response Criteria in Solid Tumors (PERCIST 1.0), incorporating the metabolic information of from FDG-PET imaging into the anatomic information of the CT to assess the tumor response.[4]

PERCIST 1.0 outlines the necessity of using consistent standardized PET protocols and recommends a normalization of SUV values from the lean body mass (SUL). The important components of the proposed PERCIST criteria include assessing normal reference tissue values in a 3-cm-diameter region of interest (ROI) in the liver, using a fixed small ROI about 1 cm^3 in volume (1.2-cm diameter), namely SUL$_{peak}$, in the most metabolically active malignant lesion (up to 5 optional foci, up to 2 foci per organ), assessing tumor size, requiring a 30% decline in SUL for response, and deferring to RECIST 1.1 in cases without FDG-avid lesions or when technically unsuitable.[10] Wahl and colleagues[10] stated that this SUL$_{peak}$ ROI should typically include the maximal SUL pixel but is not necessarily centered on the maximal SUL pixel. In addition, tumor sizes should be recorded and should be 2 cm or larger in diameter. Similarly, each pretreatment baseline tumor SUL peak must be 1.5 times the mean liver SUL + 2 standard deviations of the mean SUL. Wahl and colleagues[10] claimed that the reason for this specific ROI is that smaller single-pixel

SUV$_{max}$ is more variable than the larger ROIs.[10] In addition, PERCIST 1.0 retained the same 4 bins of response classification that were established in RECIST, but amended their respective specifications (see **Table 1**). Because of the limitations of anatomic imaging criteria, the proposed PERCIST 1.0 criteria evaluate response to therapy as a continuous variable and percentage change in SUL$_{peak}$ between the pretreatment and posttreatment scans. With the numerous approaches to assessing tumor response to treatment, PERCIST is a step toward creating a standard for comparison of PET treatment response studies around centers (**Fig. 1**).

Comparison between the different response assessment criteria has also been addressed. In this setting, Shang and colleagues[15] prospectively studied 35 patients with non–small cell lung cancer receiving standard chemotherapy, concluding that EORTC criteria and PERCIST 1.0 were more sensitive and accurate than RECIST 1.1 for the detection of early therapeutic response. Similarly, in a recent retrospective study, including 66 patients with solid tumors, Aras and colleagues[16]

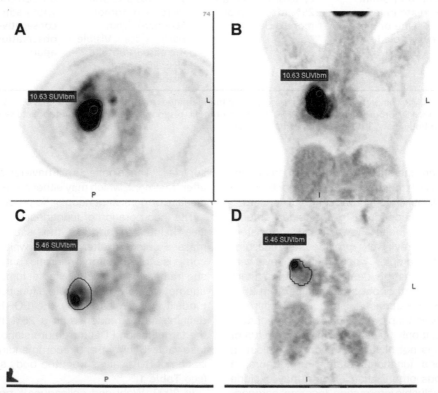

Fig. 1. PERCIST 1.0. Partial metabolic response: a 59-year-old woman diagnosed with T4N2M0 right lung adenocarcinoma treated with chemotherapy with pemetrexed and carboplatin for 3 months. Baseline FDG-PET images in axial (*A*) and coronal (*B*) projections showed a large, intense FDG-avid lung mass (SUV$_{peak}$ 10.6). Posttherapy FDG-PET/CT (*C*, *D*) images show an interval decrease of 47.1% of the FDG metabolic tumor (SUV$_{peak}$ 5.4) compatible with partial metabolic response. SUVlbm, lean body mass-based standardized uptake value.

compared WHO, RECIST 1.1, EORTC, and PER-CIST criteria for the evaluation of treatment response in malignant solid tumors and found significant agreement.

In the setting of personalized cancer treatment, Skougaard and colleagues[17] prospectively studied 61 patients with colorectal cancer receiving phase II trial therapy with a combination of irinotecan and cetuximab, concluding that EORTC and PERCIST criteria gave similar responses and overall survival outcomes with good agreement. Similarly, Goshen and colleagues[18] investigated the value of FDG-PET in the response evaluation of patients with colorectal cancer with liver metastasis treated with bevacizumab and irinotecan, concluding that FDG-PET correlated better than CT with disorder, and better indicated pathologic changes. Puranik and colleagues[19] conducted a retrospective study including 31 patients with positive epidermal growth factor receptor (EGFR) metastatic non–small cell lung carcinoma (NSCLC) on targeted therapy with gefitinib; investigators concluded that the metabolic PET criteria using EORTC were able to accurately predict response as well as disease progression early in the course of targeted therapy, compared with morphologic criteria with RECIST 1.1. More importantly, early metabolic response assessment could predict refractoriness of therapy.

STANDARDIZED QUALITATIVE PET THERAPY RESPONSE ASSESSMENT CRITERIA

In addition to the quantitative methods specified earlier, several qualitative criteria have been proposed to evaluate the treatment effectiveness in specific cancers using FDG-PET/CT imaging. The use of PET in these criteria has been proved to enhance previously underestimated values and allows more accurate survival prognostication. The most commonly used cancer-specific criteria are summarized here.[7,8,11]

Lugano Classification

FDG-PET/CT imaging has been adopted for staging and therapy response assessment of Hodgkin lymphoma (HL) and certain types of non-Hodgkin lymphoma (NHL) for nearly a decade.[20] Several unique anatomic criteria have historically been used to assess tumor response in patients with lymphoma. The first 3 staging classifications were proposed by Peters (1950), Rye (1966), and Ann Arbor (1971).[7,20] In 1999, NHL criteria were integrated with HL criteria as the International Workshop Group (IWG) response criteria. IWG anatomic response criteria proposed 5 categories of clinical response based on CT imaging of lesion size. Response was defined as lymph node size less than 1.5 cm or greater than 75% reduction in tumor size after treatment. The guidelines for categorizing tumor were established as complete remission, partial remission, stable disease, relapsed disease, and progressive disease (PD), and complete remission unconfirmed (CRu).[21] The CRu category was applied to residual adenopathy when lymph node percentage shrinkage was high but nodes remained enlarged and bone marrow was indeterminate. Residual masses are common in lymphoma after therapy in 80% of patients with HL and in 40% of patients with DLBCL; however, less than half of these masses contain malignant disease.[12] The inability of CT to distinguish a residual fibrotic mass from a malignant viable tumor is the main problem with the CT-only tumor response criteria. This issue led to the integration of the new technology of PET for tumor response assessment for patients with lymphomas. In 2005, Juweid and colleagues[22] integrated the originally CT-based IWC with FDG-PET to create the IWC + PET criteria, initially for NHL and subsequently validated for HL.[23] Subsequently, in 2007, Cheson and colleagues[24] and Juweid and colleagues[25] updated the existing IWG + PET response criteria, recommending their use in the response assessment of both HL and NHL, as the International Harmonization Project.

In 2009, in the first International Workshop on PET in Lymphoma, in Deauville, France, a simple 5-point scale called the Deauville criteria was proposed, incorporating the use of FDG-PET/CT in interim therapy response assessment of patients with lymphoma.[20,26] These visual interpretation criteria grade the FDG avidity of lymphoma compared with the FDG uptake in 2 reference organs: the mediastinum (blood pool) and the liver. The 5-point scale was as follows[20,27]: score 1 (no uptake), score 2 (tumor uptake ≤ mediastinum), score 3 (tumor uptake > mediastinum ≤ liver), score 4 (moderate increase in tumor uptake > liver), score 5 (marked increase in tumor uptake > liver and/or any new lesion sites), score X^{26} (any lesion not overtly attributable to lymphoma) (Table 2).

After a widespread discussion, the standardized Lugano classification for lymphoma tumor assessment was proposed in the 11th International Conference on Malignant Lymphoma in Lugano, Switzerland, in June 2011.[26] The Lugano classification became the standard criteria for staging, interim, and end-of-treatment response assessment in patients with lymphoma.[20] The Lugano guidelines recommend the routine use of FDG-PET/CT imaging as a gold standard for staging of FDG-avid lymphomas, including HL, diffuse large

Table 2
Hopkins therapy assessment criteria and Lugano classification for therapy response assessment

Hopkins Criteria	
CMR	Score 1 Focal uptake less than reference blood pool (IJV, mediastina)
Likely CMR	Score 2 Focal uptake greater than the reference blood pool but less than liver
Likely postradiation inflammation	Score 3 Diffuse uptake greater than the reference blood pool and liver
Likely residual tumor	Score 4 Focal uptake greater than the reference blood pool and liver
Residual tumor	Score 5 Focal and intense uptake (2–3 times) greater than the reference blood pool and liver
Lugano Classification	
CMR	Score 1: no uptake Score 2: uptake < mediastinum Score 3: uptake > mediastinum but < liver No evidence of FDG-avid disease in marrow
PMR	Score 4: uptake moderately > liver Score 5: uptake higher than liver ± new lesions Residual BM uptake higher than normal but reduced from baseline
SMD	Score 4: uptake moderately > liver Score 5: uptake higher than liver ± new lesions No change in BM uptake
PD	Score 4: uptake moderately > liver Score 5: uptake higher than liver ± new lesions Increase in intensity + new uptake foci

Abbreviations: BM, bone marrow; IJV, internal jugular vein.

B-cell lymphoma, follicular lymphoma, and mantle cell lymphoma, and have eliminated the need for bone marrow biopsies in HL and most diffuse large B-cell lymphomas. Contrast-enhanced CT is recommended for staging patients with low or variable FDG-avid histology, including chronic lymphocytic leukemia, small lymphocytic leukemia, mycosis fungoides, and marginal zone lymphoma. For therapy assessment, the Lugano classification outlined 4 categories of response using the 5-point criteria (see **Table 2**). **Figs. 2** and **3** show examples of complete response and partial response to chemotherapy in patients with HL using Lugano classification.

Hopkins Criteria

The Hopkins Criteria are a new, simple FDG-PET–based qualitative imaging tool for therapy response assessment for human solid tumors, which was first proposed for therapy response assessment of head and neck cancers.[8] Three studies have evaluated the applicability of Hopkins Criteria for therapy response assessment in head and neck cancer, lung cancer, and locally advanced

pancreatic adenocarcinoma.[8,9,28] These studies proposed the Hopkins Criteria as an effective method for evaluation of therapy response assessment with substantial inter-reader agreement in patients with head and neck cancer and lung cancers.[8,9] These interpretation criteria are a 5-point scale against which therapy response is assessed based on the intensity and pattern of FDG-PET uptake using the activity in the internal jugular vein (head and neck cancers) or mediastinal blood pool (lung cancer) as a reference background[8,9,28] (see **Table 2**). Focal FDG uptake less than or equal to the reference blood pool was scored 1, consistent with complete metabolic response. Focal FDG uptake less than the liver but greater than the reference blood pool was scored 2, and likely represents complete metabolic response. Score 3 represents diffuse FDG uptake greater than the reference blood pool or liver, and likely indicates inflammatory changes. Focal FDG uptake greater than the liver was scored 4, likely indicating residual tumor. Focal and intense FDG uptake 2 to 3 times greater than liver was scored 5, consistent with residual tumor. Scores of 1, 2, or 3 are considered negative for residual tumors,

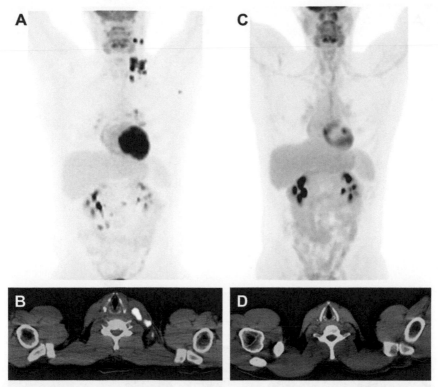

Fig. 2. Lugano classification. Complete metabolic response: 33-year-old man with history of nodular sclerosing HL. Baseline maximum intensity projection (MIP) PET (*A*) and axial (*B*) FDG-PET/CT showed intense FDG-avid laterocervical and mediastinal lymphadenopathy. FDG-PET/CT scan after 4 cycles of chemotherapy showed no suspicious FDG-avid foci (Deauville score 1), compatible with complete metabolic response (*C, D*).

whereas scores of 4 or 5 are regarded as positive for residual tumors.[8]

In a large retrospective, Marcus and colleagues[8] investigated 214 patients with primary head and neck cancers, who were scanned with FDG-PET/CT at baseline and between 5 and 24 weeks after competition of radiation therapy/chemoradiotherapy, concluding that the Hopkins Criteria had high negative predictive value of 91.1% and could predict overall survival and progression-free survival outcomes in these patients. In addition, investigators found that Hopkins Criteria added value to posttherapy clinical assessment by identifying residual disease in patients without prior clinical suspicion and excluding disease in patients suspected of residual disease.

In another retrospective study, including 201 patients with lung cancer with therapy assessment using FDG-PET/CT within 6 months of treatment completion, Sheikhbahaei and colleagues[9] found that Hopkins scoring had high accuracy (86.7%) and could significantly predict survival independently of disease stage, tumor histology, and primary treatment. Furthermore, the Hopkins scoring system for therapy response assessment

added value to prior clinical assessment, leading to a change in the therapy planning in more than two-thirds of the patients with lung cancer. A similar retrospective study was done using the Hopkins Criteria and quantitative analysis to interpret primary treatment response to chemotherapy plus or minus radiotherapy in 42 patients with locally advanced pancreatic adenocarcinoma.[28] Investigators concluded that Hopkins Criteria could not predict the overall survival of these patients, possibly because of the small pool of selected patients. However, when combined with a quantitative scoring system considering FDG avidity and total tumor burden, it was helpful for risk grouping patients after treatment completion.[28]

Overall, the use of a simple, standardized qualitative scoring system (Hopkins Criteria) has been shown to be beneficial in head and neck cancers and lung cancer. The Hopkins Criteria for locally advanced pancreatic cancer showed some advantages but only when combined with a quantitative scoring system. More studies are needed to validate and confirm their significance in other human solid tumors. **Figs. 4** and **5** show examples of cases with complete response and partial response to treatment using the Hopkins Criteria.

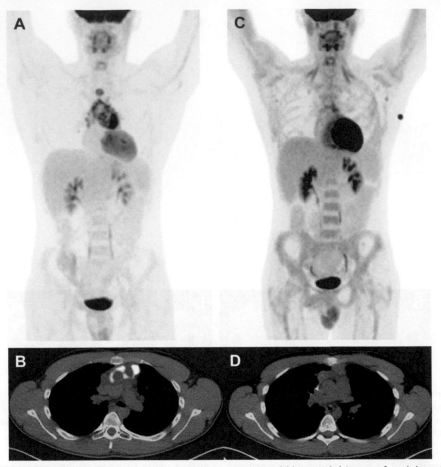

Fig. 3. Lugano classification. Partial metabolic response: a 17-year-old boy with history of nodular sclerosing HL. Baseline FDG-PET/CT scan showed intense FDG-avid superior mediastinal mass (*A, B*). FDG-PET/CT scan after completion of 4 cycles of chemotherapy showed interval decrease of the FDG avidity (Deauville score 4), compatible with partial metabolic response (*C, D*).

This response assessment method is currently being used in a multicenter randomized trial in patients with locoregionally advanced oropharyngeal cancer conducted by the NCI.[29]

Immune-related Response Criteria

Immune checkpoint inhibitors have emerged as important therapeutic modalities for the treatment of several cancers.[11] Ipilimumab, a fully human

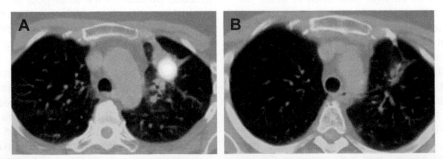

Fig. 4. Hopkins Criteria. Complete metabolic response: a 66-year-old woman with a history of EGFR mutation (+) left upper lung lobe well-differentiated adenocarcinoma. Baseline fused FDG-PET/CT (*A*) image shows intense hypermetabolic activity fusing to a 5 × 3 cm spiculated lung mass within the left upper lobe (SUV$_{max}$ of 4.6) (*A*). Post-treatment FDG-PET/CT scan (*B*) after a combination of 8 cycles of treatment with erlotinib plus bevacizumab shows near-complete metabolic response with minimal linear FDG avidity within the left upper lobe (SUV$_{max}$ of 1.5).

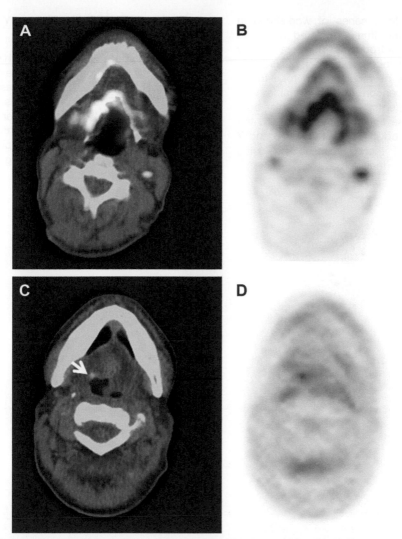

Fig. 5. Hopkins Criteria. Partial metabolic response (score 4): a 54-year-old man with stage IV base of tongue squamous cell carcinoma. Staging FDG-PET/CT scan showed an intense FDG-avid right tongue base tumor extending into the right epiglottis with bilateral intense level 2 and 3 cervical lymph nodes (*A, B*). Posttherapy FDG-PET/CT scan 3-months after completion of chemoradiation therapy shows resolution of the bilateral cervical lymph nodes with residual FDG uptake in the right tongue base (*arrow*) compatible with partial metabolic responses (*C, D*).

monoclonal antibody that blocks cytotoxic T-lymphocyte–associated protein 4, was the first US Food and Drug Administration (FDA)–approved immune checkpoint inhibitor that prolongs overall survival in patients with metastatic melanoma.[30] Inhibitors of programmed death receptor 1 (PD-1) and one of its ligands, PD-L1, represent the next generation of checkpoint inhibitors that have shown significant anticancer activity. These inhibitors are under clinical development for more than 30 tumor types, including hematologic malignancies. The FDA approved 3 PD-1 inhibitors, pembrolizumab, nivolumab, and atezolizumab, for the treatments of metastatic melanoma, non–small cell lung cancer (squamous and adenocarcinoma), renal cell cancer, bladder cancer, and HL.[31–35]

Antitumor responses to immunotherapies are unique in that lesions may enlarge before shrinking, response can be seen in spite of the presence of new lesions, and lesions may remain stable or slowly regress over time, which may take longer than cytotoxic therapies. These effects raise concerns about the use of existing response interpretation criteria, including WHO, RECIST, or PERCIST criteria.[11] Thus, there is a need for defining new standard response criteria to assess response to these novel immunotherapies. In a series of workshops in 2004 and 2005, the immune-related response criteria (IrRC) were introduced. The core novelty of the IrRC is the incorporation of measurable new lesions into a new concept of total tumor burden and comparison of this variable with baseline measurements. The IrRC consider both time point response and tumor burden, and the details are discussed in **Table 1**. **Figs. 6** and **7** show examples of therapy assessment using IrRC in patients with melanoma.

NOVEL PET METRICS FOR THERAPY RESPONSE ASSESSMENT

The therapy response assessment with PET imaging is currently based on tumor uptake change by measuring SUV_{max} or SUL_{peak}, as described for the EORTC and PERCIST criteria. This value may reflect the change of a small number of voxels (1 voxel for SUV_{max}) within the tumor. More recently, new methods have been proposed using PET volumetric parameters, including metabolic

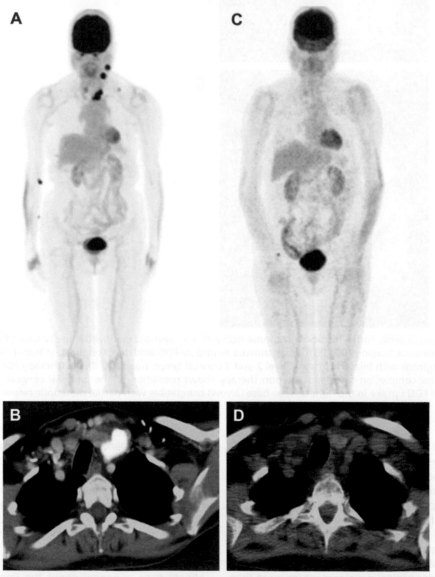

Fig. 6. IrRC. Complete metabolic response: anterior MIP (*A*), axial FDG-PET and fused FDG-PET/CT (*B*) images of a 68-year-old woman with metastatic melanoma who underwent a restaging FDG-PET/CT study. The PET/CT study shows multiple FDG-avid cervical lymph node metastases. After 2 months of receiving therapy with ipilimumab, the restaging FDG-PET/CT scan, including anterior MIP (*C*), axial FDG-PET and fused FDG-PET/CT (*D*) images, shows complete resolution of the previously seen FDG-avid metastatic foci.

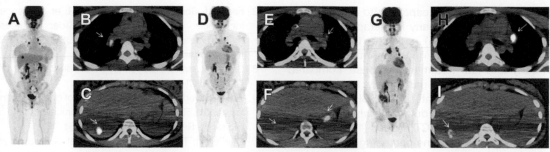

Fig. 7. IrRC. Partial metabolic response: anterior MIP (*A*), axial fused FDG-PET/CT images (*B, C*) of a 16-year-old girl with history of melanoma of the right ankle, postsurgical excision. The study shows metabolically active, metastatic mediastinal lymphadenopathy and liver lesions (*arrows*). She underwent therapy with interleukin-2 and interferon. Anterior MIP (*D*), axial fused FDG-PET/CT images (*E, F*) of a restaging PET/CT scan show partial metabolic response to treatment (*arrows*). She completed treatment and the anterior MIP (*G*) and axial fused FDG-PET/CT (*H, I*) images of the restaging PET/CT show metabolic disease progression (*arrows*).

tumor volume (MTV) and total lesion glycolysis (TLG), and these are under investigation. Both are reliable indicators of viable tumor bulk.[36] TLG is the product of mean SUV value and MTV. An automated tumor delineation is highly desired to improve quantification and for objective patient monitoring. However, the segmentation requires a time-consuming analysis contouring all the tumor lesions, compared with the analytical measurement of SUV$_{max}$, and can be challenging when several lesions coalesce in a single bulky tumor mass. Multiple studies have addressed the utility of the volumetric PET biomarkers as prognostic indicators in several malignancies[37–40]; however, there is still no consensus about the preferred segmentation methodology and response criteria for these metrics.

A new class of metrics has also recently emerged in PET imaging and is currently being clinically investigated. Those metrics are intended to quantify the heterogeneous intratumoral uptake, which has been shown to correlate with clinical outcome. Tumor heterogeneity may be seen in different subtypes of a particular malignancy, within the same subtype of a malignancy, and also within a single tumor mass. FDG uptake can vary markedly within the same tumor mass.[41] Significant tumor heterogeneity affects treatment strategies, therapy response, and patient outcomes and is one of the most important factors in personalized oncologic treatment,[42] especially for identifying therapy resistance leading to failure. Even a small subpopulation of tumor cells with unfavorable genotypic and phenotypic characteristics may lead to eventual treatment failure. Tumor heterogeneity is determined by environmental and individual molecular and genetic factors, such as regional blood flow and angiogenesis, hypoxia and necrosis, extracellular matrix, cellular proliferation and growth rate,

gene mutation, and expression of specific receptors.[41,42]

The novel PET metrics quantifying the heterogeneous intratumoral uptake are calculated on reconstructed images and are often referred to as textural features. The growing field of texture analysis is based on the assumption that the macroscopic inhomogeneity displayed on current imaging modalities corresponds with the microscopic internal structure of the tumor.[43] Recent developments in texture analysis have established strong correlation between image features and tumor heterogeneity for several imaging modalities, such as CT[44,45] and PET.[43,46–48] The homogeneity in the image data set is quantified by assessing the distribution of texture coarseness and irregularity within a structure. In PET imaging, textural feature analysis is based on statistical approaches, and several steps are required, including tumor segmentation, derived ROI content resampling, desired matrix computation (co-occurrence matrix, gray-level run length matrix, neighborhood gray-level different matrix, or gray-level zone length matrix), and associated textural indices computation.[49]

Several studies have reported that pretreatment tumor heterogeneity on FDG-PET/CT could be used as a reliable prognostic factor in different cancers, including lung cancer,[50] colorectal cancer,[51] breast cancer,[46] and head and neck cancer.[29,52]

Several recent studies have suggested that percentage change in tumor heterogeneity following treatment has the capability to predict treatment response and survival.[53–55] Bundschuh and colleagues[53] investigated textural parameters in FDG-PET/CT for their predictive and prognostic capabilities in 27 patients with rectal cancer using histopathology as the gold standard. The textural parameter, coefficient of variance defined as standard deviation divided by the mean value of the activity concentration in the tumor volume, had a statistically significant capability to assess histo-pathologic response early in therapy (sensitivity, 68%; specificity, 88%) and after therapy (79% and 88%, respectively) and was more accurate in early and late treatment response, compared with conventional PET parameters. In a prospective cohort of 47 patients with NSCLC, Cook and colleagues[54] sought to determine whether textural features on FDG-PET/CT images (1) at baseline, (2) at 6 weeks, or (3) the percentage change between baseline and 6 weeks could predict response or survival in patients treated with erlotinib. The investigators concluded that response to erlotinib was associated with reduced heterogeneity of FDG-PET. The evaluation of tumor heterogeneity using methods such as PET/CT textural analysis shows great promise in providing additional information to assess the aggressiveness of the primary tumor, to assess the tumor response, and to predict recurrence and survival outcomes. However, the clinical significance of these parameters is yet to be established and there is a need for larger prospective studies to validate these parameters.

FUTURE TRENDS

With the advances in molecular medicine in the era of personalized medicine, the ultimate goal is to tailor the treatment of specific cancer tumor types and patients. Treatment response criteria should be chosen based on the treatment delivered to the patient, and on the cancer type. Although advanced imaging techniques and parameters are under active investigation, standardization and validation of imaging biomarkers are essential before these can be incorporated into routine clinical practice and compared across institutions worldwide. RECIST criteria are simple, have wide applicability and practicality, and remain the primary criteria for response assessment in clinical practice and clinical trials, despite the significant shortcomings. Advanced and novel PET imaging techniques will be used to study the specific biological behavior of cancer during a specific therapy, and tumor response assessment should evolve in parallel with the advances in novel targeted therapeutic agents.

ACKNOWLEDGMENTS

The authors would like to thank Monica Taneja and Joby Tsai for their contributions to this article.

REFERENCES

1. Fitzmaurice C, Dicker D, Pain A, et al. The global burden of cancer 2013. JAMA Oncol 2015;1:505–27.

2. Ferlay J, Soerjomataram I, Dikshit R, et al. Cancer incidence and mortality worldwide: sources, methods and major patterns in GLOBOCAN 2012. Int J Cancer 2015;136:E359–86.

3. Siegel RL, Miller KD, Jemal A. Cancer statistics. CA Cancer J Clin 2016;2016(66):7–30.

4. Ziai P, Hayeri MR, Salei A, et al. Role of optimal quantification of FDG PET imaging in the clinical practice of radiology. Radiographics 2016;36:481–96.

5. Chalian H, Tore HG, Horowitz JM, et al. Radiologic assessment of response to therapy: comparison of RECIST Versions 1.1 and 1.0. Radiographics 2011; 31:2093–105.

6. Evangelista L, Cervino AR, Michieletto S, et al. Staging of locally advanced breast cancer and the prediction of response to neoadjuvant chemotherapy: complementary role of scintimammography and 18F-FDG PET/CT. Q J Nucl Med Mol Imaging 2014. [Epub ahead of print].

7. Johnson SA, Kumar A, Matasar MJ, et al. Imaging for staging and response assessment in lymphoma. Radiology 2015;276:323–38.

8. Marcus C, Ciarallo A, Tahari AK, et al. Head and neck PET/CT: therapy response interpretation criteria (Hopkins Criteria)–interreader reliability, accuracy, and survival outcomes. J Nucl Med 2014; 55:1411–6.

9. Sheikhbahaei S, Mena E, Marcus C, et al. 18F-Fluorodeoxyglucose PET/CT: therapy response assessment interpretation (Hopkins criteria) and survival outcomes in lung cancer patients. J Nucl Med 2016;57(6):855–60.

10. Wahl RL, Jacene H, Kasamon Y, et al. From RECIST to PERCIST: evolving considerations for PET response criteria in solid tumors. J Nucl Med 2009; 50(Suppl 1):122S–50S.

11. Wolchok JD, Hoos A, O'Day S, et al. Guidelines for the evaluation of immune therapy activity in solid tumors: immune-related response criteria. Clin Cancer Res 2009;15:7412–20.

12. Gallamini A, Zwarthoed C, Borra A. Positron emission tomography (PET) in oncology. Cancers (Basel) 2014;6:1821–89.

13. Patel CN, Goldstone AR, Chowdhury FU, et al. FDG PET/CT in oncology: raising the bar. Clin Radiol 2010;65:522–35.

14. de Wit M, Bumann D, Beyer W, et al. Whole-body positron emission tomography (PET) for diagnosis of residual mass in patients with lymphoma. Ann Oncol 1997;8(Suppl 1):57–60.

15. Shang J, Ling X, Zhang L, et al. Comparison of RECIST, EORTC criteria and PERCIST for evaluation of early response to chemotherapy in patients with non-small-cell lung cancer. Eur J Nucl Med Mol Imaging 2016;43(11):1945–53.

16. Aras M, Erdil TY, Dane F, et al. Comparison of WHO, RECIST 1.1, EORTC, and PERCIST criteria in the

evaluation of treatment response in malignant solid tumors. Nucl Med Commun 2016;37:9–15.

17. Skougaard K, Nielsen D, Jensen BV, et al. Comparison of EORTC criteria and PERCIST for PET/CT response evaluation of patients with metastatic colorectal cancer treated with irinotecan and cetuximab. J Nucl Med 2013;54:1026–31.

18. Goshen E, Davidson T, Zwas ST, et al. PET/CT in the evaluation of response to treatment of liver metastases from colorectal cancer with bevacizumab and irinotecan. Technol Cancer Res Treat 2006; 5(1):37–43.

19. Puranik AD, Purandare NC, Shah S, et al. Role of FDG PET/CT in assessing response to targeted therapy in metastatic lung cancers: morphological versus metabolic criteria. Indian J Nucl Med 2015;30:21–5.

20. Cheson BD. Staging and response assessment in lymphomas: the new Lugano classification. Chin Clin Oncol 2015;4:5.

21. Ben-Haim S, Ell P. 18F-FDG PET and PET/CT in the evaluation of cancer treatment response. J Nucl Med 2009;50:88–99.

22. Juweid ME, Wiseman GA, Vose JM, et al. Response assessment of aggressive non-Hodgkin's lymphoma by integrated international workshop criteria and fluorine-18-fluorodeoxyglucose positron emission tomography. J Clin Oncol 2005;23:4652–61.

23. Brepoels L, Stroobants S, De Wever W, et al. Hodgkin lymphoma: response assessment by revised international workshop criteria. Leuk Lymphoma 2007;48:1539–47.

24. Cheson BD, Pfistner B, Juweid ME, et al. Revised response criteria for malignant lymphoma. J Clin Oncol 2007;25:579–86.

25. Juweid ME, Stroobants S, Hoekstra OS, et al. Use of positron emission tomography for response assessment of lymphoma: consensus of the imaging subcommittee of international harmonization project in lymphoma. J Clin Oncol 2007;25:571–8.

26. Barrington SF, Mikhaeel NG, Kostakoglu L, et al. Role of imaging in the staging and response assessment of lymphoma: consensus of the international conference on malignant lymphomas imaging working Group. J Clin Oncol 2014;32:3048–58.

27. Meignan M, Gallamini A, Haioun C. Report on the first international workshop on interim-pet-scan in lymphoma. Leuk Lymphoma 2009;50:1257–60.

28. Sheikhbahaei S, Wray R, Young B, et al. 18F-FDG-PET/CT therapy assessment of locally advanced pancreatic adenocarcinoma: impact on management and utilization of quantitative parameters for patient survival prediction. Nucl Med Commun 2016;37:231–8.

29. Kwon SH, Yoon JK, An YS, et al. Prognostic significance of the intratumoral heterogeneity of (18) F-FDG uptake in oral cavity cancer. J Surg Oncol 2014;110:702–6.

30. Hodi FS, O'Day SJ, McDermott DF, et al. Improved survival with ipilimumab in patients with metastatic melanoma. N Engl J Med 2010;363:711–23.

31. Vouk K, Benter U, Amonkar MM, et al. Cost and economic burden of adverse events associated with metastatic melanoma treatments in five countries. J Med Econ 2016;19(9):900–12. [Epub ahead of print].

32. Strohlein MA, Lordick F, Ruttinger D, et al. Immunotherapy of peritoneal carcinomatosis with the antibody catumaxomab in colon, gastric, or pancreatic cancer: an open-label, multicenter, phase I/II trial. Onkologie 2011;34:101–8.

33. Grimm MO, Winkler Y, Fetter I, et al. Renaissance of immuno-oncology for urological tumors: Curr status. Urologe A 2016;55(5):621–6 [in German].

34. Barbee MS, Ogunniyi A, Horvat TZ, et al. Current status and future directions of the immune checkpoint inhibitors ipilimumab, pembrolizumab, and nivolumab in oncology. Ann Pharmacother 2015;49:907–37.

35. Carbognin L, Pilotto S, Milella M, et al. Differential activity of nivolumab, pembrolizumab and mpdl3280a according to the tumor expression of programmed death-ligand-1 (pd-l1): sensitivity analysis of trials in melanoma, lung and genitourinary cancers. PLoS One 2015;10:e0130142.

36. Tylski P, Stute S, Grotus N, et al. Comparative assessment of methods for estimating tumor volume and standardized uptake value in (18)F-FDG PET. J Nucl Med 2010;51:268–76.

37. Winther-Larsen A, Fledelius J, Sorensen BS, et al. Metabolic tumor burden as marker of outcome in advanced EGFR wild-type NSCLC patients treated with erlotinib. Lung Cancer 2016;94:81–7.

38. Liu FY, Lai CH, Yang LY, et al. Utility of F-FDG PET/CT in patients with advanced squamous cell carcinoma of the uterine cervix receiving concurrent chemoradiotherapy: a parallel study of a prospective randomized trial. Eur J Nucl Med Mol Imaging 2016;43(10):1812–23.

39. Pak K, Cheon GJ, Nam HY, et al. Prognostic value of metabolic tumor volume and total lesion glycolysis in head and neck cancer: a systematic review and meta-analysis. J Nucl Med 2014;55:884–90.

40. Zhang H, Seikaly H, Nguyen NT, et al. Validation of metabolic tumor volume as a prognostic factor for oral cavity squamous cell carcinoma treated with primary surgery. Oral Oncol 2016;57:6–14.

41. Rahim MK, Kim SE, So H, et al. Recent trends in PET image interpretations using volumetric and texture-based quantification methods in nuclear oncology. Nucl Med Mol Imaging 2014;48:1–15.

42. O'Connor JP, Rose CJ, Waterton JC, et al. Imaging intratumor heterogeneity: role in therapy response, resistance, and clinical outcome. Clin Cancer Res 2015;21:249–57.

43. Chicklore S, Goh V, Siddique M, et al. Quantifying tumour heterogeneity in 18F-FDG PET/CT imaging

by texture analysis. Eur J Nucl Med Mol Imaging 2013;40:133–40.

44. Gerlinger M, Rowan AJ, Horswell S, et al. Intratumor heterogeneity and branched evolution revealed by multiregion sequencing. N Engl J Med 2012;366: 883–92.

45. Win T, Miles KA, Janes SM, et al. Tumor heterogeneity and permeability as measured on the CT component of PET/CT predict survival in patients with non-small cell lung cancer. Clin Cancer Res 2013;19:3591–9.

46. Soussan M, Orlhac F, Boubaya M, et al. Relationship between tumor heterogeneity measured on FDG-PET/CT and pathological prognostic factors in invasive breast cancer. PLoS One 2014;9:e94017.

47. Tixier F, Le Rest CC, Hatt M, et al. Intratumor heterogeneity characterized by textural features on baseline 18F-FDG PET images predicts response to concomitant radiochemotherapy in esophageal cancer. J Nucl Med 2011;52:369–78.

48. Tixier F, Hatt M, Valla C, et al. Visual versus quantitative assessment of intratumor 18F-FDG PET uptake heterogeneity: prognostic value in non-small cell lung cancer. J Nucl Med 2014;55:1235–41.

49. Carlier T, Bailly C. State-of-the-art and recent advances in quantification for therapeutic follow-up in oncology using PET. Front Med (Lausanne) 2015;2:18.

50. Pyka T, Bundschuh RA, Andratschke N, et al. Textural features in pre-treatment [F18]-FDG-PET/ CT are correlated with risk of local recurrence and disease-specific survival in early stage NSCLC patients receiving primary stereotactic radiation therapy. Radiat Oncol 2015;10:100.

51. Han YH, Jeong HJ, Sohn MH, et al. Clinical value of intratumoral metabolic heterogeneity in [18F]FDG PET/CT for prediction of recurrence in patients with locally advanced colorectal cancer. Q J Nucl Med Mol Imaging 2016. [Epub ahead of print].

52. Cheng NM, Fang YH, Chang JT, et al. Textural features of pretreatment 18F-FDG PET/CT images: prognostic significance in patients with advanced T-stage oropharyngeal squamous cell carcinoma. J Nucl Med 2013;54:1703–9.

53. Bundschuh RA, Dinges J, Neumann L, et al. Textural parameters of tumor heterogeneity in 18F-FDG PET/ CT for therapy response assessment and prognosis in patients with locally advanced rectal cancer. J Nucl Med 2014;55:891–7.

54. Cook GJ, O'Brien ME, Siddique M, et al. Non-small cell lung cancer treated with erlotinib: heterogeneity of (18)F-FDG Uptake at PET-association with treatment response and prognosis. Radiology 2015; 276:883–93.

55. van Gool MH, Aukema TS, Sinaasappel M, et al. Tumor heterogeneity on (18)F-FDG-PET/CT for response monitoring in non-small cell lung cancer treated with erlotinib. J Thorac Dis 2016;8:E200–3.

Molecular Imaging and Precision Medicine in Dementia and Movement Disorders

Atul K. Mallik, MD, PhD[a], Alexander Drzezga, MD[b],
Satoshi Minoshima, MD, PhD[a],*

KEYWORDS

- Molecular imaging • Precision medicine • Alzheimer disease • Parkinson disease • Dementia
- Movement disorder • PET • SPECT

KEY POINTS

- Despite a lack of established preventive and disease-modifying interventions for neurodegenerative disorders, molecular imaging (MI) is being used in precision medicine approaches.
- For Alzheimer disease (AD) and Parkinson disease (PD), MI of amyloid and dopamine transporters identifies "at-risk" subjects who may potentially benefit from proposed preventive interventions.
- MI is being used in clinical trials to monitor disease progression and evaluate therapeutic interventions for both neurodegenerative dementia and movement disorders (MD).
- MI has the ability to guide management for patients with neurodegenerative dementia or MD in diagnostically challenging cases, including for nonspecific parkinsonism, drug-induced parkinsonism, and dementia with Lewy bodies.
- The advent of new MI techniques, specifically tau MI, provides new and increased opportunities for precision medicine in AD, frontotemporal dementia (FTD), and atypical parkinsonism syndrome (APS).

INTRODUCTION

Overview of Dementia

Dementia affects more than 35 million people worldwide. In the United States, nearly 15% of people age 70 and older are estimated to have dementia.[1–3] Primary neurodegenerative disorders (NDD) are the leading cause of dementia, characterized by accumulating damage to neuronal structures causing memory loss and progressive impairment of higher cognitive functions.

Alzheimer disease (AD) is the most common cause of dementia, and the fifth leading cause of death in individuals older than 65 years in the United States.[4] Vascular dementia, resulting from cerebrovascular disease and resultant vascular brain injury, is also a common cause of dementia.[5] The next most common neurodegenerative dementias are dementia with Lewy bodies (DLB) and frontotemporal dementia (FTD) syndromes, the latter of which are associated with frontotemporal lobar

Dr A. Mallik has nothing to disclose. Dr A. Drzezga: Avid Radiopharmaceuticals - Scientific Study/Trial, Consultant/Advisor; GE Healthcare - Scientific Study/Trial, Consultant/Advisor; Piramal Imaging - Scientific Study/Trial, Consultant/Advisor; Siemens Healthcare Scientific Study/Trial, Consultant/Advisor. Dr S. Minoshima: GE Healthcare - Royalty; Hitachi Medical - Scientific Study/Trial; Niphon Medi-Physics Co, Ltd - Scientific Study/Trial.
^a Department of Radiology and Imaging Sciences, School of Medicine, University of Utah, Room: 1A71, 30 North 1900 East, Salt Lake City, UT 84132, USA; ^b Department of Nuclear Medicine, University Hospital of Cologne, Kerpener Street 62, Cologne 50937, Germany
* Corresponding author.
E-mail address: sminoshima@hsc.utah.edu

PET Clin 12 (2017) 119–136
http://dx.doi.org/10.1016/j.cpet.2016.08.003
1556-8598/17/© 2016 Elsevier Inc. All rights reserved.

degeneration (FTLD) atrophy patterns and comprise multiple subtypes with distinct clinical manifestations and biomarkers.[6] As will be described herein, some of the less common NDDs, such as posterior cortical atrophy (PCA) and corticobasal degeneration (CBD), have been associated with AD or FTD neuropathology, and have also been evaluated with MI.[7,8]

Overview of Molecular Imaging in Dementia

Even before recent increased interest in precision medicine (PM), the promise of MI has been to provide quantitative information about pathophysiology, to diagnose conditions at early stages, to monitor disease progression, as well as to plan and assess the response to medical and surgical interventions. For example, there is a wealth of research about how molecular imaging can be used for the diagnosis of NDD (and movement disorders [MD]), especially in diagnostically challenging cases.[9–11] A brief overview of key MI techniques applied in NDD is provided next.

PET and SPECT (single-photon emission computed tomography) comprise the MI techniques of exogenous radiolabeled agents used to evaluate NDD and MD.[12–14] In general, PET techniques have better spatial resolution and sensitivity than SPECT, but require radioisotopes such as carbon-11 and fluorine-18 that have relatively short half-lives and require a nearby cyclotron and radiochemistry facility. In contrast, SPECT uses radioisotopes such as iodine-123 or Technecium-99m that have longer half-lives and can be distributed easily from commercial radiopharmacies, making SPECT more readily available than the PET techniques. However, this situation is changing due to the development of commercial PET radiopharmacy networks.[15]

PET with 2-(F-18)fluoro-2-deoxy-D-glucose

PET with 2-(F-18)fluoro-2-deoxy-D-glucose (FDG) is a widely available imaging modality for the diagnosis of NDD, capable of suggesting a differential diagnosis as well as detecting the early stages of certain disease processes.[16–20] Characteristic patterns of altered metabolism seen on FDG-PET are thought to reflect synaptic/neuronal dysfunction and allow earlier and reliable diagnosis of specific types of dementia, such as AD, FTD, and DLB, although some of the imaging findings can overlap. An essentially normal or preserved cerebral uptake pattern also can help suggest potentially reversible disorders, such as depression from a primary NDD.[21,22]

Regional cerebral blood flow (perfusion) SPECT has also been used to identify regional hypoperfusion patterns associated with various dementias. Although perfusion SPECT provides similar diagnostic information, comparative studies have demonstrated that FDG-PET is probably superior to perfusion SPECT in the evaluation of NDD.[23] This may be because metabolic changes are more closely tied to the pathologic changes in neurodegeneration than blood flow changes, and because PET has higher spatial resolution and sensitivity relative to SPECT.

Aβ molecular imaging agents

Extracellular amyloid plaques and intraneuronal neurofibrillary tangles (NFT) are the initially described pathologic hallmarks of AD that have since been identified as insoluble aggregated forms of 2 misfolded proteins, Aβ and hyperphosphorylated species of the microtubule-associated protein tau (p-tau), respectively.[24–26] Although the molecular pathophysiology of how Aβ and NFT pathology are related to neurodegeneration is not completely understood, the development of noninvasive imaging agents that selectively target Aβ deposits, and more recently tau, are providing more insight.[27]

Aβ PET imaging using [C-11]Pittsburgh compound B (PiB) can be considered the current gold standard of amyloid MI. Since the first study in humans published in 2004,[28] this tracer has been extensively applied to evaluate Aβ accumulation. Since then, several other clinically viable Aβ imaging agents have been developed with relatively longer-lived radionuclides, such as F-18 to facilitate regional distribution from a central nuclear pharmacy.[29] Three F-18–labeled Aβ PET imaging agents are approved by the Food and Drug Administration in the United States and worldwide: florbetapir, flutemetamol, and florbetaben. These 3 agents demonstrate different kinetic behaviors, varying levels of specific Aβ and off-target (white matter) binding and different interpretation methodologies.[30,31] Although these and other Aβ imaging agents have provided similar qualitative information for the clinical evaluation of regional brain Aβ deposition, quantitative assessments for research studies of regional Aβ load have been more variable. While there are attempts to standardize quantitative Aβ imaging measurements,[32] this has raised some concern for their use as outcome measures.[33]

Aβ imaging is a key biomarker in several large-scale, multisite studies, including the Alzheimer's Disease Neuroimaging Initiative (ADNI) and the Dominantly Inherited Alzheimer Network (DIAN, see later in this article).[34–36] These and other Aβ imaging studies have relied to some extent on the "amyloid cascade" hypothesis, which implicates the abnormal accumulation of Aβ plaques and oligomeric species as the initiating event in a pathologic cascade that ultimately leads to neurodegeneration and the clinical syndrome of AD.[37] This is supported by the fact that Aβ imaging can have an important diagnostic and prognostic role in the evaluation of AD, especially in early AD. Aβ-positivity in combination with neurodegenerative measures of neuronal injury, such as glucose hypometabolism (via FDG-PET) or cerebral atrophy (via structural MRI), is predictive of a rapid progression to dementia.[38–42] Also, because Aβ deposition appears to occur many years before the onset of dementia, amyloid PET imaging is being used in PM approaches to identify patients more likely to develop AD later in their lives (**Fig. 1**). We will discuss these applications below.

However, a number of findings regarding Aβ and other AD clinical findings and biomarkers have required a refinement of the "amyloid cascade" hypothesis. For example, levels of cortical Aβ deposition appear to plateau relatively early in the course of the disease, which may explain why the pathologic Aβ load is poorly correlated with the degree of cognitive symptoms.[38,43,44] Instead, neurofibrillary tangles and levels of potentially neurotoxic soluble Aβ-oligomers appear to be better correlated with cognitive symptoms.[27,45] In addition, Aβ is not synonymous with AD pathology. Neurodegeneration-first, pathologic changes without elevated Aβ have recently been demonstrated, termed "suspected nonamyloid pathology" (SNAP), and may ultimately lead to AD or other forms of dementia. Significant Aβ deposition has also been seen in other NDDs such as DLB.[46] Both these findings require a more nuanced understanding of the role of Aβ in the pathophysiology of AD.[47–49] Altogether, recent evidence

suggests Aβ deposition may become decoupled from the processes that mediate neurodegeneration in AD, perhaps in subclinical disease phases.[50] This is consistent with the overall findings that Aβ has some diagnostic utility and can predict progression to AD, but does less well predicting the time course of progression to AD or the degree of cognitive impairment.[45,50–56]

Tau imaging agents

Cortical NFTs with tau deposition, the second pathologic hallmark of AD, are more tightly correlated with AD disease progression than Aβ plaques.[57–62] Also, the time course and distribution of tau deposits are differentially associated with normal aging and disease, as deposits limited to the transentorhinal cortex (Braak stages I and II) are associated with normal aging, whereas neocortical tau deposition is associated with dementia.[63–69] These findings and other described limitations of Aβ imaging have driven efforts to develop tau MI radiotracers. Development of tau agents has been complicated because concentrations of tau deposition are much lower than Aβ and the tau protein can exist in 6 different isoforms based on the number of repeats of its microtubule binding domain.[70] Furthermore, tau is located intraneuronally in AD, which requires the tracer to not only cross the blood-brain barrier but also enter the neuron for binding its target. Depending on the disorder, tau aggregates also can be found in the glial cells.[71] In addition, tau can be found in different forms of aggregations (eg, paired helical filaments, straight filaments, coiled bodies) and tau can occur in phosphorylated and nonphosphorylated forms.[72,73] Finally, tau pathology is not a hallmark of one particular disease but of several different NDDs,

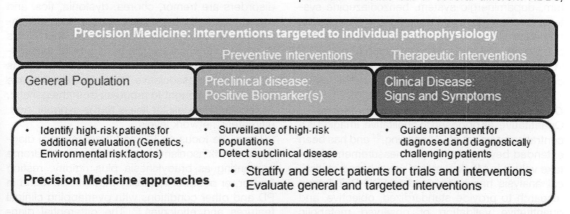

Fig. 1. Precision medicine approaches for evaluation of NDD and MD. Precision medicine involves interventions targeted to individual pathophysiology (*upper box*), which are under development but not yet available for NDDs and MDs. However, key elements used in the execution of PM[2] (Precision Medicine Approaches, *lower box*) are being applied in NDD and MD. MI is best suited to applications in the preclinical and clinical phases, including detection and stratification of preclinical disease and monitoring and evaluation of treatment response in clinical disease (see text and **Table 1**).

termed "tauopathies,"[74] including some FTDs and the atypical parkinsonian syndrome, progressive supranuclear palsy (PSP).

Several potential tau imaging agents are undergoing validation and development in both preclinical and human studies, with human research studies currently just being completed.[45] Among the promising tau imaging agents are (F-18)T807 (also known as [F-18]AV-1451),[75,76] (C-11) PBB3,[77] and (F-18)THK-5351.[70,78–80]

Although the clinical value of tau PET is not yet established, it will potentially impact the evaluation of AD. Given that NFTs are tightly associated with the degree of cognitive decline, measurement of neocortical tau is a proposed targeted biomarker of therapeutic efficacy and tau PET is already being used in AD clinical trials. For example, postmortem evaluation of the halted Phase III AD clinical trial subjects with the anti-Aβ antibody AN-1792 showed significant cortical Aβ clearance, but extensive tau deposition remained.[81,82] Increased understanding of the mechanism of tau effects on neurodegeneration has also led to research on anti-tau therapeutic agents, including approaches to reduce tau, reduce tau aggregation, and stimulate immune response to specific putative pathogenic tau species. Altogether, the use of tau PET in combination with Aβ imaging could provide the clinician with a more complete pathophysiological context to better diagnose AD and be valuable in PM approaches, as described in this article.

Other radiotracers used in dementia

Numerous radiotracers have been developed for the investigation of dementia and various neurochemical systems have been evaluated in humans. These include radiotracers for the cholinergic system, dopaminergic system, benzodiazepine system, serotonergic system, and neuroinflammation pathways. In particular, dopamine imaging has been used clinically in the evaluation of dementia in Europe and Asia, specifically when DLB is considered in the differential diagnosis.[83]

Quantification of neuroimaging biomarkers

Quantitative, as opposed to qualitative, imaging is a central component of PM imaging,[84] and has been extended beyond the simple measurement of uptake values in MI. Automated voxel-based statistical analysis has been used in FDG-PET–based research to provide standardized, objective, and quantitative validation of observed metabolic changes.[17] When applied with computer-assisted diagnosis algorithms, these techniques have demonstrated an equivalent performance to experienced readers for the diagnosis of NDD and have also improved the learning of beginning

readers.[85,86] "Three-Dimensional Stereotactic Surface Projections" (3D-SSP),[17] a widely used quantitative method for brain PET and SPECT, combines an image database, computer processing, and statistical assessment. This method creates quantitative statistical 3D maps of 2D cross-sectional images. As a result, a large amount of information is condensed into a few hemispheric surface images on which the diffuse or regional statistical deviation from the "normal" database can be overlaid. The use of automated voxel-based statistical mapping facilitates pattern recognition, thereby increasing diagnostic accuracy.[87] Although initially applied to FDG-PET and AD, 3D-SSP is now being used to visualize many different radiotracers for diagnoses and in research related to multiple disease processes.[88,89]

Also, given the differences in individual Aβ tracers described previously, the Centiloid project was established to help standardize quantitative Aβ imaging outcomes to a common scaled unit, termed "centiloids," that are independent of the individual Aβ tracer used.[32]

Finally, as will be described later in this article, quantitative analysis plays an important role in dopamine MI to normalize nonselective radiotracer binding and to better isolate specific basal ganglia changes related to movement-related symptoms.

Brief Overview of Movement Disorders: Parkinson Disease and Its Differential Diagnosis

MDs can be categorized as either hyperkinetic or hypokinetic, with either an excess or paucity of movements.[90] The most common hyperkinetic disorders are tremor, chorea, dystonia, tics, and myoclonus. In the hypokinetic group, the parkinsonian syndromes are the most frequent. Many MDs are related to basal ganglia or cerebellar dysfunction, or abnormal connections from those regions to primary or associative motor cortices. These changes are thought to progress from the genetic, molecular, and cellular levels to the synaptic and, ultimately, network levels.

Here, we focus on PD and its differential diagnosis. "Parkinsonism" is a hypokinetic syndrome presenting as bradykinesia plus rigidity, resting tremor, or postural instability that can be found in PD and other conditions with overlapping clinical features and etiologies.[91] The differential diagnosis includes PD, essential tremor (ET), adult-onset dystonic tremor, DLB, and some atypical parkinsonian syndromes (APS). ET is a common disorder characterized by bilateral, symmetric postural and kinetic tremor, more pronounced in the hands. Although less common, adult-onset dystonic tremor, with asymmetric resting arm tremor and impaired arm swing as well as cogwheel rigidity, can also be confused with PD.[92] APSs are a heterogeneous group of diseases, including multiple system atrophy and PSP, each of which can demonstrate distinct clinical features in addition to parkinsonian features, but can be difficult to distinguish in early stages. Corticobasal syndromes, including CBD, are also clinically classified as APS, but are more recently classified as FTDs based on pathologic findings.[93]

The classic histopathology of PD is Lewy bodies and Lewy neurites, which are intraneuronal aggregations of α-synuclein. An added layer of complexity is that the spectrum of Lewy body diseases includes PD, PD with mild cognitive impairment (PD-MCI), PD with dementia (PDD), and DLB. (Although differences between PDD and DLB have been demonstrated and diagnostic criteria have been adopted, the practical differentiation between these 2 disease entities is a point of continued discussion.)[94,95] Even if DLB is excluded, PD is a phenotypically heterogeneous disorder that can be described as having a classic parkinsonian motor phenotype with varying amounts of cognitive impairment. In addition, there is overlap and potential synergy between pathologic findings in PD and AD, as well with DLB, that are not fully understood.[46,96,97]

Overview of Molecular Imaging in Movement Disorders

Dopaminergic imaging and PET with 2-(F-18) fluoro-2-deoxy-ᴅ-glucose

Dopamine imaging was one of the first reported neurochemical PET procedures.[98,99] An extensive literature describes a robust model for the MI approach to MD. This includes imaging presynaptic dopamine synthetic capacity (AA/DOPA decarboxylase; ie, [F-18]FDOPA PET), presynaptic terminal transporters (dopamine and monoamine; ie, [I-123]FP-CIT [2-β-carbomethoxy-3-β-(4-iodophenyl)-N-(3- fluoropropyl) nortropane] and [I-123]β-CIT [2-carboxymethoxy-3β-(4-iodophenyl) tropane] SPECT); (C-11)methylphenidate PET, and (C-11)DTBZ (dihydrotetrabenazine) PET, and presynaptic and postsynaptic dopaminergic enzyme receptors (D1, D2, and other subtypes; ie, [C-11]NNC [(+)-8-chloro-5-(7- benzofuranyl)-7-hydroxy-3-methyl-2,3,4,5-tetra-hydro-IH-3-benzazepine] and [C-11]raclopride). Dopamine imaging was initially applied to PD,[100–103] confirming the nigrostriatal degeneration and dopamine deficits previously described by postmortem investigations. A reproducible dopamine MI

observation is that patients with PD demonstrate decreased striatal dopamine function relative to human controls, which has been demonstrated with MI of presynaptic dopamine synthetic capacity, presynaptic terminal transporters and, with lesser specificity, dopamine receptors.[104–107]

MI of presynaptic dopamine transporter (DAT) function and FDG-PET may be the most clinically relevant techniques for differentiating PD from its differential diagnoses, with the best results for ET.[83] In fact, DAT MI distinguishes PD from ET but, although it may have some value in distinguishing PD from PSP,[108] generally does not reliably distinguish PD from APS in a clinical setting.[7,109] Early on, semiquantitative evaluation of the DAT radiotracer caudate-putamen uptake ratio combined with an MI estimate of postsynaptic D2 dopamine receptor density was found to be informative in diagnostically challenging cases.[110] But later findings demonstrated that FDG-PET is superior to D2 receptor imaging for differentiating PD from APS. Consistent with these findings, a common MI approach to assist in the evaluation of parkinsonism is the joint use of FDG-PET and DAT SPECT imaging.

Other radiotracers in movement disorders

Notably, there is currently no clinically viable radiotracer for evaluating α-synuclein or Lewy body aggregates found in PD, DLB, and other α-synuceinopathies.[111,112] MI of many other neurotransmitters and molecules of interest have been used to evaluate MDs.[113,114] Additional movement disorder movement tracers will be described in relation to specific PM efforts.

Precision Medicine

PM is a patient management framework in which prevention and treatment strategies are tailored to individuals.[1] In other words, PM takes into account disease variability across patients to provide the *right intervention* to the *right person* at the *right time*.[115] In addition, 3 key elements of PM for NDD have been proposed: comprehensive risk assessment; preclinical detection of pathophysiologic processes; and interventions tailored to the molecular pathophysiology of an individual's disease.[2] These elements can be seen as part of PM approaches to NDD, even if interventions have not yet been fully realized.

Molecular Imaging and Precision Medicine in Alzheimer Disease

In AD, MI has been applied to detecting preclinical disease processes[116–118] and evaluating interventions tailored to an individual's disease (**Table 1**),

Table 1
MI in PM approaches to NDD and MD: AD, PD, and DLB

PM MI Approaches	Preclinical Detection of Pathophysiologic Processes	Interventions Tailored to the Molecular Pathophysiology of an Individual's Disease

AD	General population
	  Morris 2009
	  Chetelat 2013
	  Villemagne 2013
	  Roe 2013
	  ADNI: Weiner 2015
	Genotypic subpopulations
	  ADAD
	  DIAN: Bateman 2012, Fagan 2014,
	    Benzinger 2013
	  APOε
	  Fleisher 2013
	  API: Reiman 2011
		Selecting patients
		  Ostrowitzki 2011
		  Rinne 2010
		Evaluating interventions (completed)
		  Cummings 2014
		  Doody 2013
		  Doody 2014
		  Ostrowitzki 2011
		  Rinne 2010
		Evaluating biomarkers and interventions (ongoing)
		  ADNI: Weiner 2015
		  API: Reiman 2011
		  DIAN-TU Mills 2013
		  A4/LEARN: Sperling 2014

PD	At-risk subpopulations
	  LLRK2 mutation: Lee 2000
	  GBA mutation: Goker-Aplian 2012
	  Idiopathic RBD: Stiasny-Kolster 2005
	  Hyposmia: Sliveria-Moriayma 2009.
	Other subpopulations
	  DIP: Tinazzi 2014
		Guide management for diagnostically challenging cases
		  CUPS trial: Catafau and Tolosa 2004
		  SWEDD: Marshall 2006
		  DIP: Tinazzi 2008, 2009
		Evaluating interventions (completed)
		  CALM-PD: Parkinson Study Group 2002
		  ELLDOPA trial: Fahn 2004
		  PRECEPT trial: Parkinson Study Group S 2007
		  Marek 2003
		  Rakshi 2002

DLB		Guide management for diagnostically challenging cases: Walker 2015

Abbreviations: AD, Alzheimer disease; ADAD, autosomal dominant AD; ADNI, AD neuroimaging initiative; API, Alzheimer's Prevention Initiative; CUPS, Clinically Uncertain Parkinsonian Syndromes; DIAN, Dominantly Inherited Alzheimer Network; DIAN-TU, DIAN trial unit; DIP, drug-induced parkinsonism; DLB, dementia of Lewy bodies; MD, movement disorder; MI, molecular imaging; NDD, neurodegenerative disorders; PD, Parkinson disease; PM, precision medicine; RBD, rapid eye movement sleep behavioral disorder; SWEDD, subjects without evidence of dopaminergic defect.

as risk assessment in NDD is focused primarily on genetic and, to a lesser extent, environmental factors. AD is a genetically diverse disorder: more than 20 genetic loci have been associated with increased risk, from mutations that confer a mild increase in risk to causative, high-penetrance mutations that result in full disease expression.[119,120] Although there may be exceptions, causative mutations are generally more rare and mutations that confer increased risk more common.[121–123]

Although environmental risk factors are less well investigated in AD, traumatic brain injury is a known epigenetic risk factor for AD.[124] Notably, chronic traumatic encephalopathy demonstrates a wide spectrum of tau pathologies including but not exclusively NFT, that are heterogeneous among individual patients.[125] Thus, one can envision tau MI

in a PM approach to stratify chronic traumatic encephalopathy (CTE) patients and identify those who might benefit from future tau-targeted interventions.

To date, the most promising biomarkers for preclinical detection in AD are those obtained from MI and cerebrospinal fluid (CSF). For example, both amyloid PET and CSF biomarkers predicted progression to cognitive impairment at least several years before dementia symptom onset in a self-described "convenience sample" population from a regional AD research center.[9] The level of accuracy was thought adequate to stratify cognitively normal individuals at risk for full clinical AD, but not for prediction of impending full clinical AD in the general population (true preclinical detection) without the incorporation of additional patient characteristics. Although high levels of Aβ deposition in cognitively healthy individuals in the community are associated with subtle progressive deficits and a higher risk of cognitive impairments, these relationships appear to be modified by lifestyle activities and cognitive reserve, as well as genetic markers.[126–128] Still, individuals without dementia but with an imaged high Aβ load are at a significantly greater risk of cognitive decline.[9,129] On the other hand, the likelihood that a cognitively unimpaired patient with low Aβ load will go on to develop AD is very low. Thus, the most recent clinical diagnostic criteria for AD require MI or CSF evidence of Aβ pathology for the diagnosis of preclinical AD.[130]

Another potential use of MI and CSF biomarkers is to establish criteria for different stages of AD,[131,132] which in turn also may be helpful for tailoring therapies.

More recently, a few ongoing multicenter studies are more in line with a PM framework for preclinical detection by evaluating biomarkers in more homogeneous subgroups of AD.[133–136] For example, the ongoing DIAN trial evaluates molecular and imaging biomarkers in patients with causative genotypes for autosomal dominant AD (ADAD), which represents approximately 1% of AD cases.[137] The 3 known allele/mutations that result in ADAD, amyloid precursor protein, presenilin 1 (PSEN1), or presenilin 2 (PSEN2), all have near 100% penetrance. Therefore, these patients all progress to full clinical AD. Although complete progression to AD means there is no need to predict impending full clinical AD in these patients, selecting these patients provides important information about the time course of Aβ deposition and other clinical manifestations in relation to disease progression.[138] Also, this homogeneous sample of asymptomatic causative mutation carriers with "preclinical AD" may allow better isolation of the prognostic utility of biomarkers, which in turn may be extensible to broader populations.

With regard to therapeutic interventions, clinical trials of promising, traditional "one treatment fits all" interventions for AD have tried and have failed to significantly alter the disease course. There is currently no fundamental cure for AD. Interventions such as reducing acetylcholine degradation or suppressing ionotropic glutamatergic signaling by memantine improve certain aspects of symptoms and are currently in use in clinical practice, but have not been shown to prevent disease or slow its progression.[139] These interventions are also not specifically targeted toward the fundamental molecular pathophysiology of AD.

A few recent and ongoing trials evaluating preventive interventions directed at the molecular pathology of AD, specifically Aβ, are more in line with the PM framework. Completed trials have failed to significantly alter disease course.[140–143] For example, the anti-Aβ antibody bapineuzumab phase II trial demonstrated an important proof of concept that lowering of cortical fibrillar Aβ with bapineuzumab can be detected with (C-11)PiB PET. But the trial was halted due to lack of improvement in clinical and functional outcomes in patients with AD even with reductions in the Aβ load.[143] In contrast, a more recent secondary outcome study has suggested a therapeutic effect of solanezubmab in a subgroup of patients with mild AD, suggesting that trials included patients in too far advanced stages.[144] It should also be noted that phase II trials of a targeted tau phosphorylation inhibitor, tideglusib, have not shown any clinical benefit in AD but have reduced the progression of brain atrophy in PSP.[145,146]

For anti-Aβ agents, large-scale clinical trials are also ongoing. One example trial is the international Alzheimer's Prevention Initiative (API), which includes registries of patients with PSEN1 causative mutations, including the world's largest known ADAD kindred, and a registry of APO4ε homozygotes (who have the highest APOE dose-dependent risk for AD).[147] The API is conducting ongoing/proposed placebo-controlled randomized control trials (RCTs) of 2 investigational anti-Aβ agents.[148] The DIAN trial unit (DIAN-TU) has also undertaken a double-blinded, placebo-controlled RCT of 2 investigational anti-Aβ agents in individuals at risk for and with ADAD.[149] The Anti-Amyloid Treatment in Asymptomatic Alzheimer's Disease (A4) trial is a placebo-controlled secondary prevention RCT using an anti-Aβ agent in clinically healthy older adults with amyloid accumulation placing them at high risk for AD.[150] Notably, at least amyloid PET, and at times FDG-PET and tau MI, are included in each study's panel of AD biomarkers to evaluate the efficacy of these agents on AD pathophysiology. The Collaboration for Alzheimer Prevention (CAP) is a consortium of these initiatives, as well as federal and private organizations, including one privately funded trial (TOMORROW study) to foster collaboration toward the goal of having the greatest impact in AD prevention.[148] To this end, targeted interventions that are successful in their ability to halt or reverse latent disease in these subsets of AD can then be advanced to larger trials. With increased power, larger studies may better evaluate therapeutic effectiveness and investigate whether these interventions can be extended to individuals with different or more heterogeneous molecular drivers, but perhaps shared disease mechanisms.

Finally, although large anti-Aβ trials have not used MI for patient selection, resulting in the inclusion of up to 30% of patients with low Aβ, SNAP,[144] some anti-Aβ trials have used Aβ MI to select patients.[143,151] Although MI would need to be applied in patient selection judiciously, a successful therapeutic trial using MI as selection criteria would be a complete PM proof of concept: an MI targeted intervention tailored to an individual's disease profile. Also, the MI phenotypic difference in patients with SNAP may provide a PM opportunity, as these patients may be stratified into different risk or disease profiles with alternative management.

Frontotemporal Dementia Syndromes

As described previously, FTD syndromes are a genetically and clinically heterogeneous group of disorders. In general, slightly less than half of the frontotemporal lobar dementias are tauopathies, such as PSP or CBD, about another half are ubiquitinopathies associated with the TDP-43 mutation, and less than 10% associated with Fused in Sarcoma RNA binding protein (FUS) inclusions.[152] Based on pathologic and clinical categorization, 6 subtypes of FTD and related syndromes exist. Many FTD syndromes have characteristic molecular and other neuroimaging characteristics that can be helpful with diagnosis.[153] In terms of PM, although the tau pathology in FTD syndromes differs from that found in AD, one can envision tau MI providing an opportunity for PM approaches similar to those described for CTE previously, but for a potentially more heterogeneous group of diseases.

Precision Medicine in Movement Disorders

As with AD, MI is most applicable to PD PM in detecting preclinical disease processes and identifying interventions tailored to an individual's disease, as risk assessment in PD is focused primarily on genetic and environmental risk (such as exposure to certain toxins like manganese).[154] Still, evaluation of genetic risk shows some promise for a precision medicine–based approach to PD. PD is genetically heterogeneous, with approximately 20 genetic loci associated with varying amounts of risk for PD,[155] and phenotypically heterogeneous as described previously. Also, the genotypes associated with classic PD motor symptoms only partially overlap with the genotypes associated with cognitive impairment and dementia in PD.[156,157] Thus, it has been proposed that genotyping may help tailor targeted therapies for parkinsonian motor, cognitive, or other atypical parkinsonian symptoms.[115,158]

MI, CSF analysis, and peripheral tissue biopsy (submandibular gland) have shown promise as biomarkers for PD PM. For example, submandibular gland biopsy has been promising for detecting "early" PD, and with further evaluation may be able to serve as a proxy for the gold standard of autopsy for confirmation of the diagnosis of PD.[159,160] In the research setting, low CSF (Aβ1-42) predicts progression to dementia in PD, whereas combined functional MRI and CSF analysis suggest that abnormal α-synuclein CSF accumulation contributes to the disruption of motor-related functional connectivity in PD,[161] demonstrating the potential value of CSF analysis in preclinical PD detection.

In terms of molecular imaging, clinical parkinsonism occurs when patients with PD have lost 40% to 50% of normal mean levels of putamen dopamine terminal function.[162] MI indicates patients with PD have a faster decline in putamen DAT binding than seen in healthy age-matched controls,[163] but there is a potential window for detecting less than 50% loss of putamen DAT binding in at-risk subjects for PD.[163] It should be noted with regard to quantitative imaging, that PET and SPECT radiotracers currently available for measuring striatal DAT binding are relatively nonselective, also binding to noradrenaline and serotonin transporters with a similar or lower nanomolar affinity.[164,165] As a result, the cerebellum is commonly used as a reference tissue for nonspecific uptake, and ratiometric analyses are used for these study findings.

Overall, these findings suggest that DAT MI striatal uptake may be helpful in screening for preclinical disease in patients with increased risk for PD. However, some practical considerations need to be addressed. In PD, there is an additional loss of DAT in remaining terminals as an adaptive mechanism to attempt to preserve synaptic dopamine levels.[166] As a result, measures of DAT availability with PET or SPECT may overestimate the degree of loss at the terminal, which may increase sensitivity and decrease specificity for PD. Also, DAT blockade with drugs such as methylphenidate increases synaptic dopamine,[167] which must also be taken into account when interpreting changes in dopamine terminal function. Another important factor is the cost of imaging. An expensive imaging test cannot be used to screen the general population. Appropriate patients need to be preselected, potentially by PM risk assessment approaches like genotyping described previously, for further screening by imaging.

Although using MI to aid diagnosis is not generally considered PM, using MI to guide management of difficult diagnostic cases is in line with a PM approach. The Clinically Uncertain Parkinsonian Syndromes (CUPS) trial was designed to evaluate the impact of initial knowledge of dopamine transporter SPECT findings on the management of patients.[11] When (I-123)FP-CIT SPECT findings were provided to clinicians, DA-deficient parkinsonian syndrome was the given diagnosis in slightly more than half the cases evaluated, and the management strategy was changed in 72% of these CUPS cases. Although there was no nonimaged control group, this study suggested that measuring striatal DAT binding in the workup of uncertain parkinsonian cases refines an individual's case management. In addition, a more recent open-label controlled study demonstrated that knowing baseline DAT status led to change of management in 50% of CUPS-like cases over 4 weeks, whereas management was changed in only 21% without DAT imaging.[168] It remains to be seen if the differences in management with baseline striatal DAT information results in changes in outcomes or quality of life, which are implicit mandates for effective PM.[169]

Recent clinical trials using dopamine terminal MI to evaluate suspected early PD report that approximately 10% of these patients demonstrate normal dopamine terminal function (striatal DAT binding).[170] The clinical significance of these findings in these "subjects without evidence of dopaminergic defect" (SWEDD) is unclear, and some patients in this category might have non-PD pathology, such as adult-onset dystonia. Generally, parkinsonian symptoms in SWEDD do not progress, with some mild exceptions,[92] and a SPECT or PET finding of normal dopamine terminal function appears to be associated with a better prognosis than for those with reduced dopamine terminal function (ELLDOPA [Earlier versus Later Levodopa Therapy in Parkinson Disease], PRECEPT [Parkinson Research Examination of CEP-1347 Trial] trials).[170,171]

Still, this MI heterogeneity in patients with PD provides another opportunity for PM. For example, a small series of patients who initially fulfilled PD diagnostic criteria and were treated with dopaminergic agents, but for whom the diagnosis of PD was subsequently questioned, were all found to have normal (I-123)FP-CIT-SPECT findings (ie, SWEDD), and the cessation of dopaminergic agents was achieved without clinical deterioration.[172] Again, the impact of these changes on outcomes is not clear, but this is another example in which dopaminergic terminal imaging may help tailor treatment for individuals.

Drug-induced parkinsonism (DIP), which may occur if striatal dopamine D2 receptor availability is reduced below 20% of normal,[173] is another opportunity for the application of PM approaches.

DIP can be caused by medications, such as neuroleptic antipsychotics, sedatives used to treat vertigo and tetrabenzamine used to reduce involuntary movements.[92] DIP is not always a diagnostic dilemma clinically but it is also possible for DIP medications to unmask preclinical PD. In these cases, DIP can be clinically indistinguishable from PD, and DAT imaging may help determine whether DIP is entirely drug induced or includes a component of otherwise preclinical PD.[174] DIP and idiopathic PD have different MI signatures, as the striatal DAT availability that is reduced in idiopathic PD is normal in DIP. Using (I-123)FP-CIT-SPECT, researchers found that approximately half of clinically indistinguishable patients who developed parkinsonism while taking neuroleptics demonstrated reduced striatal DAT binding, suggesting that this DAT-deficient half of the patients had a component of preclinical PD.[174] In a related study, abnormal FP-CIT uptake in the putamen and caudate predicted motor impairment and response to L–DOPA treatment in patients with schizophrenia chronically exposed to antipsychotics.[175] Thus, DAT MI may be used in a PM approach to identify which subgroup of patients with DIP might benefit from dopamine (levodopa) therapy.

Striatal DAT imaging is also well positioned for quantitative monitoring of PD progression and for monitoring the efficacy of neuroprotective agents,[176,177] as amyloid and tau imaging are being used in AD. Results with general dopamine agonists used in clinical practice have been promising, but mixed from a PM standpoint. A large study using serial striatal (I-123)β-CIT uptake to evaluate the effects of pramipexole versus levodopa demonstrated slower decline of striatal DAT function with pramipexole, but mixed clinical changes with these medications: dyskinesias were reduced with pramipexole but improvement in the United Parkinson Disease Rating Scale (UPDRS) score was greater with levodopa.[178] The differences in clinical and imaging findings are not well understood. In addition, a slower reduction in DAT binding is difficult to interpret, and may reflect a neuroprotective effect of pramipexole, toxicity of levodopa, or might reflect adaptive downregulation of DAT after chronic exposure to levodopa.[92]

The ELLDOPA trial compared the rate of DAT function reduction and parkinsonian clinical progression in patients treated with levodopa or placebo, also with some mixed results. As expected, levodopa improved locomotor function in a dose-dependent fashion relative to placebo. However, at the highest doses, one-third of patients treated with levodopa developed fluctuating treatment responses, and nearly one-fifth developed dyskinesias.[179] Also, striatal DAT function with high levodopa doses was actually more reduced than with placebo. However, this was thought to be due to compensatory downregulation of DAT binding from chronic levodopa exposure because the clinical benefits of levodopa treatment persisted after 2 weeks of medication "washout."

In a proposed PM intervention targeted at molecular pathophysiology, the PRECEPT trial assessed the disease-modifying potential of the c-Jun N-terminal kinase (JNK) inhibitor CEP-1347 versus placebo in early PD cases. Evidence has suggested that the JNK pathway plays an important role in the neurotoxicity seen in PD.[180] Unfortunately, no clinical or imaging differences were seen between the JNK inhibitor and placebo and the study was stopped early.[181] In fact, CEP-1347 unexpectedly caused mild downregulation of striatal DAT function, which is incompletely understood and again demonstrates some challenges that can arise with MI evaluation of PM approaches.

As has been the case for AD, MI has been successfully applied in PD PM approaches to detect preclinical disease in subgroups of patients with genotypes conferring increased risk or causative mutations. For PD, glucocerebrosidase (GBA) mutations are the most common genetic determinant of PD and up to 30% of "sporadic" PD cases are heterozygous carriers of GBA mutation (homozygous GBA mutation carriers develop Gaucher disease).[156] A specific point mutation of the leucine-rich repeat kinase 2 (LRRK2) is the second most common genetic cause of dominantly inherited PD, although there are some geographic differences in the prevalence of these mutations.[157] Mutations in α-synuclein are perhaps the most well-known genetic cause of PD, but are much more rare than GBA and LRRK2 mutations.[182]

In any case, dopamine PET and SPECT are able to detect subclinical loss of DAT binding in LRRK2 and GBA mutation carriers, thereby identifying patients for potential secondary prevention trials similar to the A4 trial for AD. One example of this has been shown in family members of an LRRK2 kindred, in which (F-18)FDOPA, (C-11)DTBZ, and (C-11)methylphenidate PET were used to assess striatal dopamine storage capacity, vesicular monoamine transporter (VMAT2) binding, and DAT binding, respectively.[183] MI was able to stratify LRRK2 family members in groups of those already affected by PD, those with preclinical disease, and those who progressed to preclinical disease over time.[166] Thus, MI identifies "at-risk" individuals who may benefit from early interventions to prevent progression to clinical disease. Similar work has been done for GBA

heterozygotes, such that (I-123)FP-CIT DAT function imaging can help identify candidates for preventive therapies.[184]

Other groups of patients who are at increased risk for PD are relatives of patients with PD who are hyposmic[185–187] and patients with idiopathic rapid eye movement sleep behavioral disorder (iRBD).[188,189] Hyposmia is suggestive of early synuclein effects in the anterior telencephalon and iRBD is highly suggestive of synucleinopathy in the ventral brainstem. In both cases, the addition of MI of DAT function increases the clinical utility of these findings. If patients at risk for or with suspected PD have normal olfactory discrimination, then a negative DAT scan demonstrating normal dopaminergic function is even more reassuring. In terms of PM approaches, patients with iRBD with reduced putaminal DAT function might benefit from existing or potential parkinsonian therapies, as opposed to treatments otherwise tailored for other synuclienopathies.

Dopamine Transporter and Other Molecular Imaging for Dementia

Lewy body pathology can lead to significant cognitive impairment if it involves limbic and associated cortical areas. Based on current criteria, if the dementia occurs before or up to 1 year after the onset of parkinsonism, the condition is termed DLB. If dementia occurs more than a year after the onset of parkinsonism, the condition is termed PDD.[94] DLB is also classically associated with fluctuating levels of cognitive arousal and visual hallucinations in addition to parkinsonian motor symptoms. In terms of molecular imaging, most cases of DLB have a significant Aβ in addition to alpha synuclein load.[46] In part because of this, DAT imaging has been the focus of diagnostic MI for DLB. In a small research sample of patients with dementia with variable etiologies, clinical consensus criteria had a baseline diagnostic sensitivity of 75% and specificity of 42%, whereas baseline (I-123)FP-CIT SPECT had a baseline diagnostic SN of 88% and SP of 100%.[190] Thus, DAT has at least a supportive role to play in classifying uncertain dementia cases, and in large-scale studies has demonstrated high specificity for DLB versus AD.[83] As noted previously, the differentiation of DLB and PDD remains a point of discussion, but DLB cases may have less of a caudate-putamen uptake ratio than PDD.[191]

In a PM approach to diagnostically challenging cases similar to that described for PD, a more recent study demonstrated that a baseline DAT scan resulted in a change in the diagnosis of nearly two-thirds of patients with possible DLB versus fewer than 5% of those who were not scanned.[10] Again, the effect of these changes on quality of life and clinical outcomes remains to be seen.

I-123 metaiodobenzylguanidine (MIBG) imaging of cardiac sympathetic innervation has also been applied for diagnosis in PD and DLB. For PD, MIBG is informative but may not have enough sensitivity to be of diagnostic value. However, MIBG may help separate PD from atypical parkinsonian disorders, in which cardiac sympathetic innervation is preserved.[192] Also, DAT and MIBG may be comparable in their ability to distinguish DLB from other dementias.[193,194] Because autonomic findings may precede central nervous system findings in PD and DLB,[195] MIBG may complement other approaches to identify preclinical disease in these disorders.[196,197]

Other Movement Disorders

The most common clinical use of MI in MDs is differentiation of PD from ET. MI, including (F-18) FDOPA PET and DAT SPECT studies, have not shown abnormalities in dopamine striatal neurotransmission in ET,[198] so that FP-CIT SPECT scans can differentiate probable PD from ET, as noted previously.[199] Because the molecular mechanisms and management of PD and ET are different, DAT SPECT provides a PM approach to the management of patients for whom PD and ET are difficult to differentiate.

Atypical Parkinsonian Syndromes

The challenges of using dopamine MI for even diagnostic differentiation of PD from APS were described above. However, tau imaging is expected to be a useful MI tool for distinguishing and characterizing the tauopathy forms of APS, such as PSP and CBD, from others and may support PM approaches to managing these patients.[200]

SUMMARY

MI is a noninvasive, quantitative imaging modality targeted to pathophysiology, and as such is ideally positioned for use in PM. Indeed, even with a lack of proven targeted preventive and therapeutic interventions, MI is already being used in PM approaches for NDD and MD.

MI can identify patients at risk for or at a very early stage of the disease to potentially benefit from proposed preventive interventions. MI is also being used to stratify patients for and monitor interventions in clinical trials. Both of these MI approaches may be best demonstrated in subgroups at increased risk to progress to full clinical disease.

These subgroups may reflect a small percentage of patients with a given disease, but evaluation of the interventions may be more straightforward in these more homogeneous populations and still be extensible to broader patient populations. There are also subsets of patients with AD and PD who display atypical MI biomarker patterns (SNAP and SWEDD, respectively), and may benefit from alternative management approaches.

Finally, MI has the ability to guide management for patients with NDD and MD with diagnostically challenging presentations, including nonspecific parkinsonism, DIP, and DLB. Here, MI can identify patients who may benefit from a change in management, or even a change in diagnosis.

With the advent and refinement of new MI techniques, most notably tau imaging, PM approaches for identifying preclinical disease, stratifying patients for clinical trials and treatments, and monitoring new potential interventions will be applied to a broader range of dementia and MDs, with great promise for improving patient care.

REFERENCES

1. Collins FS, Varmus H. A new initiative on precision medicine. N Engl J Med 2015;372(9):793–5.
2. Montine TJ, Montine KS. Precision medicine: clarity for the clinical and biological complexity of Alzheimer's and Parkinson's diseases. J Exp Med 2015;212(5):601–5.
3. Plassman BL, Langa KM, Fisher GG, et al. Prevalence of dementia in the United States: the aging, demographics, and memory study. Neuroepidemiology 2007;29(1–2):125–32.
4. Murphy SL, Xu J, Kochanek KD. Deaths: final data for 2010, vol. 61. Hyattsville (MD): Statistics NCfH; 2013.
5. Sonnen JA, Santa Cruz K, Hemmy LS, et al. Ecology of the aging human brain. Arch Neurol 2011; 68(8):1049–56.
6. Snowden JS, Thompson JC, Stopford CL, et al. The clinical diagnosis of early-onset dementias: diagnostic accuracy and clinicopathological relationships. Brain 2011;134(Pt 9):2478–92.
7. Plotkin M, Amthauer H, Klaffke S, et al. Combined 123I-FP-CIT and 123I-IBZM SPECT for the diagnosis of parkinsonian syndromes: study on 72 patients. J Neural Transm (Vienna) 2005;112(5):677–92.
8. Ishii K. Clinical application of positron emission tomography for diagnosis of dementia. Ann Nucl Med 2002;16(8):515–25.
9. Roe CM, Fagan AM, Grant EA, et al. Amyloid imaging and CSF biomarkers in predicting cognitive impairment up to 7.5 years later. Neurology 2013; 80(19):1784–91.

10. Walker Z, Moreno E, Thomas A, et al. Clinical use-fulness of dopamine transporter SPECT imaging with 123I-FP-CIT in patients with possible dementia with Lewy bodies: randomised study. Br J Psychiatry 2015;206(2):145–52.

11. Catafau AM, Tolosa E, DaTSCAN Clinically Uncertain Parkinsonian Syndromes Study Group. Impact of dopamine transporter SPECT using 123I-Ioflupane on diagnosis and management of patients with clinically uncertain parkinsonian syndromes. Mov Disord 2004;19(10):1175–82.

12. Hammoud DA, Hoffman JM, Pomper MG. Molecular neuroimaging: from conventional to emerging techniques. Radiology 2007;245(1):21–42.

13. Niethammer M, Eidelberg D. Metabolic brain networks in translational neurology: concepts and applications. Ann Neurol 2012;72(5):635–47.

14. Price JC. Molecular brain imaging in the multimodality era. J Cereb Blood Flow Metab 2012;32(7):1377–92.

15. Cerone AW. Decision making and clinical nuclear medicine: a Canadian pharmacists' perspective. Society of Nuclear Medicine Annual Meeting, Toronto, ON, Canada, June 15, 2009.

16. Kuhl DE. Imaging local brain function with emission computed tomography. Radiology 1984;150(3):625–31.

17. Minoshima S, Frey KA, Koeppe RA, et al. A diagnostic approach in Alzheimer's disease using three-dimensional stereotactic surface projections of fluorine-18-FDG PET. J Nucl Med 1995;36(7):1238–48.

18. Minoshima S, Giordani B, Berent S, et al. Metabolic reduction in the posterior cingulate cortex in very early Alzheimer's disease. Ann Neurol 1997;42(1):85–94.

19. Bohnen NI, Minoshima S. FDG-PET and molecular brain imaging in the movement disorders clinic. Neurology 2012;79(13):1306–7.

20. Brown RK, Bohnen NI, Wong KK, et al. Brain PET in suspected dementia: patterns of altered FDG metabolism. Radiographics 2014;34(3):684–701.

21. Dolan RJ, Grasby PM, Bench C, et al. Pharmacological challenge and PET imaging. Clin Neuropharmacol 1992;15(Suppl 1 Pt A):216A–7A.

22. Rasgon NL, Kenna HA, Geist C, et al. Cerebral metabolic patterns in untreated postmenopausal women with major depressive disorder. Psychiatry Res 2008;164(1):77–80.

23. Yeo JM, Lim X, Khan Z, et al. Systematic review of the diagnostic utility of SPECT imaging in dementia. Eur Arch Psychiatry Clin Neurosci 2013;263(7):539–52.

24. Perl DP. Neuropathology of Alzheimer's disease. Mt Sinai J Med 2010;77(1):32–42.

25. Mirra SS, Heyman A, McKeel D, et al. The Consortium to Establish a Registry for Alzheimer's Disease (CERAD). Part II. Standardization of the neuropathologic assessment of Alzheimer's disease. Neurology 1991;41(4):479–86.

26. Hyman BT, Phelps CH, Beach TG, et al. National Institute on Aging-Alzheimer's Association guidelines for the neuropathologic assessment of Alzheimer's disease. Alzheimers Dement 2012;8(1):1–13.

27. Wang L, Benzinger TL, Hassenstab J, et al. Spatially distinct atrophy is linked to beta-amyloid and tau in preclinical Alzheimer disease. Neurology 2015;84(12):1254–60.

28. Klunk WE, Engler H, Nordberg A, et al. Imaging brain amyloid in Alzheimer's disease with Pittsburgh Compound-B. Ann Neurol 2004;55(3):306–19.

29. Mathis CA, Mason NS, Lopresti BJ, et al. Development of positron emission tomography beta-amyloid plaque imaging agents. Semin Nucl Med 2012;42(6):423–32.

30. Landau SM, Thomas BA, Thurfjell L, et al. Amyloid PET imaging in Alzheimer's disease: a comparison of three radiotracers. Eur J Nucl Med Mol Imaging 2014;41(7):1398–407.

31. Villemagne VL, Mulligan RS, Pejoska S, et al. Comparison of 11C-PiB and 18F-florbetaben for Abeta imaging in ageing and Alzheimer's disease. Eur J Nucl Med Mol Imaging 2012;39(6):983–9.

32. Klunk WE, Koeppe RA, Price JC, et al. The Centiloid Project: standardizing quantitative amyloid plaque estimation by PET. Alzheimers Dement 2015;11(1):1–15.e1–4.

33. Villemagne VL. Amyloid imaging: past, present and future perspectives. Ageing Res Rev 2016. [Epub ahead of print].

34. Weiner MW, Veitch DP, Aisen PS, et al. 2014 Update of the Alzheimer's Disease Neuroimaging Initiative: a review of papers published since its inception. Alzheimers Dement 2015;11(6):e1–120.

35. Wang F, Gordon BA, Ryman DC, et al. Cerebral amyloidosis associated with cognitive decline in autosomal dominant Alzheimer disease. Neurology 2015;85(9):790–8.

36. Jagust WJ, Landau SM, Koeppe RA, et al. The Alzheimer's Disease Neuroimaging Initiative 2 PET Core: 2015. Alzheimers Dement 2015;11(7):757–71.

37. Hardy JA, Higgins GA. Alzheimer's disease: the amyloid cascade hypothesis. Science 1992;256(5054):184–5.

38. Jack CR Jr, Knopman DS, Jagust WJ, et al. Hypothetical model of dynamic biomarkers of the Alzheimer's pathological cascade. Lancet Neurol 2010;9(1):119–28.

39. Jack CR Jr, Wiste HJ, Vemuri P, et al. Brain beta-amyloid measures and magnetic resonance imaging atrophy both predict time-to-progression from mild cognitive impairment to Alzheimer's disease. Brain 2010;133(11):3336–48.

40. Prestia A, Caroli A, Herholz K, et al. Diagnostic accuracy of markers for prodromal Alzheimer's disease in independent clinical series. Alzheimers Dement 2013;9(6):677–86.

41. Jagust WJ, Landau SM, Shaw LM, et al. Relationships between biomarkers in aging and dementia. Neurology 2009;73(15):1193–9.

42. Shaffer JL, Petrella JR, Sheldon FC, et al. Predicting cognitive decline in subjects at risk for Alzheimer disease by using combined cerebrospinal fluid, MR imaging, and PET biomarkers. Radiology 2013;266(2):583–91.

43. Jack CR Jr, Holtzman DM. Biomarker modeling of Alzheimer's disease. Neuron 2013;80(6):1347–58.

44. Jack CR Jr, Wiste HJ, Lesnick TG, et al. Brain beta-amyloid load approaches a plateau. Neurology 2013;80(10):890–6.

45. Brier MR, Gordon B, Friedrichsen K, et al. Tau and Abeta imaging, CSF measures, and cognition in Alzheimer's disease. Sci Transl Med 2016;8(338): 338ra366.

46. Gomperts SN, Rentz DM, Moran E, et al. Imaging amyloid deposition in Lewy body diseases. Neurology 2008;71(12):903–10.

47. Jack CR Jr, Knopman DS, Weigand SD, et al. An operational approach to National Institute on Aging-Alzheimer's Association criteria for preclinical Alzheimer disease. Ann Neurol 2012;71(6):765–75.

48. Jack CR Jr, Wiste HJ, Weigand SD, et al. Amyloid-first and neurodegeneration-first profiles characterize incident amyloid PET positivity. Neurology 2013;81(20):1732–40.

49. Murray J, Tsui WH, Li Y, et al. FDG and amyloid PET in cognitively normal individuals at risk for late-onset Alzheimer's disease. Adv J Mol Imaging 2014;4(2):15–26.

50. Ossenkoppele R, van der Flier WM, Verfaillie SC, et al. Long-term effects of amyloid, hypometabolism, and atrophy on neuropsychological functions. Neurology 2014;82(20):1768–75.

51. Wirth M, Villeneuve S, Haase CM, et al. Associations between Alzheimer disease biomarkers, neurodegeneration, and cognition in cognitively normal older people. JAMA Neurol 2013;70(12): 1512–9.

52. Wirth M, Madison CM, Rabinovici GD, et al. Alzheimer's disease neurodegenerative biomarkers are associated with decreased cognitive function but not beta-amyloid in cognitively normal older individuals. J Neurosci 2013;33(13):5553–63.

53. Tateno A, Sakayori T, Kawashima Y, et al. Comparison of imaging biomarkers for Alzheimer's disease: amyloid imaging with [18F]florbetapir positron emission tomography and magnetic resonance imaging voxel-based analysis for entorhinal cortex atrophy. Int J Geriatr Psychiatry 2015;30(5): 505–13.

54. Rowe CC, Ellis KA, Rimajova M, et al. Amyloid imaging results from the Australian Imaging, Biomarkers and Lifestyle (AIBL) study of aging. Neurobiol Aging 2010;31(8):1275–83.

55. Landau SM, Mintun MA, Joshi AD, et al. Amyloid deposition, hypometabolism, and longitudinal cognitive decline. Ann Neurol 2012;72(4):578–86.

56. Furst AJ, Rabinovici GD, Rostomian AH, et al. Cognition, glucose metabolism and amyloid burden in Alzheimer's disease. Neurobiol Aging 2012;33(2):215–25.

57. Arriagada PV, Growdon JH, Hedley-Whyte ET, et al. Neurofibrillary tangles but not senile plaques parallel duration and severity of Alzheimer's disease. Neurology 1992;42(3 Pt 1):631–9.

58. Nelson PT, Alafuzoff I, Bigio EH, et al. Correlation of Alzheimer disease neuropathologic changes with cognitive status: a review of the literature. J Neuropathol Exp Neurol 2012;71(5):362–81.

59. Guillozet AL, Weintraub S, Mash DC, et al. Neurofibrillary tangles, amyloid, and memory in aging and mild cognitive impairment. Arch Neurol 2003;60(5): 729–36.

60. Gold G, Kovari E, Corte G, et al. Clinical validity of a beta-protein deposition staging in brain aging and Alzheimer disease. J Neuropathol Exp Neurol 2001;60(10):946–52.

61. Nagy Z, Esiri MM, Jobst KA, et al. Relative roles of plaques and tangles in the dementia of Alzheimer's disease: correlations using three sets of neuropathological criteria. Dementia 1995;6(1):21–31.

62. Giannakopoulos P, Gold G, Kovari E, et al. Assessing the cognitive impact of Alzheimer disease pathology and vascular burden in the aging brain: the Geneva experience. Acta Neuropathol 2007; 113(1):1–12.

63. Knopman DS, Parisi JE, Salviati A, et al. Neuropathology of cognitively normal elderly. J Neuropathol Exp Neurol 2003;62(11):1087–95.

64. Bennett DA, Schneider JA, Arvanitakis Z, et al. Neuropathology of older persons without cognitive impairment from two community-based studies. Neurology 2006;66(12):1837–44.

65. Braak H, Braak E. Neuropathological stageing of Alzheimer-related changes. Acta Neuropathol 1991;82(4):239–59.

66. Braak H, Braak E. Frequency of stages of Alzheimer-related lesions in different age categories. Neurobiol Aging 1997;18(4):351–7.

67. Tomlinson BE, Blessed G, Roth M. Observations on the brains of non-demented old people. J Neurol Sci 1968;7(2):331–56.

68. Ball MJ. Neuronal loss, neurofibrillary tangles and granulovacuolar degeneration in the hippocampus with ageing and dementia. A quantitative study. Acta Neuropathol 1977;37(2):111–8.

69. Crary JF, Trojanowski JQ, Schneider JA, et al. Primary age-related tauopathy (PART): a common pathology associated with human aging. Acta Neuropathol 2014;128(6):755–66.

70. Villemagne VL, Fodero-Tavoletti MT, Masters CL, et al. Tau imaging: early progress and future directions. Lancet Neurol 2015;14(1):114–24.

71. Wang Y, Mandelkow E. Tau in physiology and pathology. Nat Rev Neurosci 2016;17(1):5–21.

72. Majounie E, Cross W, Newsway V, et al. Variation in tau isoform expression in different brain regions and disease states. Neurobiol Aging 2013;34(7): 1922.e7-12.

73. Houlden H, Baker M, Morris HR, et al. Corticobasal degeneration and progressive supranuclear palsy share a common tau haplotype. Neurology 2001; 56(12):1702–6.

74. Lee VM, Goedert M, Trojanowski JQ. Neurodegenerative tauopathies. Annu Rev Neurosci 2001;24: 1121–59.

75. Chien DT, Bahri S, Szardenings AK, et al. Early clinical PET imaging results with the novel PHF-tau radioligand [F-18]-T807. J Alzheimers Dis 2013; 34(2):457–68.

76. Xia CF, Arteaga J, Chen G, et al. [(18)F]T807, a novel tau positron emission tomography imaging agent for Alzheimer's disease. Alzheimers Dement 2013;9(6):666–76.

77. Maruyama M, Shimada H, Suhara T, et al. Imaging of tau pathology in a tauopathy mouse model and in Alzheimer patients compared to normal controls. Neuron 2013;79(6):1094–108.

78. Okamura N, Harada R, Furumoto S, et al. Tau PET imaging in Alzheimer's disease. Curr Neurol Neurosci Rep 2014;14(11):500.

79. Okamura N, Harada R, Furukawa K, et al. Advances in the development of tau PET radiotracers and their clinical applications. Ageing Res Rev 2016. [Epub ahead of print].

80. Watanabe H, Ono M, Saji H. Novel PET/SPECT probes for imaging of tau in Alzheimer's disease. ScientificWorldJournal 2015;2015:124192.

81. Nicoll JA, Wilkinson D, Holmes C, et al. Neuropathology of human Alzheimer disease after immunization with amyloid-beta peptide: a case report. Nat Med 2003;9(4):448–52.

82. Patton RL, Kalback WM, Esh CL, et al. Amyloid-beta peptide remnants in AN-1792-immunized Alzheimer's disease patients: a biochemical analysis. Am J Pathol 2006;169(3):1048–63.

83. Kantarci K, Lowe VJ, Boeve BF, et al. Multimodality imaging characteristics of dementia with Lewy bodies. Neurobiol Aging 2012;33(9): 2091–105.

84. Herold CJ, Lewin JS, Wibmer AG, et al. Imaging in the age of precision medicine: summary of the proceedings of the 10th biannual symposium of the International Society for Strategic Studies in radiology. Radiology 2016;279(1):226–38.

85. Markiewicz PJ, Matthews JC, Declerck J, et al. Robustness of correlations between PCA of FDG-PET scans and biological variables in healthy and demented subjects. Neuroimage 2011;56(2): 782–7.

86. Markiewicz PJ, Matthews JC, Declerck J, et al. Alzheimer's disease neuroimaging I. Verification of predicted robustness and accuracy of multivariate analysis. Neuroimage 2011;56(3):1382–5.

87. Hosaka K, Ishii K, Sakamoto S, et al. Validation of anatomical standardization of FDG PET images of normal brain: comparison of SPM and NEUROSTAT. Eur J Nucl Med Mol Imaging 2005;32(1): 92–7.

88. Bohnen NI, Koeppe RA, Minoshima S, et al. Cerebral glucose metabolic features of Parkinson disease and incident dementia: longitudinal study. J Nucl Med 2011;52(6):848–55.

89. Kono AK, Ishii K, Sofue K, et al. Fully automatic differential diagnosis system for dementia with Lewy bodies and Alzheimer's disease using FDG-PET and 3D-SSP. Eur J Nucl Med Mol Imaging 2007; 34(9):1490–7.

90. Lizarraga KJ, Gorgulho A, Chen W, et al. Molecular imaging of movement disorders. World J Radiol 2016;8(3):226–39.

91. Fereshtehnejad SM, Romenets SR, Anang JB, et al. New clinical subtypes of Parkinson disease and their longitudinal progression: a prospective cohort comparison with other phenotypes. JAMA Neurol 2015;72(8):863–73.

92. Brooks DJ. Molecular imaging of dopamine transporters. Ageing Res Rev 2016. [Epub ahead of print].

93. Levin J, Kurz A, Arzberger T, et al. The differential diagnosis and treatment of atypical parkinsonism. Dtsch Arztebl Int 2016;113(5):61–9.

94. McKeith IG, Dickson DW, Lowe J, et al. Diagnosis and management of dementia with Lewy bodies: third report of the DLB Consortium. Neurology 2005;65(12):1863–72.

95. Gomperts SN. Lewy body dementias: dementia with Lewy bodies and Parkinson disease dementia. Continuum (Minneap Minn) 2016;22(2 Dementia): 435–63.

96. Dugger BN, Serrano GE, Sue LI, et al. Presence of striatal amyloid plaques in Parkinson's disease dementia predicts concomitant Alzheimer's disease: usefulness for amyloid imaging. J Parkinsons Dis 2012;2(1):57–65.

97. Irwin DJ, White MT, Toledo JB, et al. Neuropathologic substrates of Parkinson disease dementia. Ann Neurol 2012;72(4):587–98.

98. Wagner HN Jr, Burns HD, Dannals RF, et al. Imaging dopamine receptors in the human brain by

positron tomography. Science 1983;221(4617): 1264–6.

99. Garnett ES, Firnau G, Nahmias C. Dopamine visualized in the basal ganglia of living man. Nature 1983;305(5930):137–8.

100. Garnett ES, Nahmias C, Firnau G. Central dopaminergic pathways in hemiparkinsonism examined by positron emission tomography. Can J Neurol Sci 1984;11(1 Suppl):174–9.

101. Leenders KL, Palmer AJ, Quinn N, et al. Brain dopamine metabolism in patients with Parkinson's disease measured with positron emission tomography. J Neurol Neurosurg Psychiatry 1986;49(8): 853–60.

102. Hagglund J, Aquilonius SM, Bergstrom K, et al. Regional kinetics of [11C]methylspiperone in the brain studied by positron emission tomography in patients with Parkinson's disease. Adv Neurol 1987;45:99–101.

103. Hagglund J, Aquilonius SM, Eckernas SA, et al. Dopamine receptor properties in Parkinson's disease and Huntington's chorea evaluated by positron emission tomography using 11C-N-methyl-spiperone. Acta Neurol Scand 1987;75(2):87–94.

104. Brooks DJ, Pavese N. Imaging biomarkers in Parkinson's disease. Prog Neurobiol 2011;95(4):614–28.

105. Bajaj N, Hauser RA, Grachev ID. Clinical utility of dopamine transporter single photon emission CT (DaT-SPECT) with (123I) ioflupane in diagnosis of parkinsonian syndromes. J Neurol Neurosurg Psychiatry 2013;84(11):1288–95.

106. Suwijn SR, van Boheemen CJ, de Haan RJ, et al. The diagnostic accuracy of dopamine transporter SPECT imaging to detect nigrostriatal cell loss in patients with Parkinson's disease or clinically uncertain parkinsonism: a systematic review. EJNMMI Res 2015;5:12.

107. Hellwig S, Amtage F, Kreft A, et al. [(1)(8)F]FDG-PET is superior to [(1)(2)(3)I]IBZM-SPECT for the differential diagnosis of parkinsonism. Neurology 2012;79(13):1314–22.

108. Messa C, Volonte MA, Fazio F, et al. Differential distribution of striatal [123I]beta-CIT in Parkinson's disease and progressive supranuclear palsy, evaluated with single-photon emission tomography. Eur J Nucl Med 1998;25(9):1270–6.

109. Pirker W, Asenbaum S, Bencsits G, et al. [123I] beta-CIT SPECT in multiple system atrophy, progressive supranuclear palsy, and corticobasal degeneration. Mov Disord 2000;15(6):1158–67.

110. Walker Z, Costa DC, Janssen AG, et al. Dementia with Lewy bodies: a study of post-synaptic dopaminergic receptors with iodine-123 iodobenzamide single-photon emission tomography. Eur J Nucl Med 1997;24(6):609–14.

111. Vernon AC, Ballard C, Modo M. Neuroimaging for Lewy body disease: is the in vivo molecular imaging of alpha-synuclein neuropathology required and feasible? Brain Res Rev 2010;65(1): 28–55.

112. Bagchi DP, Yu L, Perlmutter JS, et al. Binding of the radioligand SIL23 to alpha-synuclein fibrils in Parkinson disease brain tissue establishes feasibility and screening approaches for developing a Parkinson disease imaging agent. PLoS One 2013; 8(2):e55031.

113. Weingarten CP, Sundman MH, Hickey P, et al. Neuroimaging of Parkinson's disease: expanding views. Neurosci Biobehav Rev 2015;59:16–52.

114. Politis M. Neuroimaging in Parkinson disease: from research setting to clinical practice. Nat Rev Neurol 2014;10(12):708–22.

115. Bu LL, Yang K, Xiong WX, et al. Toward precision medicine in Parkinson's disease. Ann Transl Med 2016;4(2):26.

116. Morris JC, Roe CM, Grant EA, et al. Pittsburgh compound B imaging and prediction of progression from cognitive normality to symptomatic Alzheimer disease. Arch Neurol 2009;66(12):1469–75.

117. Chetelat G, La Joie R, Villain N, et al. Amyloid imaging in cognitively normal individuals, at-risk populations and preclinical Alzheimer's disease. Neuroimage Clin 2013;2:356–65.

118. Villemagne VL, Burnham S, Bourgeat P, et al. Amyloid beta deposition, neurodegeneration, and cognitive decline in sporadic Alzheimer's disease: a prospective cohort study. Lancet Neurol 2013; 12(4):357–67.

119. Lambert JC, Ibrahim-Verbaas CA, Harold D, et al. Meta-analysis of 74,046 individuals identifies 11 new susceptibility loci for Alzheimer's disease. Nat Genet 2013;45(12):1452–8.

120. Nalls MA, Pankratz N, Lill CM, et al. Large-scale meta-analysis of genome-wide association data identifies six new risk loci for Parkinson's disease. Nat Genet 2014;46(9):989–93.

121. Guerreiro R, Wojtas A, Bras J, et al. TREM2 variants in Alzheimer's disease. N Engl J Med 2013;368(2): 117–27.

122. Schellenberg GD, Montine TJ. The genetics and neuropathology of Alzheimer's disease. Acta Neuropathol 2012;124(3):305–23.

123. Verstraeten A, Theuns J, Van Broeckhoven C. Progress in unraveling the genetic etiology of Parkinson disease in a genomic era. Trends Genet 2015;31(3):140–9.

124. Fleminger S, Oliver DL, Lovestone S, et al. Head injury as a risk factor for Alzheimer's disease: the evidence 10 years on; a partial replication. J Neurol Neurosurg Psychiatry 2003;74(7):857–62.

125. Armstrong RA, McKee AC, Stein TD, et al. A quantitative study of tau pathology in eleven cases of chronic traumatic encephalopathy. Neuropathol Appl Neurobiol 2016. [Epub ahead of print].

126. Mosconi L, Rinne JO, Tsui WH, et al. Amyloid and metabolic positron emission tomography imaging of cognitively normal adults with Alzheimer's parents. Neurobiol Aging 2013;34(1):22–34.

127. Vemuri P, Lesnick TG, Przybelski SA, et al. Effect of lifestyle activities on Alzheimer disease biomarkers and cognition. Ann Neurol 2012;72(5):730–8.

128. Kemppainen NM, Aalto S, Karrasch M, et al. Cognitive reserve hypothesis: Pittsburgh Compound B and fluorodeoxyglucose positron emission tomography in relation to education in mild Alzheimer's disease. Ann Neurol 2008;63(1):112–8.

129. Resnick SM, Sojkova J, Zhou Y, et al. Longitudinal cognitive decline is associated with fibrillar amyloid-beta measured by [11C]PiB. Neurology 2010;74(10):807–15.

130. Sperling RA, Aisen PS, Beckett LA, et al. Toward defining the preclinical stages of Alzheimer's disease: recommendations from the National Institute on Aging-Alzheimer's Association workgroups on diagnostic guidelines for Alzheimer's disease. Alzheimers Dement 2011;7(3):280–92.

131. Albert MS, DeKosky ST, Dickson D, et al. The diagnosis of mild cognitive impairment due to Alzheimer's disease: recommendations from the National Institute on Aging-Alzheimer's Association workgroups on diagnostic guidelines for Alzheimer's disease. Alzheimers Dement 2011;7(3): 270–9.

132. McKhann G, Drachman D, Folstein M, et al. Clinical diagnosis of Alzheimer's disease: report of the NINCDS-ADRDA Work Group under the auspices of Department of Health and Human Services Task Force on Alzheimer's Disease. Neurology 1984;34(7):939–44.

133. Bateman RJ, Xiong C, Benzinger TL, et al. Clinical and biomarker changes in dominantly inherited Alzheimer's disease. N Engl J Med 2012;367(9): 795–804.

134. Fagan AM, Xiong C, Jasielec MS, et al. Longitudinal change in CSF biomarkers in autosomal-dominant Alzheimer's disease. Sci Transl Med 2014;6(226):226ra230.

135. Benzinger TL, Blazey T, Jack CR Jr, et al. Regional variability of imaging biomarkers in autosomal dominant Alzheimer's disease. Proc Natl Acad Sci U S A 2013;110(47):E4502–9.

136. Fleisher AS, Chen K, Liu X, et al. Apolipoprotein E epsilon4 and age effects on florbetapir positron emission tomography in healthy aging and Alzheimer disease. Neurobiol Aging 2013;34(1):1–12.

137. Moulder KL, Snider BJ, Mills SL, et al. Dominantly inherited Alzheimer network: facilitating research and clinical trials. Alzheimers Res Ther 2013; 5(5):48.

138. Su Y, Blazey TM, Owen CJ, et al. Quantitative amyloid imaging in autosomal dominant Alzheimer's disease: results from the DIAN study group. PLoS One 2016;11(3):e0152082.

139. Zemek F, Drtinova L, Nepovimova E, et al. Outcomes of Alzheimer's disease therapy with acetylcholinesterase inhibitors and memantine. Expert Opin Drug Saf 2014;13(6):759–74.

140. Doody RS, Farlow M, Aisen PS. Alzheimer's disease cooperative study data a, Publication C. Phase 3 trials of solanezumab and bapineuzumab for Alzheimer's disease. N Engl J Med 2014; 370(15):1460.

141. Doody RS, Raman R, Farlow M, et al. A phase 3 trial of semagacestat for treatment of Alzheimer's disease. N Engl J Med 2013;369(4):341–50.

142. Doody RS, Thomas RG, Farlow M, et al. Phase 3 trials of solanezumab for mild-to-moderate Alzheimer's disease. N Engl J Med 2014;370(4): 311–21.

143. Rinne JO, Brooks DJ, Rossor MN, et al. 11C-PiB PET assessment of change in fibrillar amyloid-beta load in patients with Alzheimer's disease treated with bapineuzumab: a phase 2, double-blind, placebo-controlled, ascending-dose study. Lancet Neurol 2010;9(4):363–72.

144. Salloway S, Sperling R, Fox NC, et al. Two phase 3 trials of bapineuzumab in mild-to-moderate Alzheimer's disease. N Engl J Med 2014;370(4): 322–33.

145. Lovestone S, Boada M, Dubois B, et al. A phase II trial of tideglusib in Alzheimer's disease. J Alzheimers Dis 2015;45(1):75–88.

146. Hoglinger GU, Huppertz HJ, Wagenpfeil S, et al. Tideglusib reduces progression of brain atrophy in progressive supranuclear palsy in a randomized trial. Mov Disord 2014;29(4):479–87.

147. Reiman EM, Langbaum JB, Fleisher AS, et al. Alzheimer's Prevention Initiative: a plan to accelerate the evaluation of presymptomatic treatments. J Alzheimers Dis 2011;26(Suppl 3):321–9.

148. Reiman EM, Langbaum JB, Tariot PN, et al. CAP-advancing the evaluation of preclinical Alzheimer disease treatments. Nat Rev Neurol 2016;12(1): 56–61.

149. Mills SM, Mallmann J, Santacruz AM, et al. Preclinical trials in autosomal dominant AD: implementation of the DIAN-TU trial. Rev Neurol (Paris) 2013; 169(10):737–43.

150. Sperling RA, Rentz DM, Johnson KA, et al. The A4 study: stopping AD before symptoms begin? Sci Transl Med 2014;6(228):228fs213.

151. Ostrowitzki S, Deptula D, Thurfjell L, et al. Mechanism of amyloid removal in patients with Alzheimer disease treated with gantenerumab. Arch Neurol 2012;69(2):198–207.

152. Bigio EH. Making the diagnosis of frontotemporal lobar degeneration. Arch Pathol Lab Med 2013; 137(3):314–25.

153. Finger EC. Frontotemporal dementias. Continuum (Minneap Minn) 2016;22(2 Dementia):464–89.

154. Kleinman M, Frank S. Epidemiology and clinical diagnosis of Parkinson disease. PET Clin 2013; 8(4):447–58.

155. Corti O, Lesage S, Brice A. What genetics tells us about the causes and mechanisms of Parkinson's disease. Physiol Rev 2011;91(4):1161–218.

156. Alcalay RN, Caccappolo E, Mejia-Santana H, et al. Cognitive performance of GBA mutation carriers with early-onset PD: the CORE-PD study. Neurology 2012;78(18):1434–40.

157. Srivatsal S, Cholerton B, Leverenz JB, et al. Cognitive profile of LRRK2-related Parkinson's disease. Mov Disord 2015;30(5):728–33.

158. Stamelou M, Bhatia KP. Atypical parkinsonism: diagnosis and treatment. Neurol Clin 2015;33(1): 39–56.

159. Beach TG, Adler CH, Serrano G, et al. Prevalence of submandibular gland synucleinopathy in Parkinson's disease, dementia with Lewy bodies and other Lewy body disorders. J Parkinsons Dis 2016;6(1):153–63.

160. Adler CH, Dugger BN, Hinni ML, et al. Submandibular gland needle biopsy for the diagnosis of Parkinson disease. Neurology 2014;82(10):858–64.

161. Campbell MC, Koller JM, Snyder AZ, et al. CSF proteins and resting-state functional connectivity in Parkinson disease. Neurology 2015;84(24):2413–21.

162. Benamer HT, Patterson J, Wyper DJ, et al. Correlation of Parkinson's disease severity and duration with 123I-FP-CIT SPECT striatal uptake. Mov Disord 2000;15(4):692–8.

163. Marek K, Innis R, van Dyck C, et al. [123I]beta-CIT SPECT imaging assessment of the rate of Parkinson's disease progression. Neurology 2001; 57(11):2089–94.

164. Fischman AJ, Bonab AA, Babich JW, et al. Rapid detection of Parkinson's disease by SPECT with altropane: a selective ligand for dopamine transporters. Synapse 1998;29(2):128–41.

165. Mozley PD, Schneider JS, Acton PD, et al. Binding of [99mTc]TRODAT-1 to dopamine transporters in patients with Parkinson's disease and in healthy volunteers. J Nucl Med 2000;41(4):584–9.

166. Lee CS, Samii A, Sossi V, et al. In vivo positron emission tomographic evidence for compensatory changes in presynaptic dopaminergic nerve terminals in Parkinson's disease. Ann Neurol 2000;47(4): 493–503.

167. Volkow ND, Wang GJ, Fowler JS, et al. Imaging the effects of methylphenidate on brain dopamine: new model on its therapeutic actions for attention-deficit/hyperactivity disorder. Biol Psychiatry 2005;57(11):1410–5.

168. Kupsch AR, Bajaj N, Weiland F, et al. Impact of DaTscan SPECT imaging on clinical management,

diagnosis, confidence of diagnosis, quality of life, health resource use and safety in patients with clinically uncertain parkinsonian syndromes: a prospective 1-year follow-up of an open-label controlled study. J Neurol Neurosurg Psychiatry 2012;83(6):620–8.

169. Kupsch A, Bajaj N, Weiland F, et al. Changes in clinical management and diagnosis following DaTscan SPECT imaging in patients with clinically uncertain parkinsonian syndromes: a 12-week follow-up study. Neurodegener Dis 2013;11(1):22–32.

170. Marek K, Seibyl J, Eberly S, et al. Longitudinal follow-up of SWEDD subjects in the PRECEPT Study. Neurology 2014;82(20):1791–7.

171. Fahn S. A new look at levodopa based on the ELL-DOPA study. J Neural Transm Suppl 2006;(70): 419–26.

172. Marshall VL, Patterson J, Hadley DM, et al. Successful antiparkinsonian medication withdrawal in patients with Parkinsonism and normal FP-CIT SPECT. Mov Disord 2006;21(12):2247–50.

173. Farde L, Nordstrom AL, Wiesel FA, et al. Positron emission tomographic analysis of central D1 and D2 dopamine receptor occupancy in patients treated with classical neuroleptics and clozapine. Relation to extrapyramidal side effects. Arch Gen Psychiatry 1992;49(7):538–44.

174. Lorberboym M, Treves TA, Melamed E, et al. [123I]-FP/CIT SPECT imaging for distinguishing drug-induced parkinsonism from Parkinson's disease. Mov Disord 2006;21(4):510–4.

175. Tinazzi M, Morgante F, Matinella A, et al. Imaging of the dopamine transporter predicts pattern of disease progression and response to levodopa in patients with schizophrenia and parkinsonism: a 2-year follow-up multicenter study. Schizophr Res 2014;152(2–3):344–9.

176. Marek K, Jennings D, Seibyl J. Imaging the dopamine system to assess disease-modifying drugs: studies comparing dopamine agonists and levodopa. Neurology 2003;61(6 Suppl 3):S43–8.

177. Rakshi JS, Pavese N, Uema T, et al. A comparison of the progression of early Parkinson's disease in patients started on ropinirole or L-dopa: an 18F-dopa PET study. J Neural Transm (Vienna) 2002; 109(12):1433–43.

178. Ahlskog JE. Slowing Parkinson's disease progression: recent dopamine agonist trials. Neurology 2003;60(3):381–9.

179. Fahn S, Oakes D, Shoulson I, et al. Levodopa and the progression of Parkinson's disease. N Engl J Med 2004;351(24):2498–508.

180. Wang W, Ma C, Mao Z, et al. JNK inhibition as a potential strategy in treating Parkinson's disease. Drug News Perspect 2004;17(10):646–54.

181. Parkinson Study Group PRECEPT Investigators. Mixed lineage kinase inhibitor CEP-1347 fails to

delay disability in early Parkinson disease. Neurology 2007;69(15):1480–90.

182. Petrucci S, Ginevrino M, Valente EM. Phenotypic spectrum of alpha-synuclein mutations: new insights from patients and cellular models. Parkinsonism Relat Disord 2016;22(Suppl 1):S16–20.

183. Adams JR, van Netten H, Schulzer M, et al. PET in LRRK2 mutations: comparison to sporadic Parkinson's disease and evidence for presymptomatic compensation. Brain 2005;128(Pt 12):2777–85.

184. Goker-Alpan O, Masdeu JC, Kohn PD, et al. The neurobiology of glucocerebrosidase-associated parkinsonism: a positron emission tomography study of dopamine synthesis and regional cerebral blood flow. Brain 2012;135(Pt 8):2440–8.

185. Ponsen MM, Stoffers D, Booij J, et al. Idiopathic hyposmia as a preclinical sign of Parkinson's disease. Ann Neurol 2004;56(2):173–81.

186. Sommer U, Hummel T, Cormann K, et al. Detection of presymptomatic Parkinson's disease: combining smell tests, transcranial sonography, and SPECT. Mov Disord 2004;19(10):1196–202.

187. Silveira-Moriyama L, Schwingenschuh P, O'Donnell A, et al. Olfaction in patients with suspected parkinsonism and scans without evidence of dopaminergic deficit (SWEDDs). J Neurol Neurosurg Psychiatry 2009;80(7):744–8.

188. Eisensehr I, Linke R, Noachtar S, et al. Reduced striatal dopamine transporters in idiopathic rapid eye movement sleep behaviour disorder. Comparison with Parkinson's disease and controls. Brain 2000;123(Pt 6):1155–60.

189. Stiasny-Kolster K, Doerr Y, Moller JC, et al. Combination of 'idiopathic' REM sleep behaviour disorder and olfactory dysfunction as possible indicator for alpha-synucleinopathy demonstrated by dopamine transporter FP-CIT-SPECT. Brain 2005;128(Pt 1):126–37.

190. Walker Z, Jaros E, Walker RW, et al. Dementia with Lewy bodies: a comparison of clinical diagnosis, FP-CIT single photon emission computed tomography imaging and autopsy. J Neurol Neurosurg Psychiatry 2007;78(11):1176–81.

191. O'Brien JT, Colloby S, Fenwick J, et al. Dopamine transporter loss visualized with FP-CIT SPECT in the differential diagnosis of dementia with Lewy bodies. Arch Neurol 2004;61(6):919–25.

192. Novellino F, Arabia G, Bagnato A, et al. Combined use of DAT-SPECT and cardiac MIBG scintigraphy in mixed tremors. Mov Disord 2009;24(15):2242–8.

193. Treglia G, Ceriani L, Giovanella L. Current role and future perspectives of radioiodinated MIBG in the evaluation of dementia with Lewy bodies. Curr Radiopharm 2014;7(1):75–8.

194. Novellino F, Bagnato A, Salsone M, et al. Myocardial (123)I-MIBG scintigraphy for differentiation of Lewy bodies disease from FTD. Neurobiol Aging 2010;31(11):1903–11.

195. Donaghy PC, O'Brien JT, Thomas AJ. Prodromal dementia with Lewy bodies. Psychol Med 2015; 45(2):259–68.

196. Yoshita M, Taki J, Yokoyama K, et al. Value of 123I-MIBG radioactivity in the differential diagnosis of DLB from AD. Neurology 2006;66(12):1850–4.

197. Estorch M, Camacho V, Paredes P, et al. Cardiac (123)I-metaiodobenzylguanidine imaging allows early identification of dementia with Lewy bodies during life. Eur J Nucl Med Mol Imaging 2008; 35(9):1636–41.

198. Antonini A, Moresco RM, Gobbo C, et al. The status of dopamine nerve terminals in Parkinson's disease and essential tremor: a PET study with the tracer [11-C]FE-CIT. Neurol Sci 2001;22(1):47–8.

199. Benamer TS, Patterson J, Grosset DG, et al. Accurate differentiation of parkinsonism and essential tremor using visual assessment of [123I]-FP-CIT SPECT imaging: the [123I]-FP-CIT study group. Mov Disord 2000;15(3):503–10.

200. Kepe V, Bordelon Y, Boxer A, et al. PET imaging of neuropathology in tauopathies: progressive supranuclear palsy. J Alzheimers Dis 2013;36(1):145–53.

Moving?

Make sure your subscription moves with you!

To notify us of your new address, find your **Clinics Account Number** (located on your mailing label above your name), and contact customer service at:

Email: journalscustomerservice-usa@elsevier.com

800-654-2452 (subscribers in the U.S. & Canada)
314-447-8871 (subscribers outside of the U.S. & Canada)

Fax number: 314-447-8029

Elsevier Health Sciences Division
Subscription Customer Service
3251 Riverport Lane
Maryland Heights, MO 63043

ELSEVIER

Moving?

Make sure your subscription moves with you!

To notify us of your new address, find your **Clinics Account Number** (located on your mailing label above your name), and contact customer service at:

Email: journalscustomerservice-usa@elsevier.com

800-654-2452 (subscribers in the U.S. & Canada)
314-447-8871 (subscribers outside of the U.S. & Canada)

Fax number: 314-447-8029

Elsevier Health Sciences Division
Subscription Customer Service
3251 Riverport Lane
Maryland Heights, MO 63043

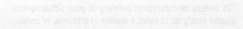

*To ensure uninterrupted delivery of your subscription, please notify us at least 4 weeks in advance of move.

Printed and bound by CPI Group (UK) Ltd, Croydon, CR0 4YY

03/10/2024

01040384-0005